T0183976

Communications
in Computer and Information Science   **1016**

Commenced Publication in 2007
Founding and Former Series Editors:
Phoebe Chen, Alfredo Cuzzocrea, Xiaoyong Du, Orhun Kara, Ting Liu,
Krishna M. Sivalingam, Dominik Ślęzak, Takashi Washio, and Xiaokang Yang

Editorial Board Members

Simone Diniz Junqueira Barbosa
   Pontifical Catholic University of Rio de Janeiro (PUC-Rio),
   Rio de Janeiro, Brazil
Joaquim Filipe
   Polytechnic Institute of Setúbal, Setúbal, Portugal
Ashish Ghosh
   Indian Statistical Institute, Kolkata, India
Igor Kotenko
   St. Petersburg Institute for Informatics and Automation of the Russian
   Academy of Sciences, St. Petersburg, Russia
Junsong Yuan
   University at Buffalo, The State University of New York, Buffalo, NY, USA
Lizhu Zhou
   Tsinghua University, Beijing, China

More information about this series at http://www.springer.com/series/7899

José García-Alonso · César Fonseca (Eds.)

Gerontechnology

First International Workshop, IWoG 2018
Cáceres, Spain, and Évora, Portugal, 14 and 17 December, 2018
Revised Selected Papers

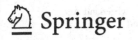 Springer

Editors
José García-Alonso
University of Extremadura
Cáceres, Spain

César Fonseca (iD)
University of Évora
Évora, Portugal

ISSN 1865-0929   ISSN 1865-0937   (electronic)
Communications in Computer and Information Science
ISBN 978-3-030-16027-2   ISBN 978-3-030-16028-9   (eBook)
https://doi.org/10.1007/978-3-030-16028-9

© Springer Nature Switzerland AG 2019
This work is subject to copyright. All rights are reserved by the Publisher, whether the whole or part of the material is concerned, specifically the rights of translation, reprinting, reuse of illustrations, recitation, broadcasting, reproduction on microfilms or in any other physical way, and transmission or information storage and retrieval, electronic adaptation, computer software, or by similar or dissimilar methodology now known or hereafter developed.
The use of general descriptive names, registered names, trademarks, service marks, etc. in this publication does not imply, even in the absence of a specific statement, that such names are exempt from the relevant protective laws and regulations and therefore free for general use.
The publisher, the authors and the editors are safe to assume that the advice and information in this book are believed to be true and accurate at the date of publication. Neither the publisher nor the authors or the editors give a warranty, expressed or implied, with respect to the material contained herein or for any errors or omissions that may have been made. The publisher remains neutral with regard to jurisdictional claims in published maps and institutional affiliations.

This Springer imprint is published by the registered company Springer Nature Switzerland AG
The registered company address is: Gewerbestrasse 11, 6330 Cham, Switzerland

Preface

The International Workshop on Gerontechnology (IWoG) aims to promote research and scientific exchange related to gerontechnology, and to bring together researchers and practitioners from various disciplines of academia, public administrations, and industry in order to tackle emerging challenges in gerontechnology and associated technologies, as well as to assess the impact of these technologies on society, media, and culture.

This volume collects the full research papers (field, statistics, technical and vision works) and short research papers presented at the First International Workshop on Gerontechnology (First IWoG), held in Cáceres (Spain) and Évora (Portugal), during December 14 and 17, 2018. The First IWoG was a multilocation workshop, a condition that further enriched its identity.

The first edition of IWoG accepted contributions related to different dimensions of gerontechnology: use of technology to improve functional ability and promote healthy aging; health interventions to support caregivers of elderly people; the effectiveness of public health initiatives and clinical interventions for prevent, reverse, or mitigate decreases in physical and mental abilities; solutions for active aging, social integration, and self-care; monitoring and management of chronic and non-chronic diseases in ambient assisted living; learning, training, and coaching systems to promote healthy life in ambient assisted living environments; smart homes and sensor networks for ambient assisted living; context-awareness in ambient assisted living environments; use of context and location information in user interfaces; elderly nutrition; health, wellness, and disease monitoring; knowledge management for health (context, cognition, behavior, and user modeling); health ecosystems (frameworks, models and methodologies); smart technologies and algorithms for health.

This workshop was organized by the Program Committee (PC), with a senior PC composed of well-known experts from the field in charge of monitoring the work and animating the discussions of the broader regular PC. This made it easier to run the virtual PC meeting of the full research papers track and the discussion about each paper.

The program for IWog 2018 was versatile and multifaceted. We selected a total of 32 papers out of 71 submissions, resulting in an acceptance rate of 45%.

This excellent and comprehensive program would not have been possible without the help of those who contributed to the success of the event. We would like to thank all the different chairs for their hard work: Javier Berrocal, Jaime Galán, Lorenzo Mariano, Enrique Moguel, Helena Arco, Rogério Ferrinho, Céu Marques, David Mendes, and Gorete Reis. Our thanks also go to Manuel Lopes, who gave the main presentation of the workshop. We would also like to thank Roberto Grilo (CCDR President), Miguel Simón Expósito (SEPAD Assistant Director), José Robalo (ARS President), and Ana Freitas (University of Evora Chancellor), who established the round table in the concluding session.

We are grateful to our local organizers, the 4IE team of the University of Extremadura and the University of Evora for their logistical support, and to Springer for publishing this volume. In addition, we want to thank the PC members, the additional reviewers, and the student volunteers for their effort to make IWoG 2018 a very special event, both in terms of academic ambition as well as practical arrangements.

Finally, we want to thank the authors and the IWoG community for taking the time and effort to participate in IWoG 2018.

December 2018

José García-Alonso
César Fonseca

Organization

Program Chairs

José García-Alonso   University of Extremadura, Spain
César Fonseca   University of Évora, Portugal

Proceedings Chair

Enrique Moguel   University of Extremadura, Spain

Program Committee

Juan Manuel Murillo	University of Extremadura, Spain
Javier Berrocal	University of Extremadura, Spain
Lorenzo Mariano Juárez	University of Extremadura, Spain
Sergio Cordovilla	University of Extremadura, Spain
Carlos Canal	University of Málaga, Spain
Manuel José Lopes	University of Évora, Portugal
David Mendes	University of Évora, Portugal
Niko Mäkitalo	University of Helsinki, Finland
César Alberto Collazos	University of Cauca, Popayán, Colombia
Julio Ariel Hurtado	University of Cauca, Popayán, Colombia
Mohamed Mohamed	Ubiquitous Platforms Almaden Research Center, San Jose, California, USA
Luca Foschini	University of Bologna, Italy
Elena Navarro	University of Castilla-La Mancha, Spain
Javier Jaén	University of Valencia, Spain
Felismina Mendes	University of Évora, Portugal
Pedro Parreira	Nursing School of Coimbra, Portugal
Ana Paula Oliveira	Polytechnic Institute of Portalegre, Portugal
Adriano Pedro	Polytechnic Institute of Portalegre, Portugal
Rogério Ferreira	Polytechnic Institute of Beja, Portugal
Ana Canhestro	Polytechnic Institute of Beja, Portugal
Lucília Nunes	Polytechnic Institute of Setubal, Portugal
Jaime Galán-Jiménez	University of Extremadura, Spain
Sergio Rico Martín	University of Extremadura, Spain

Sponsors

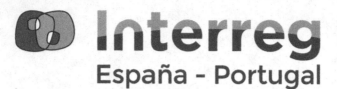

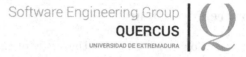

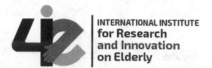
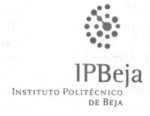

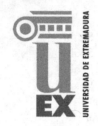

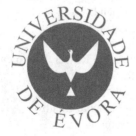
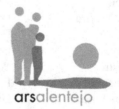

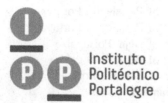

Contents

Solutions for Active Aging, Social Integration and Self-care

Knowledge Management for Health: Context, Cognition, Behavior and User Modeling

Complex Event Processing for Health Monitoring

Alejandro Pérez-Vereda[1]($\boxtimes$), Daniel Flores-Martín[2], Carlos Canal[1],
and Juan M. Murillo[2]

[1] University of Malaga, Malaga, Spain
apvereda@uma.es, canal@lcc.uma.es
[2] University of Extremadura, Cáceres, Spain
{dfloresm, juanmamu}@unex.es

Abstract. The increase of the life expectancy has become a challenge in regions with a low population density. This fact is caused by the existence of small towns all far from one another and with the peculiarity of many elders with special health care living there. This situation increases in a high percentage the health costs of the region having to attend daily all these elders who need a close monitoring. We live in a IoT era with a huge quantity of new connected devices with lots of sensors. Taking advantage of this, it is possible to monitor these elders from the distance without having to cover the complete area of the region every day. This way, our approach is using a mobile centric architecture that permits the elders having a device which infers a health virtual profile of them with data from its sensors and from other smart devices like bands with pulsometers. At this point we propose using Complex Event Processing techniques to combine the data coming from all sources and analyze it to extract meaningful information for the doctors and caregivers and even detect important events like falls in real time.

Keywords: Internet of Things · Internet of People · People as a Service · Virtual user profiles · Complex Event Processing · Elders · Gerontechnology

1 Introduction

Nowadays, the index of life expectancy has become higher than ever. Far from being a problem, this is good news, as we live longer and in better conditions. However, there is a side effect of this fact: There are more elders in today's society. These elders have special health care conditions. Usually, they need more revisions, more examinations, therapies or treatments. This involves a notable increment of the costs allocated for health funds in almost every government.

Going further, apart from having an elder population, there are specific regions which also have a lower population density. The European Union mean for population density is 113 hb/Km^2, but there are regions with numbers even bellow 4 hb/Km^2[1]. This fact joined with a high geographic dispersion lets a situation with small rural

---

[1] https://population.un.org/wpp/DataQuery/.

© Springer Nature Switzerland AG 2019
J. García-Alonso and C. Fonseca (Eds.): IWoG 2018, CCIS 1016, pp. 3–14, 2019.
https://doi.org/10.1007/978-3-030-16028-9_1

towns being all far from the other and with quite little people living there. This poses a challenge for the health department of the region needing to get to all these towns wasting lots of resources.

A solution to this problem comes with the hardware advances in the creation of new chips to include in almost every device. We are assisting to the development of smart things, capable of sense and interact with each other and with the people who use or are just near them. Indeed, by 2020, there will be 50 to 100 billion devices connected to the Internet [1]. With all these devices and sensors with internet connection, we have the opportunity to help the elders without having to get there. There is research work on solutions for monitoring lots of aspects of the elder's life, like nutrition, exercises, moves… This way, and with communication methods like videocalls, it is possible to monitor the everyday life of this people, reducing in a high percentage the health costs in displacements, little hospitals maintenance and so on.

Actually, health monitoring has become one of the biggest areas in the technology industry, developing many smart devices like watches or bands with pulsometer and other more specific sensors. Then, health apps use these sensors plus the GPS of the mobile phone to identify the daily activity and make suggestions on how to improve it to have a healthier life [2]. Others use the same sensors to alert us from air quality [3] or even use the camera to detect some skin diseases [4].

In previous works, the authors of this paper advocated for the use of a mobile computation architecture called People as a Service (PeaaS) [5] based on the creation of virtual profiles of people inferred by their own smartphones. This approach comes hand in hand with these solutions as we can obtain health profiles of the elders based on the information coming from all the sensors available in the smartphone and connected wearables. Our work differs from the mentioned existing applications using a decentralized architecture. Furthermore, all the data is processed and stored only in the smartphone, not in a server, giving its owner the opportunity of managing it and control the third parties access to it. This permits the users being the owners of their health information to be capable of sharing it with their doctors.

The problem we have to face here is the inferring of the virtual profile to extract meaningful information from all the data coming from different sources, combining and analyzing it. For that purpose, in this paper we propose empowering the PeaaS architecture with a Complex Event Processing (CEP) [6] engine to recognize patterns and extract all the important events occurring in the everyday life of the elders in real time. To better illustrate our proposal and validate the results we selected the following case of study.

In a small village located in a rural and depopulated region like the above mentioned lives Mary. He is 70 years old and lives alone with his children living away. Until now there was no problem for visiting the doctor by himself in the nearest town to control his diabetes, but Mary is starting to lose things and forget some appointments and his children start to worry on him moving alone.

In order to avoid having to visit the doctor that often, the health system provides Mary some devices like a glucometer and a smart band that connects via Bluetooth with the smartphone he usually uses to speak with his grandchildren. This way, the measurements and records of the new devices are stored in Mary's smartphone with other relevant information like proximity detections of family or friends acquired by the smartphone itself using the Bluetooth too. Now Mary's family and doctor are aware of his health conditions and location. For example, abnormal levels of sugar in blood. Also, if he gets lost in his daily way to the groceries in the morning, is detected in real time by the CEP engine available in his smartphone. If something seems to be wrong the smartphone can alert his children or the doctor to send there someone for help.

In this case of study the smartphone plays a key role collecting, processing and storing information about Mary coming from different sensors like GPS signal, and health devices. All this data as well the inferred information composes Mary's virtual profile.

The structure of this paper is as follows. Section 2 discusses the state of the art and some related works found in the recent literature. Next, Sect. 3 introduces our proposal and presents the architecture of system, together with the technologies that support it. In Sect. 4, we develop a proof of concept to show the main features of our proposal. Finally, Sect. 5 presents the conclusions and briefly discusses future work.

2 Related Work

With the number of sensors available today embedded in the smartphones, wearables and other devices in our everyday environment, it is easy to get access to lots of data about the users and their context. In this sense, Ambient Intelligence has emerged as a discipline for making everyday environments sensitive and responsive to people's needs [7]. Aiming to obtain a complex virtual profile with high level information about health and habits, we propose in this paper the integration of PeaaS and CEP. CEP is a technology enabling the analysis of big amounts of data coming from different sources for detecting meaningful information and reacting to the new situation in real time. Indeed, from its beginnings, CEP engines were executed in servers or even desktop computers for the detection of domain specific critical situations. Nevertheless, with the computing capacity and pervasive presence of the smartphones today, the previously proposed PeaaS architecture suggests moving this processing tasks to the smartphone itself, empowering it with the ability of analyze the information it receives from the user and her environment. This approach is denoted as mobile CEP [8] and has implicit advantageous characteristics, as there is no need of implementing a communication between the engine and the sensors, everything lays in the smartphone, giving the system privacy and correlation of the information.

The main goal of gathering information about the users of a system is learning from them, and proactively, meet their needs trying to reduce their manual intervention to the minimum. Contextual data are used to infer virtual profiles with more concrete in- formation about the users [9, 10]. These profiles may then be exploited to know important aspects of the everyday life of the user like her diet, movements, exercise habits, and more specific health information like heart rate or blood pressure or sugar measures. Currently, there are different approaches to create these virtual profiles [11–13].

If we review existing solutions related with elders' health monitoring, a big part of them are related only with the elder geopositioning. Keruve [http://www.keruve.es/] and Neki [https://neki.es/] are two of the most known enterprise solutions enabling the caregiver to locate the patient in real time. Even so, the GPS devices these and other companies sell are quite expensive and out of many family's budget. In the research environment, we find similar solutions like The Escort System [14]. But it has the same problems as the others. Also, there are solutions based on mobile applications like Cerqana [https://cerqana.com/] and Tweri [http://www.tweri.com/].

The major issue here is that neither of them offer in any case more information than GPS positioning. Considering all the information about routines, movements or health about the user that can be inferred from the monitoring of the sensors in their smartphones and wearables they carry and from other smart devices they interact with, it is possible to provide more information, considering more specific data and giving higher level appreciations. For example, there are studies [15–17] relating the realization of outdoor activities, the smartphone use, and sleep routines with the probability of suffering depression. All of these indicators could be extracted from the data recollected by the sensors available.

3   Architecture of the Proposal

Smartphones are evolving in terms of internal storage and computing capacity and can be now used as little computers with help of some gadgets for power supply. So, researchers are now realizing that smartphones are able to run tasks which were executed in computers or servers before. In this section, we detail the architecture proposed for the integration of the PeaaS model with the CEP technology for its execution in mobile phones. CEP acts as an inference engine to create a health profile of the user and alert of important events. As a consequence of this, the profile, engine, and data producers are all together in the smartphone.

One distinctive of the system is that it is designed for a mobile computing architecture. For that, we take advantage of our experience in previous work and use the PeaaS approach already mentioned in preceding sections. PeaaS endows the smartphone with the capability of storing, updating and of course sharing a virtual profile of its owner. Hence, the smartphone becomes a proxy or interface of its user with the rest of the world, in particular with smart devices in the environment.

The software architecture of the proposal for integrating the CEP technology in the PeaaS model is shown in Fig. 1. As it was expected, all the modules and components of the architecture are inside the smartphone itself following the PeaaS philosophy. So, the smartphone plays the central role and the virtual profile is only stored in it, third parties will be able to use it externally. The traditional server idea disappears with a decentralized architecture with each node acting as if they were one server.

The architecture is composed of five components or modules. The mobile resources, the virtual profile, the communications module, the execution core and the inference engine. Due to the operative systems restrictions, the system must be deployed at the application level. So, all modules lay on it to access specific functionalities or resources.

The Mobile Device Resources layer represent all the sensors available in the smartphone to whom we have access from it (accelerometer, GPS…). The sensors from wearables and other devices connected to the smartphone are not represented here but they will be accessible anyway through the External Services module.

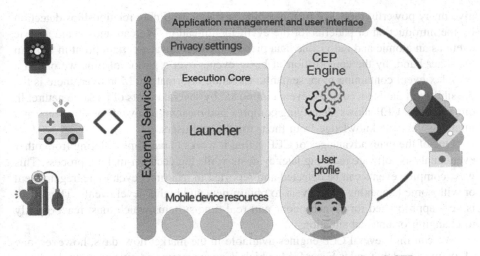

Fig. 1. Software components architecture of the integration PeaaS-CEP

The key element of the whole system is the virtual profile. Here is where all the information about the user is stored. This information contains both the historic of interesting events detected chronologically ordered and also the high level profile containing meaningful information about the user. For our use case, this information will be related with health aspects, like blood pressure, exercise time, or even often moves and companion. Then the profile is offered as a service, permitting third parties or other applications installed in the phone using it attending to privacy considerations. These rules of privacy are stablished by the user and stored in the Privacy Settings module. This module controls the access to the profile by any other apart from the CEP engine. For example, Mary's doctor will have access only to the parts of the profile concerning to health issues, not to his daily moves.

The External Services module give support to the interactions of the smartphone with other external sources of information. These sources are external devices like wearables, home assisting ones or public web services offering contextual information like weather, public transport, air quality, etc. Furthermore, this module manages the communications with third parties when an important or critical event is detected in real time by the CEP engine. For example, when detecting a sudden Mary's blood pressure increment, this module will manage the communications of what is happening to the emergencies service.

The Execution Core is where the front-end application is running. The application is the one containing the domain specific inference event patterns. The application running provide the CEP engine with the necessary patterns to obtain the required information and also provides the External Services layer the access information of the devices it wants to use.

Finally, the inference engine component is implemented by a CEP module. Complex Event Processing [6] is a cutting-edge technology providing an architecture and mechanisms permitting to discover complex events or situations by analyzing and correlating data coming from different sources and other basic or complex events. CEP give many powerful tools like membership, causality, or timing relationships detection by the introduction of patterns for the event identification. We can understand a basic event as an atomic and indivisible data piece which occurs at a certain point in time, in the other hand, by the composition of basic events over a period of time we obtain a complex event containing more semantic meaning information. Moreover, there is the possibility of having a complex event composed by several events of its same nature. In one sentence, CEP allows identifying complex and meaningful events or situations, and inferring valuable knowledge from them for the end users.

One of the main advantages of CEP is that it works in real time differing from other event analysis software reducing latency costs while the decision-making process. This way, complex events can be detected and reported in real time, even to aggregate them or with some happening basic event to obtain new and higher-level events. Thus, CEP is very appropriated for asynchronous and real time systems which must react quickly to changing or unusual situations.

We can find several CEP engines available in the market nowadays, however, one of the most widely used is Esper [18], which is open source and give many tools like an online engine, a Java and .NET API, and an event processing language (Esper EPL) for the patterns' definition. Esper also have an Android version for its engine called Asper [19], but unlikely this project is discontinued nowadays, so by the moment for our implementation we use the Java API. The system works as stated in Fig. 2.

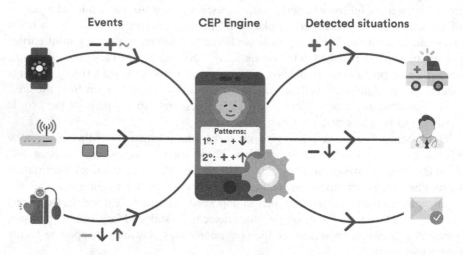

Fig. 2. Mobile CEP system overview

The CEP module interacts with the virtual profile of the user, updates and completes it with new information extracted from incoming events and also uses the information stored to infer higher level knowledge from its combination and patterns detection. The incoming events can be received from two different points: from the local resources or sensors allocated in the smartphone, or from the peripheral sensors in the smartwatch or other devices connected through the External Services module. As remarked before, the engine has two main tasks: the information extraction, and the inference of higher level knowledge. From the first task, we can detect interesting pieces of information we want to store for later analysis or detect specific situations or conditions to derive some actions or changes. For example, if Mary gets lost, the smartphone will immediately alert the caregiver. The inference task consists on the analysis of the detected and stored information, combining it with new appreciations stored or with happening incoming events, this way we can know the Mary's usual moves and paths and the places he visits to even predict where she will be at certain moment. This high level contextual information of the user is stored back in the profile to permit other apps or third parties like a doctor use it and control the daily activity of the elder regarding the privacy settings stablished.

4   Moves Detection

One of the objectives of this paper is to validate the proposal developing a proof of concept application for our case of study concerning the health of old people. In order to better show how the proposal works, we focus our analysis on data coming only from the smartphone, concretely on GPS data, to extract information about the paths the user is following during her daily moves outside. Nevertheless, the approach could be used for any other data even coming from other devices to infer the indoor activity, or other health information like sleep quality, mood, or wellness parameters like blood pressure or sugar in blood levels.

Then, for this paper we develop an Android application with a GPS monitoring process and with a CEP engine to analyze the locations and obtain the moves made by the user, her most visited places and even part of her timetable. This way we can predict future moves or detect a move that the user should be doing at a point in time.

4.1   Data Recollection

The application developed uses the google maps services just to obtain location timestamps and store them with the date and time they were picked. The app monitors the GPS sensor of the smartphone and stores the latitude and longitude every time the user moves. We established a configurable 35 meters' threshold so, each time the user moves this limit away, we collect the GPS position and also speed measurements, as shown in Fig. 3.

As it can be seen, this way of monitoring the GPS sensor of the smartphone give us several conveniences to detect when the user starts a move or finishes it and the speed at which she is moving. When there is any timestamp detected, the user is stopped, and while we are collecting new ones, depending on the frequency of the measures, means that is moving slower or faster, for example to detect the mean of transport being used. Also, this implementation gives us the opportunity of implementing an energy saving application, being idle while the user is not making a move.

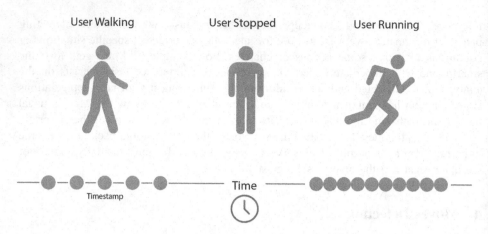

Fig. 3. Location timestamps recollection over time

4.2   Patterns Recognition

The CEP engine needs a stream of incoming events, not raw data directly. So, we defined a basic event to represent each timestamp and to be the input the engine needs. This has to be done for each kind of information entity we want the engine to process.

For our case of study, we just needed to define one basic event. The basic event we use in this case is called *Point* and has properties to store the *latitude*, *longitude*, *speed* and *time*. It is important to remark that the conversion from the raw data to the *Points* has a little implication to consider. It cannot be delayed from their detection for the system to interpret the frequency between them and process time operations over the flow. This is done as the basic events are going to be created just when they are detected permitting the system to actuate in real time.

With the sequence of conversed basic events, we just need to define the patterns we want it to recognize and the actions to tackle when detecting each pattern. For the sake of the validation of the proposal we designed 4 patterns just trying to identify the moves done by the user and the places visited along the day with those moves. For the pattern definition, the Esper CEP engine provides an Event Processing Language (EPL) as a declarative language to work with high frequency time-based events. EPL is SQL-92 standard compliant and includes extended tools for dealing with events series and time.

First of all, the easiest pattern to detect, considering how the data is being collected, is a stop. The only thing to take into account is the elapsed time between two successive *Points*. We consider a time window of 150 s (configurable) to identify a move stop. The EPL rule for this event stays as follows.

```
insert into MoveStop
select p1.latitude as latitude,
        p1.longitude as longitude ,
        p1.timestamp as timestamp
from pattern [every p1 = Point -> (timer:interval(150 seconds)
and not p2 = Point)];
```

The result of the above rule is another event called *MoveStop* with *latitude, longitude* and *timestamp* properties. When an event is detected it is important to throw it to the flow immediately to be able of being part of another more complex event.

Once we have detected the stops, the start of the moves are detected immediately. The point in which the move starts is the next one to the stop, as while we are stopped in the same place, no timestamped *Point* is collected. The following rule shows how we obtain the *MoveStarts*.

```
insert into MoveStart
select p2.latitude as latitude,
        p2.longitude as longitude ,
        p2.timestamp as timestamp
from pattern [every p1 = MoveStop -> p2 = Point];
```

At this point, we have identified the main points of interest for detecting moves. Now, we proceed joining these two kinds of points to categorize the gaps between them. From a *MoveStart* to a *MoveStop* what we have is the *Move* itself. In addition, if we make the join by the other side, from a stop to a start, we detect the staying in a *Place*. We define these rules below.

```
insert into Move
select p1.latitude as latitude_start,
        p1.longitude as longitude_start,
        p1.timestamp as start,
        p2.latitude as latitude_end,
        p2.longitude as longitude_end,
        p2.timestamp as end
from pattern [every (e1 = MoveStart -> e2 = MoveStop)];

insert into Place
select p1.latitude as latitude,
        p1.longitude as longitude,
        p1.timestamp as start,
        p2.timestamp as end
from pattern [every (p1 = MoveStop -> p2 = MoveStart)];
```

As a result and using the previous patterns, we can test the application recording geopositioning data during a move and see what the engine recognizes and stores as the events detected. In Fig. 4 we can observe two captions. The first one shows an example of a path followed during the move as the smartphone collected it. It was a move in which we stopped at a bakery in Hilera street, near Andalucía avenue. Then, in the second caption, we can observe the same map but only with the events detected by the CEP engine that correspond correctly with the start and end of the move and with the mentioned bakery. This work is completely reproducible, and the necessary tools with the application are available on GitHub[2].

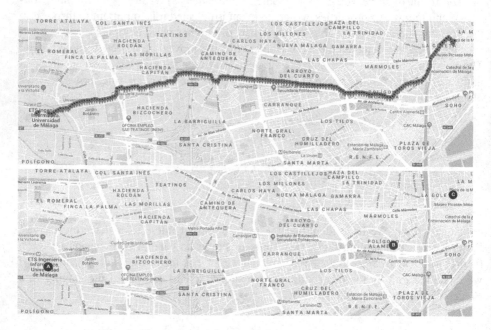

Fig. 4. Test path stopping at a bakery and results obtained

5   Conclusions and Future Work

In previous works we advocated for the use of the smartphones to infer a virtual profile of their users. These virtual profiles are the key for a world in which the users are the owners of their own data and decide who have access to it. This way, our information will only be stored at one place and the companies, applications and other people will interact with it for consulting or updating it.

We proposed in this paper the use of CEP technology to infer this virtual profile inside the smartphone. With the integration of CEP in the model, we are enabling the smartphone to interact with all the other peripheral devices and wearables. The purpose

---

[2] GitHub: https://github.com/aperezvereda/PeaaS-CEP.

is to join all the different data provided an obtain knowledge from its composition and analysis. This approach is especially interesting for e-health applications as we can obtain directly a patient's clinic profile and make a daily monitoring of the more quotidian routines of exercise, mood, moves, etc., share this information in real time with the doctor, and also detect critical situations.

The only inconvenient we found here was the discontinuity of the Asper CEP engine for Android so we decided to use the actual Java implementation of Esper engine in a desktop computer but using the real data the smartphone is storing. However, the final objective is to have a complete mobile version so, when we came with a mobile CEP engine in the future, this could be migrated to the smartphone and use the same rules that we use today in the desktop version. As a consequence, we prepared the Android application for data collection to export the data to a file. Then, the desktop application is able to receive that file, read it, and obtain the simple events contained in it.

For future work, we must face the lack of an updated mobile CEP engine and also perform further analysis on it with more complex rules and joining data from different sources to even detect more points of interest but during the move, for example, turns or speed changes to infer more information about the path and how is the move made. For this purpose, all the architecture must be deployed on a smartphone connected with other devices. In addition, the rules presented in this work are not fault tolerant. They work fine but, in special situations obtaining wrong timestamp points due to GPS signal lost indoors we had some bad detections of *MoveStart*. So, a filtering task should be done to obtain correct and precise results.

Another task to develop is the need of defining the structure of the virtual profiles, making them extensible and of course implement security and privacy protocols. The profile must be scalable to contain information from different and new data sources and permit controlling the access to the profile and how it is made.

Acknowledgments. This work has been partially financed by the Spanish Government through projects TIN2015-67083-R and TIN2015-69957-R (MINECO/FEDER, UE), by the 4IE project 0045-4IE-4-P funded by the Interreg V-A España-Portugal (POCTEP) 2014–2020 program, and by the Regional Government of Extremadura (project GR15098).

References

1. Perera, C., Liu, C.H., Jayawardena, S., Chen, M.: Context-aware computing in the internet of things: a survey on internet of things from industrial market perspective. CoRR (2015)
2. Do, T.M., Loke, S.W., Liu, F.: Healthylife: an activity recognition system with smartphone using logic-based stream reasoning. In: Mobile and Ubiquitous Systems: Computing, Networking, and Services, pp. 188–199. Springer, Heidelberg (2013)
3. de Prado, A.G., Ortiz, G., Boubeta-Puig, J.: CARED-SOA: a context-aware event-driven service-oriented architecture. IEEE Access **5**, 4646–4663 (2017)
4. Kassianos, A., Emery, J., Murchie, P., Walter, F.: Smartphone applications for melanoma detection by community, patient and generalist clinician users: a review. Br. J. Dermatol. **172**(6), 1507–1518 (2015)

5. Guillen, J., Miranda, J., Berrocal, J., Garcia-Alonso, J., Murillo, J.M., Canal, C.: People as a service: a mobile-centric model for providing collective sociological profiles. IEEE Softw. **31**(2), 48–59 (2014)
6. Luckham, D.: Event Processing for Business: Organizing the Real-Time Enterprise. Wiley, Hoboken (2011)
7. Marzano, S.: The New Everyday: Views on Ambient Intelligence. 010 Publishers, Rotterdam (2003)
8. Dunkel, J., Bruns, R., Stipkovic, S.: Event-based smartphone sensor processing for ambient assisted living. In: IEEE Eleventh International Symposium on Autonomous Decentralized Systems (ISADS), pp. 1–6 (2013)
9. Bellavista, P., Corradi, A., Fanelli, M., Foschini, L.: A survey of context data distribution for mobile ubiquitous systems. ACM Comput. Surv. **44**(4), 1–45 (2012)
10. Raskino, M., Fenn, J., Linden, A.: Extracting value from the massively connected world of 2015 (2015)
11. Park, H.S., Oh, K., Cho, S.B.: Bayesian network-based high-level context recognition for mobile context sharing in cyber-physical system. Int. J. Distrib. Sens. Networks **7**(1) (2011). https://doi.org/10.1155/2011/650387
12. Gronli, T.M., Ghinea, G., Younas, M.: Context-aware and automatic configuration of mobile devices in cloud-enabled ubiquitous computing. Pers. Ubiquit. Comput. **18**(4), 883–894 (2014)
13. Makris, P., Skoutas, D.N., Skianis, C.: A survey on context-aware mobile and wirelessnetworking: on networking and computing environments' integration. IEEE Commun. Surv. Tutorials **15**(1), 362–386 (2013)
14. Taub, D., Lupton, E., Hinman, R., Leeb, S., Zeisel, J., Blackler, S.: The escort system: a safety monitor for people living with alzheimer's disease. IEEE Pervasive Comput. **10**(2), 68–77 (2011)
15. Saeb, S., et al.: Mobile phone sensor correlates of depressive symptom severity in daily-life behavior: an exploratory study. J. Med. Internet Res. **17**(7), e175 (2015)
16. Muhlfeit, J., Melina, C.: The Positive Leader. Pearson Education Limited, Kustantaja (2012)
17. Murphy, M.J., Peterson, M.J.: Sleep disturbances in depression. Sleep Med. Clin. **10**(1), 17–23 (2015)
18. EsperTech – Esper (2017). http://www.espertech.com/esper/
19. Eggum, M.: Asper - Esper for Android (2014). https://github.com/mobile-event-processing/Asper

Facial Recognition of Emotions with Smartphones to Improve the Elder Quality of Life

Sheila Bonilla(✉), Enrique Moguel, and Jose Garcia-Alonso

University of Extremadura, Cáceres, Spain
{shbonillap,enrique,jgaralo}@unex.es

Abstract. The increase in the elderly population today is a fact. This group of people needs day-to-day care due to their age and, in addition, they often have health problems. Technology can be used to mitigate these problem. However, it must be beared in mind that most of this population is currently unable to get the most out of electronic devices. To help elders benefit from these devices systems adapted to their needs and preferences are needed. In particular, systems that use the elders contextual information to integrate several aspects of eldercare and adapt them to each elder would provide significant benefits. In this paper, we propose to use smartphones as the device who centralizes contextual information of the elders, focusing on emotion recognition. These emotions will be used to recognize to what extent an elderly person needs care at certain times of the day and to adapt surrounding IoT systems to their needs and moods.

Keywords: IoT · Facial recognition of emotion · Smartphone · Elderly

1 Introduction

Today, thanks to advances in technology, one of the fastest advancing electronic devices is the mobile phone. Nowadays, a large part of the population uses their mobile phones to communicate, search information, socialize, etc. Even in the context of elder population, there has been an increase in the uses of smartphones in recent years [14].

Most of the population in developed countries is formed by elder people (65 years of older). It is estimated that by 2030 this age group may reach 26% of the population [13]. In Spain, since 2012, 75.9% of people over the age of 65 use a mobile phone and, in addition, the use of this device has become a daily habit for them [14].

In order to help this sector of the population, in addition to using mobile phones, more IoT (Internet of Things) devices are used everyday. These devices are connected to everyday objects through the Internet to add new or improved functionalities to them. Frequently, the elderly tend to use this type of device

© Springer Nature Switzerland AG 2019
J. García-Alonso and C. Fonseca (Eds.): IWoG 2018, CCIS 1016, pp. 15–25, 2019.
https://doi.org/10.1007/978-3-030-16028-9_2

without being aware of it. For example, through medical care in intelligent homes, where the main objective of these systems is to have better control over the patient's health care, reducing hospital visits and improving their quality of life. Another example in which IoT devices are used is the intelligent medication service, since the success in the treatment of any person depends to a great extent on taking the prescribed medicines at the right time. Due to this, smart pillbox or even smart pharmaceutical packaging were created [12]. These devices need technical skills, since the must be initially configured so that they know how to satisfy their owners needs, for example the time at which the elderly should take their medicines. However, if these needs changes, the devices must be reprogrammed.

Having this into account, the emotional state of the users is usually overlooked when gathering contextual information. However, the emotions displayed by user when performing certain action are of great interest to improve the systems behaviour.

According to [8] there are six basic types of emotions, which are: joy, sadness, surprise, fear, disgust and anger. Being able to identify these emotions will help improve the contextual information gathered, and therefore, obtain systems better adapted to the needs and moods of their owners. In the context of the elder population, this technique could be used to perform actions like detecting if the person has a problem at a certain moment of the day or even quite the opposite, due to the fact that this person has a positive emotional state.

For emotion recognition, numerous techniques are currently used, such as facial recognition through images or videos [16], but as far as the authors know it has not been studied how to include this in the everyday life of elderly people. In this paper, we present a technique to analyse the emotional state of the elderly, through facial recognition of emotions and the subsequent use of this information as part of the Situational Context, which allows for a better adaptation of IoT systems to the emotional state of elderly people.

In order to present our proposal, the rest of paper is structured as follows: In Sect. 2, we will detail the background of this work focusing on emotion recognition and adaptation techniques based on contextual information; in Sect. 3, we will describe our proposal in which we will highlight the architecture and two case studies. In Sect. 4, we will summarize the most relevant related works focusing on the use of emotion recognition. Finally, in the last Section we will show the conclusions and future works.

2   Background

Every year the number of IoT devices grows faster [15], but the way to interconnect these devices does not change. Because of this, interconnection is a problem that exists today, so it is not possible to squeeze its full potential [4]. This work address such situations. With the help of facial recognition of emotions and the use of the Situational Context to gather information of the devices and adapt their behaviour to the users needs, we will be able to integrate different IoT devices with which to help improve the emotional state and quality of life of the elderly. In the following sections we will show the possible techniques for facial recognition of emotions and then how we can adapt these techniques to other IoT devices through the virtual profile.

2.1 Techniques for the Recognition of Emotions

The field of research related to facial recognition of emotions, currently presents a large number of studies [6] aimed at proving in some way, the detection of emotions. The mobile phone has a great influence on this part, as it helps to take videos or even photos that can help to detect them. Most of the emotions recognition models follow a set of techniques, steps or even categorizations. Next, some of the most relevant will be detailed.

This study use the detection of emotions through images [9]. Its purpose is to present a system that detects the face of a person and classify it according to facial expression. In addition, it follows a set of very detailed techniques with which they can detect the face of the person, extract their discriminatory information and finally, be able to classify the expressions obtained.

Continuing with the recognition of images, we also find this relevant work [8]. Its objective is to analyze a possible facial image processing system based on people's emotions, following a specific structure and detailed step by step to reach the best possible solution.

In the field of detection of emotions through videos, we highlight the following article [1]. Anubhad consists of a preliminary prototype designed to recognize facial expressions through videos in real time or even videos stored on the device itself (this includes a version for Windows and Android). The features used for facial expression recognition are based on two categories: geometric and appearance. Thanks to this categorization, as a result, a high percentage is obtained in the recognition of the six basic emotions mentioned above and the recognized emotions can be stored in the device themselves or they can be exported to be used by other systems or devices.

Of all the works previously analyzed, the one that best suits our objectives is Anubhad [1]. This prototype gathers a great number of characteristics that we were looking for such as the following: it is developed in Android, its operation has been tested, it detects the emotional feeling of the person and also, stores the video by which we have detected the emotion.

2.2 Adaptation Techniques/Virtual Profile

In order to adapt the needs of the elderly to IoT devices, we use the virtual profile. This profile is based on the Situational-Context paradigm focused on analyzing the conditions that exist in places where there are Internet of Things systems. This model is used to gather all the information about the elder available in their devices and systems that interact in their normal lives. Using the Situational-Context, the information gathering is transparent to people which implies that they do not need any technical knowledge or skill. Before this study, the Situational Context did not have information related to emotions. Therefore, thanks to this study, we have incorporated the information of the emotional state of a person at certain times of the day. This can help to enrich the context as well as being able to help it. Through the information obtained, virtual profiles are generated that can be used to automatically adapt the behavior of IoT devices to the needs and preferences of each elder [5]. For example, when a person is found to be sad, they are in their living room and it is also 5:00pm. We can put on the television program that this elder likes the most since his retransmission is currently being broadcasted.

Elderly people want to keep their autonomy, so that, whenever possible, they adapt their routines by adding new elements to their homes and/or using new technologies that facilitate the performance of their daily tasks and, at the same time, allow caregivers not to have to constantly accompany them [2]. By adding more IoT devices, we will capture more information in the virtual profile, which will make richer information so we can provide more efficient solutions to suit the elderly.

The authors of this paper previously presented a technological solution to make life easier for patients with dementia [2]. Smartphones, smart clocks and other devices were used to control the location and vital symbols of a person with dementia. Caregivers could therefore be alerted when a parameter deviated from its normal values, for example, when the heart rate exceeded the values set by the caregiver, or when the affected person was in an area that the caregiver had not marked as safe.

From this, they developed a mobile application to monitor elderly people with cognitive impairment with a certain degree of autonomy. The objective of this system is to detect the different daily routines of the user (schedules, movement patterns, etc.). Then, the smartphone monitors the user's daily activities and acts if any deviation is detected (for example, guiding the elderly to finish an activity or alerting their relatives). The identification of routines is based on all available contextual information, such as time, location (indoors or outdoors), biometric data, family members or caregivers accompanying the elderly or the weather. The analysis of this information makes it possible to detect a wide variety of recurrent activities, along with all the contextual information associated with those activities. Identified routines are stored along with their contextual information and the transitions between them that the user follows. Finally, they defined an algorithm to identify deviations from routines, and to detect when, depending on the Situational Context it is necessary to activate an alert. All this allows us to identify a greater number of activities, better control the conditions in which each activity must be carried out and detect which deviations from the routines must trigger an alert.

Our virtual profile was initially composed of: a basic profile with the information of the elder, a social profile that stores high level information about the basic profile, goals which are deduced from the basic and social profile and finally, the skills to make decisions and changes in the environment [11]. But if, in addition to these components, we add to this profile the daily routines of an elderly and, based on these routines, a facial emotion detector through which we store the emotional feeling of the elderly, we will achieve the objective of making them richer in information, which will lead to IoT systems able to react to emotional changes in the elder.

3   Improving the Elderly Quality of Life by Using Emotion Recognition

As we have previously said, an increasing percentage of the population uses electronic devices more easily. Thanks to the Situational Context paradigm, it is not necessary for elder to have a great deal of knowledge about electronic devices to take advantage of their capabilities.

The proposal presented here is an application capable of recognizing the emotional state of a person. This information is stored together with the existing virtual profiles proposed by the Situational Context. Using Anubhav [1] we recognize the six types of basic emotions using a video stored on the smartphone or capturing it in real time. In addition, we have the possibility to export this information to other devices. Our proposal includes the possibility of linking emotions with other contextual information.

The information obtained about emotions is later used to simplify or automate the interactions of the elder with different IOT devices. For example, notifying family members of a sudden change in the emotional state.

Additionally, the proposed application will stored in a timeline the videos collected by the device alongside the emotional feeling and the time at which this recognition has been made. This will allow the system to monitor the usual emotional state of the elders and to detect a change in the elders daily routine and what may have caused this change according to the emotions detected combined with the rest of contextual information.

3.1   Architecture of the Proposal

We have developed an architecture with which we intend to achieve the detection of emotions together with a better interconnection between different IoT devices and thus be able to get the maximum benefit. This architecture implies the interaction of different entities and the use of context information.

The components developed for the architecture detailed in Fig. 1 are as follows:

- **Connectivity Manager:** Establishes the physical connection between entities. Sends and receives information regarding skills, needs, personal information, etc.
- **Context Manager:** Responsible for creating and updating contextual information. Contains the information of the entities belonging to the same situation in a given instant of time.
- **Profile:** Union of the Basic and Social Profile of the entity.

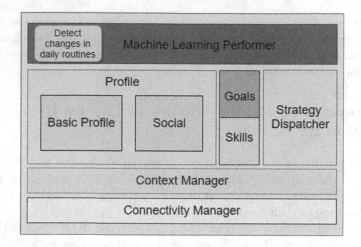

Fig. 1. Developed architecture to add change detection in a daily routine elderly

- **Basic Profile:** Basic Profile: It is the basic information that identifies the entity (Personal Information). It also contains raw data about the history of interaction with other entities (Raw Data History).
- **Social Profile:** Stores the set of all data inferred by the basic profile (Inferred Data History).
- **Skills:** Functionalities of the entity. It produces a change in the context that is not possible with its own needs.
- **Strategy Dispatcher:** Devices can detect what needs there are in the context, and which ones can solve their skills, so a strategy is solved when there is a skill that can cover the need of an entity. The complexity of strategies lies in the collaboration of entities to identify and solve needs.
- **Machine Learning Performer:** Analyzes the history of activities of the entity to detect patterns and learn from it, with the aim of automating tasks in the future.
  - **Detect changes in daily routines:** It analyzes the daily routines that have been detected through the patterns of machine learning and, when a change occurs in these, proceeds to the detection of emotions.

The facial recognition through the smartphone will be made daily a minimum of three times. These three recognitions will always be done at the same time interval and are as follows:

- First recognition will be done early in the morning when it is detected that the elderly has woken up. The recognition will be made when the elderly takes the mobile for the first time in the day.
- Second recognition, just after the midday meal. Through the daily routines we will detect at the hour that the elder usually takes her lunch, for this reason we will have a stored hourly interval. After this interval, the first time the elderly person picks up the phone, the recognition will be made.

– Third recognition will take place after dinner. As in the second recognition, the elderly will have stored the time interval of his dinner. Therefore, after the interval, the first time the elderly picks up the mobile phone, the emotional recognition will be stored.

This architecture achieves an interconnection of IoT devices at the functional level. As the flow diagram in Fig. 2 shows, the interconnection is based on relating an entity's daily routines to their owner emotions. In this case, when a change in a routine is detected the system will proceed to perform a facial recognition through a video of a total of ten seconds since the person takes his device. This video will be stored in the Raw Data History. Information about the emotion and date will be stored in Personal Information. When the emotion is detected and everything is stored in the device, the change of routine will be notified to a relative/caregiver of the elderly, indicating through a text message/email that this person has not performed a daily routine and also indicating their emotional state. If the elder at the time of recognition does not take the smartphone and the period of recognition ends. This information is not stored in the device so as not to cause an error.

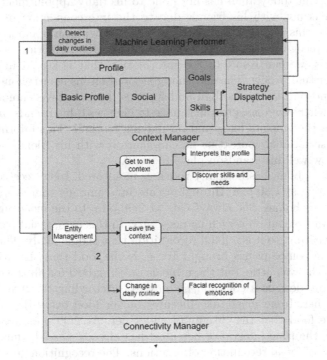

Fig. 2. Context manager flowchart

3.2 Case Studies

As we know, facial recognition of emotions can be quite useful in helping the elderly. With the designed architecture, we will be able to facilitate the elderly daily life. By detecting a change in their daily routine, we can know their emotional state and depending on the state in which the person is, act on it. In order to explain in more detail the situations of help for the elderly, two examples will be given below based on the following context:

The elderly mostly carry out daily routines such as going to buy bread, doing household chores, going out with friends to their usual park or even sitting in their village square to tell each other anecdotes. These routines are monitored, a change in these can indicate a change in your health or mood among others. On this basis, we will develop two examples:

- Juan has his daily routines monitored as discussed above. This person has his own mobile phone with which he makes calls and even communicates through social networks with his friends, who also have smartphones. Through monitoring we can control when a routine is not performed in the usual range of hours. Juan, usually goes out with his friends to his village square around 12:00 a.m. But today Juan has not gone to his daily appointment. We know that Juan is not with his friends due to the interconnection of his smartphones. For this reason, the process of facial recognition of emotions begins. Once this recognition is over, it shows us that Juan emotion is happiness. Having this, we can resort to the information that is stored in the device with the virtual profile. The last change stored on his smartphone is a video of his grandson playing football and for this, he has stayed home watching it. Later, when Juan goes to the square to chat with his friends, he wants to show them the video of his grandson playing football. This information is in the same situational context so he can share it with his friends so they can also see how well his grandson plays football.

- Irene, just as Juan, has her daily routines monitored. Irene receives her food every morning at 1:30 p.m. through a catering company that travels daily to these people's homes. She always eats at 2:00 p.m. In the meantime, she sets the table and prepares everything necessary. In this case, facial recognition is done after eating, so it is a fixed recognition that is done daily. The food that the catering company has brought Irene, is the food that she has liked the least since she was little, but these meals are standard for all the elderly and the company designs a common menu daily. According to what her doctor has asked her, Irene must take pictures of her food every day in order to control the food that the caterer provides her. At 2:30 p.m Irene picks up her phone, the time interval of her meal has already passed, thus activating the process of facial recognition of emotions. The recognition gets the feeling of anger because she didn't like the food. Joining the photo together with Irene's feeling of anger and the tastes we have stored in our paradigm, we can see that the food she has been brought to eat today is the food she likes the least. Faced with this situation, Irene's mobile phone automatically sends a message to the catering company in which it shows that the food served to her today does not please her and with it she manages not to have this type of food sent to her in the future.

4 Related Works

Facial recognition of emotions is a technique used in multiple investigations. Next, we will categorize the different uses of emotion recognition in elderly person:

- As we can see in paper [10], they have developed an application for the recognition of emotions in elderly people from their facial expression, using a webcam. They are able to distinguish the six types of basic emotions (joy, sadness, surprise, fear, disgust and anger) and also the neutral expression. These six emotions are grouped into three categories: happiness, negative emotion and surprise. They have applied their technology in homes, placing a webcam in front of the elder and asking the person to simulate the facial expression associated with an emotion. The best results they obtained were in surprise and happiness. In this paper, they aim to make the most of facial recognition of emotions by helping older people to detect anomalies in mood and be able to improve it through external stimuli. The main difference in the hardware used between this paper and ours is that they use a camera to detect emotions, while we have it integrated into the smartphone itself. On the other hand, their main objective is related to the elders being able to help them through external stimuli as we do, from their emotional state and with the virtual profile.
- In this next study (as in ours), they have thought of a very important aspect: the need for a high level of care due to the loss of autonomy. Motivated by this, they propose a facial recognition of emotions through video in Alzheimer's patients [3]. By testing these patients, their methods come to detect four different facial expressions which are: neutral, smile, sadness and speech. They hope that their benefit will be in the face of positive emotions in which knowing their cause could be determined and replicated to increase the standard of living of the patients and that also leads to a delay in the development of Alzheimer's disease.
- In this last study, they combine the facial recognition of emotions with other techniques, as we pretend with the Situational Context. This paper [7] combines cloud computing with the development of cloud-based healthcare systems and services. Cloud computing has inspired healthcare professionals to remotely monitor patients' health while they are at home. To that end, this document proposes a cloud assisted voice and facial recognition framework for elderly health monitoring, where portable devices or video cameras collect voice along with facial images and are delivered to the cloud server for possible analysis and classification. The patient status recognition system extracts speech characteristics and texture descriptors from facial images. It then classifies them. The status that has been recognized is then sent to the remote

care center, health professionals, and providers to provide the necessary services to provide uninterrupted health monitoring.

These three paper pursue the same goal: to make life easier for the elderly through intelligent devices, whether IoT, smartphone or both. However, as far as the authors know, there is no work using the facial emotions of the elderly to adapt IoT systems to their needs and moods.

5   Conclusions and Futures Works

After different searches of the literature, nothing was found that was completely adapted to the objectives we were looking for. Because of this, we developed our proposal. With the previously developed Situational Context, we have added a new functionality that helps to enrich it. This new function is the facial recognition of emotions, through which we can detect the emotional feeling of the elderly using a smartphone. With this recognition, we obtain the emotional state of the person, which can be: joy, sadness, surprise, fear, disgust and anger. With our idea, we are able to improve the quality of life of the elderly through the recognition of emotions and we can act on this, sending notifications to family members or caregivers so they know how that person is at a certain time of day and because of what may be so.

Following this line, several validations are currently being carried out. Firstly, tests are being carried out on the smartphone's battery consumption. On the other hand, we are looking at the level of data consumption. Finally, and most importantly, we seek the acceptance of the elderly to be able to record videos and thus reach our goal of recognizing emotions.

In future works we will extend our proposal of facial recognition of emotions. The application will be developed for any Android device in which we can do tests on elderly people and that, correcting the flaws that may be in the categorization of emotions, we can detect the emotion as accurately as possible. On the other hand, following with the Virtual Profile, we will continue enriching this profile adding new functionalities, besides integrating a greater number of IoT devices with which we can capture information and, to have in a more precise way the cause by which the old man changes his emotion in a certain moment of the day.

Acknowledgements. This work was supported by 4IE project (0045-4IE-4-P) funded by the Interreg V-A España-Portugal (POCTEP) 2014–2020 program, by the Spanish Ministry of Economy, Industry and Competitiveness (TIN2014-53986-REDT and TIN2015-69957-R (MINECO/FEDER)), by the Department of Economy and Infrastructure of the Government of Extremadura (GR15098), and by the European Regional Development Fund.

References

1. Agarwal, S., Santra, B., Mukherjee, D.P.: Anubhav: recognizing emotions through facial expression. Vis. Comput. **34**(2), 177–191 (2018)
2. Berrocal, J., Garcia-Alonso, J., Murillo, J.M., Canal, C.: Rich contextual information for monitoring the elderly in an early stage of cognitive impairment. Pervasive Mob. Comput. **34**, 106–125 (2017)
3. Dantcheva, A., Bilinski, P., Broutart, J.C., Robert, P., Bremond, F.: Emotion facial recognition by the means of automatic video analysis. Gerontechnol. J. (2016)
4. Flores-Martin, D., Pérez-Vereda, A., Berrocal, J., Canal, C., Murillo, J.M.: Coordinación de Dispositivos IoT mediante Web Semántica y Ontologías en Situational-Context. JISBD (2018)
5. Garcia-Alonso, J., Berrocal, J., Murillo, J.M., Mendes, D., Fonseca, C., Lopes, M.: Situational-context for virtually modeling the elderly. In: Novais, P., et al. (eds.) ISAmI 2018. AISC, vol. 806, pp. 298–305. Springer, Cham (2019). https://doi.org/10.1007/978-3-030-01746-0_35
6. Goyal, S.J., Upadhyay, A.K., Jadon, R.S., Goyal, R.: Real-life facial expression recognition systems: a review. In: Satapathy, S.C., Bhateja, V., Das, S. (eds.) Smart Computing and Informatics. SIST, vol. 77, pp. 311–331. Springer, Singapore (2018). https://doi.org/10.1007/978-981-10-5544-7_31
7. Hossain, M.S., Muhammad, G.: Cloud-assisted speech and face recognition framework for health monitoring. Mob. Netw. Appl. **20**(3), 391–399 (2015)
8. Kulkarni, A., Shendge, A., Varma, V., Kimmatkar, N.V.: Intelligent emotion detection system using facial images (2018)
9. Li, H., Buenaposada, J.M., Baumela, L.: Real-time facial expression recognition with illumination-corrected image sequences. In: 8th IEEE International Conference on Automatic Face & Gesture Recognition, FG 2008, pp. 1–6. IEEE (2008)
10. Lozano-Monasor, E., López, M.T., Vigo-Bustos, F., Fernández-Caballero, A.: Facial expression recognition in ageing adults: from lab to ambient assisted living. J. Ambient Intell. Humanized Comput. **8**(4), 567–578 (2017)
11. Moguel, E., et al.: Enriched elderly virtual profiles by means of a multidimensionalidad integrated assessment platform (2018)
12. Núñez, C.A.V., Mendoza, P.S., Hernández, K.A., Molinares, D.J.: Internet de las cosas y la salud centrada en el hogar. Salud Uninorte **32**(2) (2016)
13. Rodrigues, R., Huber, M., Lamura, G., et al.: Facts and figures on healthy ageing and long-term care. European Centre for Social Welfare Policy and Research, Vienna (2012)
14. Sánchez López, M.A., Fernández Alemán, J.L., Toval, A., Carrillo de Gea, J.M.: Teléfonos inteligentes para la tercera edad: una revisión de aplicaciones móviles de salud (2015)
15. Stergiou, C., Psannis, K.E., Kim, B.G., Gupta, B.: Secure integration of IoT and cloud computing. Future Gener. Comput. Syst. **78**, 964–975 (2018)
16. Suk, M., Prabhakaran, B.: Real-time mobile facial expression recognition system—a case study. In: Proceedings of the IEEE Conference on Computer Vision and Pattern Recognition Workshops, pp. 132–137 (2014)

Toward Privacy-Aware Healthcare Data Fusion Systems

Isam Mashhour Al Jawarneh[1](✉) (iD), Paolo Bellavista[1] (iD),
Luca Foschini[1] (iD), Rebecca Montanari[1], Javier Berrocal[2] (iD),
and Juan M. Murillo[2] (iD)

[1] Dipartimento di Informatica – Scienza e Ingegneria, University of Bologna,
Viale Risorgimento 2, 40136 Bologna, Italy
isam.aljawarneh3@unibo.it
[2] Escuela Politécnica, Universidad de Extremadura,
Avda. De la Universidad s/n, 10003 Cáceres, Spain

Abstract. Mobile wearable and sensor-enabled devices offer an opportunity for deluging unprecedented amount of health-related data that is beneficial in health and caregiving research. Fusing data ingested throughout various heterogeneous channels is essential for better provisioning novel healthcare solutions. However, this is typically challenged by privacy-awareness. For example, the European Commission throughout its call-for-proposals always stresses a requirement that provisioned solutions should consider privacy and should boost security- and privacy-awareness in cloud computing environments. Current solutions either do not consider privacy requirements or provide solutions that are mostly ad hoc and patch efforts. In this position paper, we motivate the adoption of Blockchain technologies for providing privacy-awareness to novel healthcare data fusion solutions. Our envisioned solution is proposed on top of current state-of-the-art blockchain and big data representatives, specifically Hyperledger Fabric and Apache Spark.

Keywords: Blockchain · Privacy-aware · Healthcare · Spark ·
Hyperledger Fabric · Context-aware

1 Introduction

The significantly elevated number of people with cognitive impairments within European communities has motivated European Commission to focus on a project entitled "smart and healthy living at home" [1] within the consortium of Horizon 2020 vision. If left unsolved, this problem poses significant challenges that negatively impacts elder people's independence and quality of life. There is an urgent need for promoting novel large-scale deployment of IT solutions that improve citizen's quality of life, thus causes significant gains in health and care delivery across Europe. The project focuses on many aspects of data privacy, including development of privacy-aware models for data fusion, thus encouraging data aggregation across different platforms and application areas. Also, the personal and sensitive nature of health data mandates to pay special attention to trust, privacy and data protection by design.

© Springer Nature Switzerland AG 2019
J. García-Alonso and C. Fonseca (Eds.): IWoG 2018, CCIS 1016, pp. 26–37, 2019.
https://doi.org/10.1007/978-3-030-16028-9_3

In addition, pilots should build upon state-of-the-art open source platforms, results from IoT-based smart living environments and clearly advance beyond current state of the art solution's capabilities.

Within this context, an interesting application that is emerging as strongly required should monitor and increase autonomy of elder people who develop cognitive impairments especially in their early stages with diseases such as Alzheimer, Parkinson, and Dementia. Such process constitutes a pipeline consisting of an integral part of a (possibly tiered) architecture that starts by acquiring (near) real time knowledge of the patient's ambient without an explicit configurational intervention on the patient's part all the way down to analyzing and discovering deep insights from such data, including a provision of customizable context-aware services tailored to those patient's needs. The importance of building such a pipeline stems from the fact that those elder people are normally accompanied by their caregivers. Increasing autonomy of those elder people means relaxing such a condition that their caregivers must always accompany them.

Elder people with cognitive impairments typically wears sensor-enabled devices that periodically capture their locational data in addition to their physical activity status (i.e., setting, walking, sleeping, etc.). An interesting application is found in a work by [2] from the relevant literature, which proposes a method for detecting disorientation from GPS trajectories, aiming at providing suitable (near-) real-time health-related services to elders who suffer impairments (physical or cognitive), such as reminders and alerts. They basically model patient's movement trajectories as a graph based on historical GPS traces, thereafter identify outlying trajectories that have a defined wandering or deviating pattern as potential instances of disorientation. However, opportunities are open for applying all kinds of deep analysis, including machine learning and deep leaning, thus promoting a better exploitation of big healthcare data. However, an obstacle that is not to be underestimated which hinders advancements in this direction is that contextually-tagged health sensitive data is typically confidential. Hence, a demand is raised for a privacy-aware health care big data management system that preserves privacy while allowing a proper circulation among permissioned parties. The two contradicting requirements (privacy-awareness, thereby data ownership, and allowing data to circulate among interesting parties) mandates the exploration of novel methods that better balance those tradeoffs in a way that is satisfying them both to a good conceivable degree. This prescription perfectly matches traits provided by such a system as Hyperledger Fabric[1] (thereafter HF for short), which is basically based on Blockchain paradigm, but at the same time introducing the metaphor of *channels* (described in a dedicated subsection thereafter). HF is not intrinsically designed for processing big data workloads. However, as ledgers are growing boundlessly there processing challenges capacities of centralized-server-based systems. Promising solutions include scaling in and scaling out. We here encourage scaling out as it is a truth that not all healthcare practitioners own private beefed-up servers and many of them depend on cloud computing premises. We specifically encourage the integration between HF and Apache Spark. Simply put, Spark plays the role of big data processor in this context.

---

[1] https://www.hyperledger.org/projects/fabric.

In this position paper, we propose an integrated distributed solution that is based on de facto solutions such as Apache Spark [3] and HF, and which are privacy-aware. The synergy that this kind of integration offers lies in the fact that they both constitute a harmonious pipeline which ensures privacy-awareness in the backend (HF-based storage) and fast insightful analysis in the front-end (Spark analytics).

The remainder of the paper is organized as follows. We first walk through a brief background that summarizes Blockchain and associated technologies, health data privacy and fusion challenges and the breeds of big data processing systems. In a later section, we define our envision for a privacy-aware cloud- and blockchain-based health data management system. In the last section, we draw conclusions and recommend future research frontiers.

2 Background

2.1 Health Data Privacy and Fusion

Interesting smart city applications rely on fusing multiple sensor data sources into cloud computing [4]. This fact seamlessly flows into the worlds of healthcare. Health problems that remain mysteries for decades may be solved by data fusion and parallel massive computing capabilities. However, the absence of relevant healthcare data fusion mechanisms that enable full exploitation of participatory big health data scenarios remains an issue. An example mystery in health domain includes the question about why elder people with specific cognitive impairments potentially develop different behaviors at later stages. Monitoring those people's everyday life and activities seems promising, but it means collecting data about them and their surrounding ambient in a manner that preserves their privacy, which at a first glance seems a façade. Elder people and their caregivers are typically sensitive when it comes to breaching their privacy. To top that off, governmental regulations exaggerate the problem by strictly prohibiting the exploitation of such data without explicit consents from their owners. Collecting and analyzing healthcare data in a participatory manner provides insightful results that normally advances research so that it unveils hidden layers of knowledge discovery. Privacy-aware healthcare data sharing is essential to promote the collaboration between healthcare stakeholders. For example, health research institutes use those fused data for facilitating treatments, drug manufacturing and recommending better hospitalization best-practices. Also, health insurance companies fuse such data for customizing health insurance plans so that they meet individual needs.

2.2 Health Data Context-Aware Analysis

In the last two decades or so, the attention of big data management has been biased toward spatio-temporal representation of data. Specifically, because data (coming from sensors) is spatially-tagged. Also, most queries seek answers that are proximity-like. For example, all restaurants or attractions that are in a specific radius around a tourist. This pattern of analysis has provided us with interesting insights for many years. However, after years of tuning and optimizations, specifically in Machine Learning

(ML) and data mining domains, it has been found that a hidden dimension plays a great role in answering personalized queries, that is known as context. In simple forms, context means any object that is affecting an entwined subject in a specific location and time [5]. Therefore, a consortium of corelated systems termed as Context-Aware Recommendation Systems (CARS) have appeared, suggesting that personalized recommendation should consider subject's surrounding ambient [6]. This is specifically gaining an unprecedented momentum in healthcare domain [7].

2.3 Blockchain

Blockchain is a novel privacy-aware technology that is gaining an additional momentum in recent years and is loosely defined as a list of records interlinked with one another and secured with cryptography. Representatives include Bitcoin [8] and Ethereum [9]. Transactions are contiguously appended to a linked-list based Blockchain, a process that is typically preceded by gathering several transactions into a single block. Every block has a unique identification hash value stored in its header. Merkle Tree [10] is normally used for representing a list of hashes for all transactions that compose the block. Each block maintains a hash of its predecessor block, manifesting itself as a chain that is interconnected up to first block (aka genesis).

Blockchains are typically manufactured within boundaries of peer-to-peer (P2P) network, where all nodes are equal, and notion of centralization thus disappears. Each node stores a local copy of Blockchain. Also, a group of nodes (known as miners in this context) regularly compete for a so-called leader election (aka proof-of-work (POW)). The winning node decides upon appending an upcoming block to Blockchain.

Blockchains (aka ledgers) that are formed traditionally by this method typically grow unbounded in a manner that requires a considerable time for new registrants to make a transaction. Also, processing that big ledger for insightful analytics exceeds normal capacities of most available software tools. To such an end, those complications constitute obstacles that hinders its adaption in interesting domains such as participatory healthcare. As such, an emerging system recently come into play, known as HF, which provides opportunities for exploiting Blockchain-based concepts in interesting domains such as e-commerce and participatory healthcare.

2.4 Hyperledger Fabric

HF is a novel Blockchain-based technology that has been coined after distributed ledger technology (DLT), constituting a platform for distributed ledger backed by a modular pluggable architecture that enforce confidentiality and privacy as main concerns [11]. Analogous with other blockchain techs, it houses a ledger, uses contracts (known as chain-codes in their parlance). However, participants in Hyperledger are responsible for managing their transactions. HF manifests a permissioned network metaphor, where members may only join through a trusted Membership Service Provider (MSP). The crux of HF that differentiate it from traditional Blockchain techs is that it allows creating special groups termed as *channels*, hosting group of members which share same ledger of transactions, and any member which is outside the loop does not has a copy of that ledger.

Swappable network elements are allowed in and out HF through its modular architecture. Attentively, this allows any big data processing engine to be plugged into any HF network. The ledger that resides in one channel can be shared across the entire network. If some organizations decide to keep their transactions confidential, a private data collection is used to separate this data and save it in a private database. A logical segregation that provides access only to a subset of organizations. In this sense, channels are designed to keep data shared only between members of the channel, whereas collections share data among only subset of channel's members. The other difference that makes it part from conventional blockchains is the fact that all participants have known identities. Networks are organized by a group of organizations rather than single one. The blockchain network is constructed from a group of peers (nodes) that belong to different organizations. Orderers are peers that are responsible for receiving transaction proposals and manage their lifecycle until commitment. Applications of an organization are connected to its peers in addition to some of those of other organizations.

Centralization is absent in this formalization, as networks does not depend on any individual organization, and will remain as long as one organization exists, even when others leave. Different organizations may contribute different applications, thus opening widely the gates for data fusion and interoperability. It totally depends on the organization's choice of how to process their copy of the ledger, thus separating application and presentation logic between organizations although they host the same ledger data.

Applications interface with peers belonging to their organization or other organizations, depending on the type of interaction with the ledger. In case of ledger-query interactions, applications normally use their own organization's peers. On the contrary, for ledger-update interactions, applications must connect to all peers for endorsing the ledger update.

2.5 Big Data Processing Engines

Shortcomings of batch data processing engines have spawned a consortium of big data processing systems that are based on parallel computing paradigm, including those that are processing oriented such as MapReduce [12] and Hadoop [13] and storage oriented such as MongoDB [14] and CouchDB [15]. For this work, we have selected Apache Spark as a representative for the overwhelming traits it provides. Spark has been coined after Hadoop's MapReduce, aiming basically at overcoming some of its shortcomings, which rationales preferring it on batch-oriented Hadoop. It is core-base is structured entirely on the so-called Resilient Distributed Datasets (RDDs) [16], which is the basic data abstraction in Spark, representing an immutable, partitioned collection of elements that can be operated on in parallel. Spark comprises a wide range of libraries and functionalities for various processing workloads (for example, GraphX, MLlib and streaming). Restated more precisely, we have opted for Spark because of Spark's generality benefits, including simplified API, easier to develop applications, efficient to combine processing workloads, and possibility of new lines of applications (such as streaming machine learning) which where intractable before. Its pluggable design and modular architecture streamline fusing new workloads in a hot-swappable manner, thus unburden heavy works from shoulders of developers and help fast-tracking new lines of research. In this paper, we focus on proposing the fusion of GraphX (a library in Spark) and use it to layer a health data processing engine atop HF blockchain, thus retrofitting HF so that it houses a Spark cluster injected within its components, and therefore bridging the gap between the two paradigms. Spark GraphX mainly works by distributing graphs as tables (RDDs in Spark parlance). HF is specifically designed for assisting in data-privacy preservation, thus respecting the "data ownership" principles. However, processing ledger's data is not supported out-of-the-box in HF. Stated in other words, HF is a privacy-aware backend storage engine that is not designed to handle processing workloads and here is where Spark comes into play. Spark is a big data processing ecosystem that works with all kinds of data models and operates on their contents parallelly. The synergy between the two paradigms offers an umbrella where privacy-awareness meets big data processing capabilities.

3 Privacy-Aware Health Data Management: Tentative Design

In this section, we propose a privacy-aware system model that basically aims at fusing health data from multiple heterogeneous sources into trusted (aka permissioned blockchain networks) channels, thus constituting a baseline for interesting ML applications that may uncover hidden insights, therefore helping in improving healthcare service provisioning. Stated in another way, interesting healthcare data is available as an asset within the proprietary of various healthcare parties that are heterogenous by nature. For example, pharmaceutical sector differs from dentists in the way they are managing their health-related data (for example, having different data models). Bringing those datasets into harmony is challenging yet important. For example, discovering which dental drugs works better in specific treatment contexts, thus assisting pharmaceutical manufacturing industry in ways that help them improve their products. Also, facilitating an investigation of effectiveness of some medical drug lines that are manufactured for some chronic diseases such as diabetes and blood pressures, thus informing the decision for their long-term adoption.

3.1 System Design

Health data generated by IoT's devices is typically tagged with contextual information such as demographic (age, companion) or vital signs (such as heart beat rate or blood pressure), which is considered private for most people. Protecting data privacy (therefore data ownership) is a priority and such data should only be shared with trusted pre-defined set of parties. This exactly matches HF feature-support by design [17]. It is specifically for this reason that we propose basing our design on HF from the privacy-awareness corner. Figure 1 elucidates a tentative modular architecture of our proposed system.

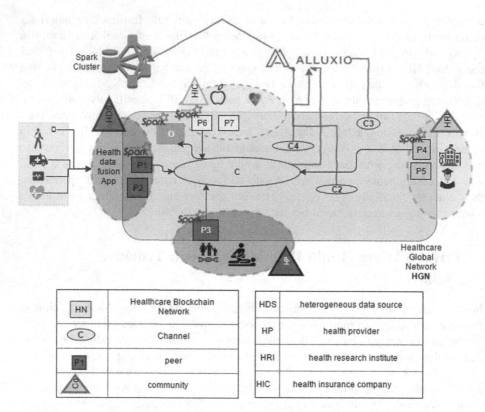

Fig. 1. A modular architecture of privacy-aware health big data management system.

It mainly encompasses the following elements:

(I) **Healthcare Global Network (HGN).** A Blockchain-based healthcare network that is composed of many communities (for which description follows) that voluntarily share some parts of their data within the boundaries of channels they join.

(II) **Px, where x is a number.** Peers analogous to those in original HF design. Those are basically nodes in the P2P network. In our proposed design, each of those hosts a Spark copy, thus acts as a worker node for the corresponding Spark cluster. There are many types of peers and we refer interested readers to [3] for further reading about the types of peers.

(III) Each **community** (schematized in Fig. 1 as a dashed elliptic shape) manifest itself from a group of parties that are either managed under an umbrella of an organizing institution (such as the ministry of healthcare), join a formed community voluntarily or are invited by some community leaders to join a community. We preliminarily define the following communities (a list that is far from being exhausted and potentially will be expanded in an upcoming related research):

- **Health Research Institutes (HRI) communities.** Constitute universities and reputable research labs in health domain. Those communities use big healthcare data for research and development. For example, studying a relationship between some variables that may affect the evolution of a specific disease during different stages.
- **Heterogeneous Data Sources (HDS) Communities.** Constitute of individual patients (or elder people) and their caregivers. Those are continuously sending their health-related data that are normally collected through mobile devices or sensors. Data collected through mobile devices include the ambient around patient at a specific moment in time and trajectories of paths that those patients take through GPS coordinates. Sensor data are collected through sensors worn by patient signifying their vital signs at different moments in time. Collection of this data is beneficial for HRI communities research and all other interested communities.
- **Health Provider (HP) communities.** Constitutes of hospitals, polyclinics, pharmaceutical industry and health recreation centers. For example, pharmaceutical industry can use patient's collective data for studying the cause/effect of a line of a manufactured drug, thus informing the decision for better manufacturing efforts.
- **Health Insurance Companies (HIC).** Constitutes parties that are managed by official standards. For example, HIC can use data from HDS in order to make personalized health insurance plans that better suits a group of patients based on their current contextual information.

(IV) **Orderes.** (schematized as rectangle with big 'O' symbol inside, with Spark icon on the left upper edge). The main job of those is exactly as described by HF, but here we add Spark master, which chiefly encapsulates queries as closures and ship them to worker nodes (hosted in peers in our design).

To take a more utilitarian perspective, the synergy we envision between Spark and HF proceeds as follows; First, HF acts as a backend privacy-aware storage that can store health data in a way that respects data ownership principles, but at the same time disseminate such data for the benefit of trusted parties that constitute a permissioned network. However, HF alone is not enough as it natively does not support processing workloads. This point witnesses the importance of integrating Spark as a front-end processing engine that compliments the pipeline. Spark acts as a machine that consumes HF's data, analyze it to get deep insights for informing policy ad decision making in healthcare landscape. A synergy that is promising because it meets two indispensable healthcare data management requirements. Those are; privacy-awareness and fast processing of big data. Stated technically, we deploy an individual Spark cluster injected within the components of an HF channel. Precisely speaking, Spark master is deployed in one of the orderer nodes (ordering services in HF parlance), while each peer of the same channel hosts a Spark worker. The distinction is important in this context because whereas peers host a ledger, orderers do not, therefore, they do not serve as worker nodes and are not used to obtain a ledger for Spark analysis. The merit of this design is two folds. First, we do not have to launch new network instances for deploying a Spark cluster, thus saving scarce bare-metal resources. Second, we avoid shuffling data throughout the network as ledgers resides locally in same nodes where Spark worker nodes are hosted. This could be even more advantageous in the sense that same data is residing at all peers (nodes), hence shuffling (which is typically the costliest process in a Spark cluster) is, theoretically speaking, totally avoided, an advantage that can provide a significant performance boost. This also means that an inherent corelated problem which use to be challenging (forming stragglers where total execution time is bounded by their finishing times) is totally avoidable herein. What's more, assets (core data representation model in HF) are represented in HF as collections of key-value pairs, a style which is isomorphic and perfectly meshes with that of Spark's RDD by design. Moreover, this design guarantees that instead of having to worry about implementing our own half-baked, custom privacy-aware processing solutions, we take advantage of all efforts that have been put into Spark's parallel processing mechanism and HF privacy-awareness. This way, HF acts as a storage backend providing a persistence layer for Spark processing frontend cluster. Since Spark will be injected within the layers of pre-existing HF channel nodes, it is unlikely to become a bottleneck at any stage throughout a full processing pipeline. A claim that is testified and borne out by a myriad of successful applications in the literature, fitting Spark to work together with other paradigms.

Typically, a channel's ledger transactions are transformed into graphs (a data representation model accepted by Spark). Stated in another way, we aim at designing interfaces that delivers ledger dialects to Spark's GraphX by converting ledger transactions into graphs, thereafter, applying any Spark workload to analyze the data, including ML, deep learning and data mining. We can for example use pageRank (provided by GraphX) on a graph that is representing a HF ledger, requesting top10 medicines in a Blockchain network.

As exemplified in Fig. 1, Spark master hosted by an Orderer (rectangular symbol with O inside), whereas each one of peer P1 from HDS community, P6 from HIC, P3 from HP and P4 from HRI hosts a Spark worker. channels C, C2, C3 and C4 of the network HN can cache some shared data through Aluxio[2] (an external caching service).

Yet remains many challenges that need attentive design for the proposed framework to work properly. For example, the essence of Spark's merit lies behind collaborative parallel computing, meaning that a set of nodes are working synchronously to finish a specific task where each node finishes its part. Having said that, and because for a HF, each channel's peer contains a full copy of ledger it is necessary to coordinate the work and disseminate among participating nodes appropriately. A tentative design we envision is that an Orderer delegates graph formation to one of the peers and then asks this peer to return a metadata describing the graph in a sufficient way that enables the Orderer to distribute graph analysis tasks among participating nodes. Consequently, every peer works locally on its subgraph applying a local copy of the algorithm in labor, thereafter sending results to the master, which performs a join process for all sub-results and return a total result to requester.

From a constellation of optimizations that we are considering, we specifically mention the case of adaptive and proactive (or reactive) response for fast arriving

---

[2] http://www.alluxio.org/.

streams and burst workloads (specifically for online stream processing scenarios), thus responding in appropriate manner that prevents those situations from becoming bottlenecks. Tentatively, we envision electing some common Orderers among all channels of the HF network so that they serve as leaders that can collects shared data that they know is common among all participating channels and cache it in an external caching solution such as Alluxio (formerly Tachyon). This allows faster data access especially in those scenarios where data processed is collected from multiple participating channels.

Another challenge is that widespread innovation of these capabilities is currently stifled by the difficulty in obtaining the contextual data, especially in health domain. For this, we are planning to employ some crawling mechanisms to scrape relevant data from social sites such as yummly[3]. For example, studying cause/effect from thousands of interactions between members and food recipes [18].

4   Related Works

Several works in the relevant literature have proposed approaches for fusing health data. Authors in [19] proposed a Healthcare Data Gateway (HGD) mobile-based application that basically aims at integrating healthcare data from the repositories of various healthcare practitioners. The essence of their work is enforcing data ownership by allowing patients to choose with whom to share their health data with. However, medical records of all kinds are always kept safe in a Blockchain and are accessed for statistical purposes by governmental authorities such as the Ministry of Healthcare. For example, for counting number of people who has specific symptoms or diseases.

In the same vein, [20] proposes MedRec as a decentralized Electronic Medical Records (EMR) system that is based on Blockchain. The participation of health practitioners is incentivized as Blockchain miners, where they need to participate in a POW competition. For prototype implementation, they employ smart contracts on Ethereum Blockchain to log patient-provider relationship. This way health providers insert new patient's records and patients are informed and thus authorize the proper circulation of their EMRs. On the downside, this means burdening their shoulders with extra processing loads that heavily taxes their system's performance. One other drawback is that their methods for handling logistics and coordination add layers of complexity to the existing overburdened system, thus challenging any processing system's capability.

5   Conclusions and Ongoing Works

Considerations for privacy of contextual data are mostly ad hoc and patch efforts. HF provides an umbrella that promotes the exploitation of permissioned networks in sharing and fusing sensitive big data among trusted stakeholders. This is beneficial in

---

[3] https://www.yummly.com/.

many real-life domains such as healthcare and may provide a boost for research and development. Specifically, the cases where monitoring patient's daily life activities encapsulates capturing some of their sensitive contextually tagged data. However, despite HF is promising and can enable the rapid revolution of privacy-aware data fusion, it is still a mean to an end, where the essence is analyzing data collectively, thus delivering a promising line of hope for solving mysteries that otherwise remain elusive, including for example, understanding the development of Alzheimer throughout different patient's life stages. Also, discovering medicines and treatments that are context-aware. For example, some blood pressure drugs may not work as expected under specific context circumstances (winter versus summer, humidity, etc.).

However, data accumulated in ledgers are expected to grow boundlessly, challenging static desk-bound computer systems, which is detrimental to real-time query performance and easily makes it laborious. Beefed-up overburdened servers are not always available as assets held-out by all practitioners. It is however possible with assistance of parallel processing ecosystems such as Spark to fast-track processing of Blockchains even in the event of fast arriving online data streams. By the framework we are proposing, we aim at taking all the aforementioned notions steps further by abstracting the underlying complexities of a modular architecture, thus allowing healthcare practitioners and stakeholders to focus on employing data for discovering deep insights rather than delving into its management's complex logistics. HF alone is not able to process big held-out data. As the ledger is growing boundlessly, ledger becomes itself a source of frustration and the challenges of programming applications atop this new paradigm begin to sink in. we aim to build precursor technologies in the next stage.

An ongoing work includes developing a layer on top of the proposed system that perform some feature engineering to discover most influential features for analysis. Also, developing a full-fledge library for interfacing Spark with HF. As a starter, developing a front-stage for converting the ledger into a graph-based data representation that is acceptable by Spark's GraphX.

References

1. E. Commission. (2017, 1/5/2018). TOPIC: Smart and healthy living at home. http://ec.europa.eu/research/participants/portal/desktop/en/opportunities/h2020/topics/dt-tds-01-2019.html
2. Lin, Q., Zhang, D., Connelly, K., Ni, H., Yu, Z., Zhou, X.: Disorientation detection by mining GPS trajectories for cognitively-impaired elders. Pervasive Mob. Comput. **19**, 71–85 (2015)
3. Zaharia, M., Chowdhury, M., Franklin, M.J., Shenker, S., Stoica, I.: Spark: cluster computing with working sets. Presented at the Proceedings of the 2nd USENIX conference on Hot topics in cloud computing, Boston, MA (2010)
4. Wang, M., Perera, C., Jayaraman, P.P., Zhang, M., Strazdins, P., Shyamsundar, R., et al.: City data fusion: sensor data fusion in the internet of things. Int. J. Distrib. Syst. Technol. (IJDST) **7**, 15–36 (2016)
5. Sezer, O.B., Dogdu, E., Ozbayoglu, A.M.: Context-aware computing, learning, and big data in internet of things: a survey. IEEE Internet Things J. **5**, 1–27 (2018)

6. Ricci, F., Rokach, L., Shapira, B., Kantor, P.B.: Recommender Systems Handbook. Springer, New York (2010). https://doi.org/10.1007/978-0-387-85820-3
7. Berrocal, J., Garcia-Alonso, J., Murillo, J.M., Canal, C.: Rich contextual information for monitoring the elderly in an early stage of cognitive impairment. Pervasive Mob. Comput. **34**, 106–125 (2017)
8. Nakamoto, S.: Bitcoin: a peer-to-peer electronic cash system (2008). https://bitcoin.org/bitcoin.pdf. Accessed Sept 2018
9. Wood, G.: Ethereum: a secure decentralised generalised transaction ledger. Ethereum Proj. Yellow Paper **151**, 1–32 (2014)
10. Merkle, R.C.: Protocols for public key cryptosystems. In: 1980 IEEE Symposium on Security and Privacy, p. 122 (1980)
11. Codd, E.F.: A relational model of data for large shared data banks. Commun. ACM **13**, 377–387 (1970)
12. Dean, J., Ghemawat, S.: MapReduce: simplified data processing on large clusters. Commun. ACM **51**, 107–113 (2008)
13. White, T.: Hadoop: The Definitive Guide. O'Reilly Media Inc., Sebastopol (2009)
14. Banker, K.: MongoDB in Action: Manning (2012)
15. Anderson, J.C., Lehnardt, J., Slater, N.: CouchDB: The Definitive Guide: Time to Relax. O'Reilly Media, Newton (2010)
16. Zaharia, M., Chowdhury, M., Das, T., Dave, A., Ma, J., McCauley, M., et al.: Resilient distributed datasets: a fault-tolerant abstraction for in-memory cluster computing. Presented at the Proceedings of the 9th USENIX conference on Networked Systems Design and Implementation, San Jose, CA (2012)
17. Hyperledger Fabric (2018). https://hyperledger-fabric.readthedocs.io/en/release-1.3/
18. Trattner, C., Elsweiler, D.: Food Recommender Systems: Important Contributions, Challenges and Future Research Directions, arXiv preprint arXiv:1711.02760 (2017)
19. Yue, X., Wang, H., Jin, D., Li, M., Jiang, W.: Healthcare data gateways: found healthcare intelligence on blockchain with novel privacy risk control. J. Med. Syst. **40**, 218 (2016)
20. Azaria, A., Ekblaw, A., Vieira, T., Lippman, A.: MedRec: using blockchain for medical data access and permission management. In: 2016 2nd International Conference on Open and Big Data (OBD), pp. 25–30 (2016)

Technologies to Increase the Quality of Life of the Elderly Population

Food and Health: Relationships Between Technology and Social Sciences

David Conde Caballero[1] , Borja Rivero Jiménez[1]([⊠]) ,
Beatriz Muñoz González[1], Carlos Alberto Castillo Sarmiento[2] ,
Carmen Cipriano Crespo[2] , and Lorenzo Mariano Juárez[1]

[1] University of Extremadura, Cáceres, Spain
{brivero,bmunoz,lorenmariano}@unex.es
[2] University of Castilla-La Mancha, Talavera de la Reina, Spain
{carlosa.castillo,mariacarmen.cipriano}@uclm.es

Abstract. Population aging constitutes one of the central issues on the political agenda of the 21st century. The social implications of these population dynamics are subject to discussion due to their evident impact on aspects such as labour relations, health and care systems, pension policy but also on family models or the social construction of feelings. In this context, the understanding of food ideologies and practices in rural populations is a crucial issue in health policies and interventions. With the traditional tools and assumptions of ethnographic fieldwork, our research is aimed at a series of objectives in order to complete the limited knowledge on these issues: (1) to know the nutritional situation of the elderly population in rural areas; (2) to describe cultural food practices and their association with ideologies, representations, supply and availability systems; and (3) to relate technological innovation with our empirical research findings. We can describe two categories of analysis on which we are working. First, the problems of access to food. The circulation of food -"the field of the eatable"- is conditioned from a structural framework. Then, is also crucial in the diagnostic phase. We work too on the mapping of study areas with a variable representation of distances and difficulties depending on factors such as functionality, but also social position or gender. The intersections between socio-cultural approaches and technology occur in the field of interventions. Technological proposals can prove successful and attractive in labs, but they need to "work" in real life.

Keywords: Aging · Anthropology · Nutrition · Technology · Health

1 Introduction

Population aging constitutes one of the central issues on the political agenda of the 21st century. Average life expectancy in Spain has been doubled in just four generations due to the intense fall in mortality during the first half of the 20th century. Improvements in nutrition and health care are cited as the

© Springer Nature Switzerland AG 2019
J. García-Alonso and C. Fonseca (Eds.): IWoG 2018, CCIS 1016, pp. 41–47, 2019.
https://doi.org/10.1007/978-3-030-16028-9_4

main factors. A century ago it was unusual to reach the age of 35; today, life expectancy continues to increase in our country and people aged 65 or over already represent 18,7%(8,701,380 people) of the entire population [25]. By the year 2064, according to the Spanish National Statistics Institute (INE) [12], more than 33% of the population of developed countries will be over the age of 65, 38,7% in the case of Spain, reaching 222,000 centenarians compared with the current 12,000 [1].

The social implications of these population dynamics are subject to discussion due to their evident impact on aspects such as labour relations, health and care systems, pension policy but also on family models or the social construction of feelings. The challenges presented by this coming scenario are formidable and aggravated in certain European regions -such as Alentejo in Portugal or Extremadura in Spain- where urban concentration movements converge in processes of depopulation of the rural environment, inhabited mainly by elderly people who are more and more alone. As an example, and according to INE [13], in 2014 elderly people represented 27,9% of the population of municipalities with less than 2000 inhabitants, reaching 40 in some towns and villages of Extremadura.

In this context, the understanding of food ideologies and practices in this type of population is a crucial issue in health policies and interventions. This is even more important if we have into account the relationship between food and well-being that is a commonly described in the scientific literature [2,21,26], and in the case of elderly people, their particular vulnerability in nutritional matters has also been underlined, which represents for some authors a major public health problem [3,7,22]. However, the literature available on aging and nutrition has been biased towards analyses of specific health problems or focused on institutionalized settings. We know very little about these practices and ideologies in elderly people living in rural areas. It should be underlined here that food and nutrition are complex and multidimensional areas. They may be defined on the basis of physical and psychological aspects, but also social and cultural ones [5,18], the final determinants of how ideologies are constructed around eating or representations of what is or is not healthy food, and which therefore emerge as primary attitudinal determinants in defining how the elderly feed themselves.

2 Objectives

Our research is aimed at a series of objectives in order to complete the limited knowledge on these issues. From sociological approaches, and articulated on the impact of culture, we intend, among others:

1. To know the nutritional situation of the elderly population in rural areas.
2. To describe cultural food practices and their association with ideologies, representations, supply and availability systems, economic issues and other elements that build food security in the areas under study.
3. To relate technological innovation with our empirical research findings, both at production or analysis levels and in the evaluation of proposed theoretical models.

3   Research/Methodology

The qualitative research presented here is linked to the traditional tools and assumptions of ethnographic fieldwork [11,24]. The group of subjects that make up the object of study is located in the southwest of Spain, specifically the towns of Campillo de Deleitosa and Casares de las Hurdes, both in the province of Cáceres, and Garlitos, Zarza-Capilla and Malcocinado belong to the province of Badajoz, all of them in the county of Extremadura. The municipalities have been selected on the basis that they have shown a population with a higher rate of ageing in contexts with difficulties in accessing public health, social services and food storage resources and that, generally, they have a small population. The research techniques we intend to apply are described below (Table 1).

Table 1. Research techniques and empirical materials.

Research technique	Typology of empirical materials
In-depth interviews	Narratives with answers from interviews according to the model of semi-structured interview worked
Interviews plus observation	Mapping and registration of supply spaces, practices on this process, storage, preparation (cooking techniques, instruments...) consumption (where, in what company...) and food consumption. Description of the scheme of the food process with emphasis on difficulties and limitations
Informal conversations	Informal conversations, not always recorded, to improve the script of the interview and provide other empirical material
Focus groups	Opinions, beliefs, perceptions, interests and attitudes regarding "appropriate" and healthy ways of eating
Questionnaires *24 h dietary recall*	Standardized questionnaire with adaptations to the particularities of the work field
Observation of food practices	Participant observation and field journal entries
Household food inventories	Description of standard diets: collection of shopping lists, refrigerators, kitchens, preparation modes

4   Technology in Socio-cultural Research

This project provides an unbeatable space for interdisciplinary-based research. As an example, we can describe here two of the categories of analysis on which we are working. First, the problems of access to food. There is consensus on defining food access and stockpiling as a central pillar of community food security [9,20]. Many studies have delimited this question to economic variables, with access restrictions based on household income calculations. This is a correct and also a valid approach in our research context, but not the only one. In the villages of our research there is a particular delineation in the supply, with places that have no stores or supermarkets. The circulation of food - "the field of the eatable" - is conditioned from a structural framework, limited to private initiatives of itinerant sale. The social construction of taste, we must keep in mind, is based on complex relationships between the ideological and the material. But structural limitations - the consumption of fresh food, such as unfrozen fish, for example-constitute a space where technological proposals must be developed. During our conversations with some of the food sellers, they admitted that they carried what they "sold", underlining the ability of buyers to delimit their sale. This is not entirely the case. The sale of non-perishable products implies a lower risk for business owners. However, we could work on systems that allow us to define shopping lists of fresh products that do not involve a risk for business investment or articulate actions from the administration to overcome these logistical problems. Technology has a lot of space to work on here.

In the same category of analysis, it should be reminded that the trips to gathering centres are usually defined in universal terms: distance from home to the store. However, these data require more particular analysis, given the specificity of the population in areas such as levels of functionality or dependence. As the figures in these domains change, so do the distance. We also need to observe statistics with a closer look. There are data available that could tell us if a family has a vehicle. But in the micro dynamics, we must know the use that the person in charge of food purchasing can make of this vehicle. In the case of the aged rural context of Extremadura, women have a much more limited capacity for use. In the fieldwork we have been able to see how the use of the vehicle for female activities -buying is still today mentioned in the responsibility of women-is subordinated to other male uses, such as going to the "bar". Statistics and figures need to incorporate the concept of agency into the equation.

In our study, interdisciplinary work is also crucial in the diagnostic phase. We work on the mapping of study areas with a variable representation of distances and difficulties depending on factors such as functionality, but also social position or gender. Our intention is to offer tools that make possible to visualize existing problems in a more accurate way. This interdisciplinary relationship between social sciences and technology can also be observed in the collaborative work on research technological tools. We are currently working on the design of an application to improve the food surveys, to speed up the collection of data, including descriptions of observation units.

Food decisions, those that have such a great impact on the health of populations, are not only constrained by material aspects. On the contrary, it is crucial to know the ideologies and their construction processes, the second major category we are dealing with here. We need to know what, but especially how and why. It has been studied, for example, how the mass media play a crucial role in this regard by disseminating information and knowledge, to the point that the dissemination of information on medicine, public health and nutrition science through them is an area of concern for many social and health scientist [8, 10, 15], in many cases contributing to myths or the spread of misconceptions.

The current sensitive level of analysis allows us to affirm that the notion of "healthy" of this population group is far from the medical and nutritional prescriptions. We need to offer data that not only show the gap, but also provide explanations to clarify the construction processes. From the analysis of ideologies and food practices we can provide an initial step to technologists to provide solutions affecting these construction processes. For instance, if a low consumption of liquids is detected and why, technologists could provide solutions that allow, for example, reminders. If we detect that health education in nutritional terms is not achieving its objective, the joint effort with technologists can delimit tools or new languages to build health education. Today it is not at all strange to talk about electronic prescriptions, while there is plenty of scientific literature on the scope of the mobile phone as a tool for communication between health professionals and the population [4,6,17,27,28]. Some studies have underlined its capacity to improve the quality of life in the elderly [19], to the extent that it has been used as a communicative tool in health education or prevention of problems associated with pathologies such as diabetes or vascular problems [16,23].

5   In Conclusion

The work on food and ageing population in rural areas seems today indissoluble from the contributions of technological innovation. We have referred here to aspects in the production of empirical materials, but social approaches and methodologies can also contribute to the analysis of technological solutions. The specific features of our study population must be taken into account in this sense, but it is also true that technological solutions must be adapted, not by delimiting themselves to the "known space", but rather to what is to come. When we conclude our research, perhaps there will be possible forms of food prescription where health professionals can monitor the diet of a family helping to choose the healthiest option.

Finally, the intersections between socio-cultural approaches and technology occur in the field of interventions. Technological proposals can prove successful and attractive in labs, but they need to "work" in real life. In this sense, the relationship between technology and society is crossed by factors such as age, rurality index or gender, and therefore a new ethnographic research will allow the analysis of microsocial contexts that provide us with information and define the possible problems derived from uses, or what it is the same, according to Lowrie [14], we will try to understand how technology is assembled within social processes and the effect it has (or could have).

Acknowledgment. This work was supported by the 4IE project (0045-4IE-4-P) funded by the Interreg V-A España-Portugal (POCTEP) 2014–2020 program.

References

1. Abellán García, A., Rodríguez-Laso, Á., Pujol Rodríguez, R., Barrios, L.: 12.000 centenarios en 2017 en España, ¿222.000 en 2066? (2017). http://envejecimientoenred.es/centenarios_en_espana/
2. Arbonés, G., et al.: Nutrición y recomendaciones dietéticas para personas mayores. Nutr. Hosp **18**(3), 109–137 (2003). https://doi.org/10.4321/S0212-71992004000600002
3. Brownie, S.: Why are elderly individuals at risk of nutritional deficiency? Int. J. Nurs. Pract. **12**(2), 110–118 (2006). https://doi.org/10.1111/j.1440-172X.2006.00557.x
4. Burdette, S.D., Herchline, T.E., Oehler, R.: Surfing the web: practicing medicine in a technological age: using smartphones in clinical practice. Clin. Infect. Dis. **47**(1), 117–122 (2008). https://doi.org/10.1086/588788
5. Chen, C.C.H., Schilling, L.S., Lyder, C.H.: A concept analysis of malnutrition in the elderly. J. Adv. Nurs. **36**(1), 131–142 (2001). https://doi.org/10.1046/j.1365-2648.2001.01950.x
6. Coiera, E
7. DiMaria-Ghalili, R.A., Amella, E.: Nutrition in older adults. Am. J. Nurs. **105**(3), 40–50 (2005)
8. Fineberg, H.V., Rowe, S.: Improving public understanding: guidelines for communicating emerging science on nutririon. Food Saf. Health **90**(3), 194–199 (1998)
9. Godfray, H.C.J., et al.: Food security: the challenge of feeding 9 billion people (2010). https://doi.org/10.1126/science.1185383
10. Hackman, E.M., Moe, G.L.: Evaluation of newspaper reports of nutrition-related research. J. Am. Diet. Assoc. **99**(12), 1564–1566 (1999). https://doi.org/10.1016/S0002-8223(99)00384-3
11. Hammersley, M., Atkinson, P.: Etnografía: métodos de investigación. Paidós, Barcelona (1994)
12. INE: Proyección de la Población de España 2014–2064: Notas de prensa. Technical report (2014). https://doi.org/10.1017/CBO9781107415324.004
13. Instituto de Mayores y Servicios Sociales (IMSERSO): Informe 2014. Las Personas Mayores en España. Technical report, Ministerio de Sanidad, Servicios Sociales e Igualdad, Madrid (2015). http://www.imserso.es/InterPresent1/groups/imserso/documents/binario/22029_info2014pm.pdf
14. Lowrie, I.: Algorithms and automation: an introduction. Cult. Anthropol. **33**(3), 349–359 (2018). https://doi.org/10.14506/ca33.3.01
15. Maheshwar, M., Narender, K., Balakrishna, N., Rao, D.R.: Teenagers Understanding and influence of media content on their diet and health-related behaviour. J. Clin. Nutr. Diet. **04**(02) (2018). https://doi.org/10.4172/2472-1921.100071
16. Melanson, D.: Sanofi-Aventis debuts iBGStar blood glucose meter for iPhone (2010)
17. Perera, C.: The evolution of e-health – mobile technology and mHealth. J. Mobile Technol. Med. **1**(1), 1–2 (2012). https://doi.org/10.7309/jmtm.1
18. Pirlich, M., Lochs, H.: Nutrition in the elderly. Bailliere's Best Pract. Res. Clin. Gastroenterol. **15**(6), 869–884 (2001). https://doi.org/10.1053/bega.2001.0246
19. Roupa, Z., et al.: The use of technology by the elderly. Health Sci. J. **2**, 118–126 (2010)
20. Schmidhuber, J., Tubiello, F.N.: Global food security under climate change. Proc. Natl. Acad. Sci. **104**(50), 19703–19708 (2007). https://doi.org/10.1073/pnas.0701976104

21. Schneider, M.: Public health and the aging population. In: Schneider, M.J. (ed.) Introduction to Public Health, 2nd edn, pp. 489–512. Jones and Barlett Publishers, Sudbury (2006)
22. Seiler, W.O.: Nutritional status of ill elderly patients. Zeitschrift fur Gerontologie und Geriatrie **32**(Suppl 1), I7–11 (1999)
23. Tucker, A.T.: Augmentation of venous, arterial and microvascular blood supply in the leg by isometric neuromuscular stimulation via the peroneal nerve. Int. J. Angiol. **19**(1), 31–37 (2010). https://doi.org/10.1055/s-0031-1278361
24. Velasco, H., De Rada, Á.D.: La lógica de la investigación etnográfica: un modelo de trabajo para etnógrafos de la escuela. Trotta, Madrid (2006)
25. Vidal Domínguez, M.J., et al.: Informe 2016: Las personas mayores en España. Datos estadísticos estatales y por comunidades autónomas, p. 540 (2017)
26. World Health Organization: Diet, nutrition and the prevention of chronic diseases. Technical report (2003)
27. Wu, R., et al.: An evaluation of the use of smartphones to communicate between clinicians: a mixed-methods study. J. Med. Internet Res. **13**(3), e59 (2011). https://doi.org/10.2196/jmir.1655
28. Wu, R.C., et al.: The use of smartphones for clinical communication on internal medicine wards. J. Hosp. Med. **5**(9), 553–559 (2010). https://doi.org/10.1002/jhm.775

Perceptions and Needs with Regard to Technologies for Professional Practice

A Prospective Qualitative Study Among Caregivers in Spain

Eulàlia Hernández-Encuentra[1](✉) [iD], Alícia Aguilar-Martínez[2] [iD],
Daniel López Gómez[3] [iD], Beni Gómez-Zúñiga[1] [iD],
Modesta Pousada[1] [iD], Israel Conejero-Arto[4] [iD],
and Francesc Saigí-Rubió[5] [iD]

[1] PSiNET Research Group, Faculty of Psychology and Education Sciences,
Universitat Oberta de Catalunya, Barcelona, Spain
{ehernandez,bgomezz,mpousada}@uoc.edu
[2] FoodLab Research Group, Faculty of Health Sciences,
Universitat Oberta de Catalunya, Barcelona, Spain
aaguilarmart@uoc.edu
[3] CareNet Research Group, Internet Interdisciplinary Institute (IN3),
Faculty of Psychology and Education Sciences,
Universitat Oberta de Catalunya, Barcelona, Spain
dlopezgo@uoc.edu
[4] eHealth Lab Research Group, Faculty of Health Sciences,
Universitat Oberta de Catalunya, Barcelona, Spain
iconejero@uoc.edu
[5] i2TIC Research Group, Faculty of Health Sciences,
Universitat Oberta de Catalunya, Barcelona, Spain
fsaigi@uoc.edu

Abstract. The purpose of the paper is to gain an understanding of the perceptions and needs of caregivers looking after the elderly or those with multiple disabilities with regard to the use of technology in the course of their work, in order to design the associated training.

A qualitative study using semi-structured interviews of 10 caregivers from different disciplines caring for the elderly or those with multiple disabilities in Spain.

Results: There is a generalized personalized use of ICT that cannot easily be transferred to caregiving duties. The difference between formal and informal care does not seem to be as important as the type of work performed: nevertheless, formal caregivers display a standardized pattern in their responses, perceiving a potential benefit and an ease in incorporating technology, but this is not accompanied by any social influence or conditions to facilitate this. With regard to the pattern of informal caregivers' responses, although the same tendency can be noted, some uncertainty can be appreciated, particularly with regard to performance expectancy.

As a conclusion, although the benefits that technology could bring to caregivers' tasks are perceived, no organizational or family-based context to

© Springer Nature Switzerland AG 2019
J. García-Alonso and C. Fonseca (Eds.): IWoG 2018, CCIS 1016, pp. 48–61, 2019.
https://doi.org/10.1007/978-3-030-16028-9_5

promote or facilitate it can be appreciated, and it is this that might be the primary target of the first stage of training. In a second phase, training for caregivers would be focused on the effective use of technology.

Keywords: Caregivers · Technology · Needs analysis

1 Introduction

The interest in technology and aging as a research area has increased in recent years, engaging researchers from different scientific fields [1]. The elderly's acceptance of innovative technology in their everyday life is a key success factor for governments, technology providers, healthcare providers, and other major players in elderly people's lives [2]. However, the biggest challenge in this regard lies in satisfying the need for holistic and comprehensive service, which means providing personalized services and adapting technology and content to different stakeholders' individual needs. A review of the literature shows that the major players in this context are the elderly themselves, their families, healthcare providers, technology providers, and the government and policymakers [2]. Here it is important to fully understand the psychological, social, ethical and legal dimensions; clinical prerequisites have to be considered, and appropriate and usable technological solutions must be developed under the watchful eye of a legal and ethical regulatory framework.

Various theoretical models have been developed, primarily based on theories in psychology and sociology, employed to explain technology acceptance and use. One of these is the unified theory of acceptance and use of technology (UTAUT) [3], which is a synthesis of previous models. From this theory, we can extract important content for major players in the technology adoption process, which clarifies the adoption process and provides critical points for technology implementation. In fact, the UTAUT model has identified critical factors and contingencies related to predicting intention-to-use behaviors and technology use itself [4]. Since it was first published, the UTAUT has served as a baseline model for a number of studies in both organizational and non-organizational settings.

The original UTAUT had four key constructs (performance expectancy, effort expectancy, social influence and facilitating conditions), which, along with their definitions, were later adapted to the technology acceptance and use context. As such, performance expectancy is defined as the degree to which using a technology will benefit users when performing certain activities. Effort expectancy is the degree of ease associated with the use of technology. Social influence is the extent to which users perceive that others holding an important place in their lives (e.g. family and friends) believe they should use a particular technology. Facilitating conditions refer to users' perceptions of the resources and support available to carry out a behavior [3, 5].

According to the UTAUT, the constructs of performance expectancy, effort expectancy and social influence affect people's intention to use technology, while this intention and facilitating conditions determine actual technology use. As a complement to the existing constructs, three other constructs were added in a second version of the model (UTAUT2). These are: hedonic or intrinsic motivation, price value, and experience and habit. Hedonic motivation is defined as the fun or pleasure derived from using a technology, and it has been shown to play an important role in determining technology acceptance and use [4, 5]. Price value is positive when the benefits of using a technology are perceived to be greater than the monetary cost. When this occurs, it has a positive impact on intention, which is why price value must be included as a predictor of behavioral intention to use a technology.

The last constructs added to the UTAUT2 are experience and habit. Although related, they are distinct. Experience reflects an opportunity to use a target technology and is typically operationalized as the time that has passed since an individual first used a type of technology [4], while habit is defined as the extent to which people tend to behave a certain way automatically because it is learned [6].

There are times, however, where it is not only the elderly who are adopting a technology: it can also be a useful tool for the caregivers themselves. The latter are, usually, younger than those they care for or, at the very least, in better physical and mental shape. In this regard, it would be useful to understand the needs they believe can be covered by technology and what use they make of it. Very little research has taken into account how elderly people's (formal or informal) caregivers use technological aids. Indeed, strictly speaking, only the paper by Yu, Li and Gagnon [7] analyses the matter, focusing specifically on the factors that help or hinder the acceptance of information and communication technologies (ICT) by those caring for the elderly.

Given the lack of scientific information on the matter, our goal here is to provide an initial approach to the particular view held of technology and ICT by caregivers looking after the elderly or those with multiple disabilities, their predisposal to using them to enhance the care they provide and their training needs with regard to these technologies.

It is our opinion that the UTAUT2 method can be useful, not only to provide an account of the adoption of technology by the elderly themselves, but also by their caregivers. So, in this regard, we have decided to use the UTAUT2 as a baseline model, as it is a proposal that integrates different theories and because it has already been well researched. Moreover, most of the topics we expect this study to focus on are covered by its constructs or can be related to one of them. Thus, this model has served as the framework for the interview guidelines and the interviews' analysis.

2 Methodology

A qualitative study was performed based on semi-structured interviews carried out in person or by telephone with different caregivers, with the aim of gathering their experiences, perceptions and opinions with regard to the use of technology in providing care and attending to the elderly. The study was performed on the basis of "key informants", defined as first-choice, accessible informants who were participating or had participated on an active basis in caring for and assisting the elderly, and who were prepared to offer their experience, opinion and knowledge for the purpose of the study. Additionally, the scope of our study was limited to Spain, for reasons of accessibility and sample control. Table 1 indicates the interview's structure.

Table 1. General script for interviews (See Appendix. Script Interview for the complete script)

Interview structure
Demographic questions (profile)
Section 1: The practical parameters that determine the patient's acceptability of ALTs (anxiety for technology, privacy versus autonomy, social stigma, cultural differences, etc.).
Section 2: The role of the caregiver in this new environment and the smooth cooperation between the caregiver and the ALTs.
Section 3: The impact assisted living technologies have on the ethical and social sphere of the beneficiaries, namely: privacy, autonomy, obtrusiveness, passivity, reliance on automation, and reduction of social interaction.

Informants were selected using the purposeful chain sampling technique (also known as "snowball sampling"), to ensure the greatest variability in professional profiles, given that caregiving is a wide-ranging multidisciplinary field. A preliminary proposed list of key informants was drawn up, and the persons included therein then contacted, explaining to them the purpose of the research, requesting their collaboration and, in turn, their recommendations for other caregivers to contact, who permitted the broadening and enhancement of the results' interpretation and who, in turn, led us to other caregivers. The interviews were deemed concluded when the information on the categories appearing in the analysis process was regarded as saturated.

All relevant procedures were implemented to protect the confidentiality of the information and the anonymity of the participants. The interviews were recorded in audio format to facilitate their subsequent analysis.

A thematic analysis was performed, grouping caregivers' responses on the basis of: (a) their relationship with technology and their willingness to adopt it, and (b) technology-related requirements and training needs to improve their work.

3   Results

Over the course of August and September 2018, we interviewed ten caregivers (five formal and five informal) working in public care facilities and in the private sphere (private nursing homes and home-based care). All of them were women with extensive experience in care work. However, the greatest difference between the two groups was the fact that informal caregivers were older and had a lower education level (see Table 2).

3.1   Relationship with the Technology and Predisposition to Its Adoption Per the UTAUT2 Model

Table 3 provides a summary of responses with regard to the model's variables and Table 4 shows representative quotes as examples.

Table 2. Demographic profiles

	Formal caregivers (n = 5)	Informal caregivers (n = 5)
Gender	100% women	100% women
Average age (years)	44	57
Level of studies	Vocational training as nursing assistant (specializing in geriatric care)	Basic
Average experience of caregiving	14 years	14 years (a perception of "lifelong" in 2 out of 5)
User	100% elderly	80% elderly 20% young people with multiple disabilities
Place of work	Barcelona (7), Valencia (1), Granada (2)	

Table 3. Summary of answers related to the UTAUT2 model's variables

	Formal caregivers	Informal caregivers
Performance expectancy	Yes	Yes/No
Effort expectancy	Yes	Yes
Social influence	No	No
Facilitating conditions of use	No	No
Hedonic motivation	No	No
Price value	Yes	Yes/Not clear
Experience of use (in general, not specifically in care activities)	Yes	Yes
Habit	Yes	Yes/Not clear

All the caregivers interviewed used digital technologies to a greater or lesser degree. Nevertheless, when asked about the use of technology within their professional environment, they regarded technology in terms of tools useful in minimizing their physical workload, rather than thinking right away of ICT. It is in this sense that technology (for bathing, transporting or movement) is perceived of as an increase in the quality of care or assistance and thus offering significant benefits for their work. In a couple of cases, these benefits were also associated with the caregiver's own quality of life and with reducing or minimizing work-related injuries.

When examining in greater depth informal caregivers' relationship with digital technologies (cameras, sensors, apps, etc.), speedy communication with healthcare professionals or support resources were considered fundamental and, to this end, the cellphone was their tool of choice. The situation was different for some formal caregivers, who were not authorized to use their cellphones at work.

Additionally, although all of them were aware of and appreciated alarm and/or remote assistance systems, the general responses obtained did not reflect a perception of the usefulness of ICT for improving quality of care. None of the caregivers mentioned having added them as a new tool at work. Neither specific care or assistance tasks (observation, monitoring, etc.) nor administrative ones (registering treatment, administration of medication doses, etc.) were carried out with digital technology: pen and paper were always used.

Despite this lack of usage at work, ICT were perceived of with a certain degree of optimism by most interviewees, although they placed on record their lack of understanding of the different options available and of how to use them. Amongst informal caregivers, the possibility of rapidly contacting a professional to resolve doubts or access new resources with information on caregiving was among some of the perceived uses. For their part, amongst formal caregivers, greater access to information on the care given and the status of the person cared for, from anywhere and consultable by any member of the care team, were some of the aspects mentioned as possibly being useful.

At the same time, but only in the case of one formal caregiver, reference was made to planned technology projects for the center to facilitate communications between professionals and family members.

Lastly, seven of the ten caregivers gave the highest score (5 on a scale from 1 to 5) to willingness to use technology and did not believe that it would be difficult to incorporate it into their professional activities, as all of them used it on a personal level (cellphones, tables, computers, email, etc.).

Together with personal factors, the model points to the importance of the surrounding environment's influence on users in the adoption and use of ICT. More specifically, recommendations made by significant others and friends (peers) or by their superiors or managers at the center where the caregivers worked could impact upon the decision to use technologies. All of the caregivers acknowledged that the influence of patients, patients' family members and professional colleagues was non-existent. Additionally, no influence was exercised by center employees or management.

Although not unanimously, no social pressure associated with professional improvement or advancement was received, nor did they feel responsible for the final decision to use ICT in their jobs. They regarded it as family members' or organization management's responsibility to implement them, and then their responsibility to use such technologies once implemented. In the case of informal caregivers, the search for technological innovations was much more dependent upon technology helping solve practical problems and really being a support in caregiving.

Difficulties in acquiring these technologies and securing the institution's permission were repeatedly highlighted by caregivers as significant limitations when it came to introducing these ICT into their work. Although the need to secure financing is indicated as a factor that could favor the use of ICT, the taking of decisions as to whether to adopt a technological device appears to be a key and prior aspect to be resolved.

Table 4. Quotes on the relationship with technology and willingness to adopt it, per UTAUT2 model

"The technologies I incorporated were aimed at solving the issue of mobility: wheelchairs, an armchair and an electronic bed that allowed me to move my husband more easily, and grab handles in the showers". (Informal caregiver 5)
"Technology could improve caregiving activities, particularly to work with less personal effort, and more comfortably, both for me and for patients". (Formal caregiver 1)
"I'm not too sure how technology could help me as a caregiver. I think that it could be useful to communicate with those I'm caring for or perhaps also with some professional so they could help me". (Informal caregiver 1)
"I think that we could use a tablet to note down everything we do to a person and be more connected. I could see everything that the physical therapist has done to them, or if they have taken their medication, from anywhere". (Formal caregiver 2)
"I think I would have an easy relationship with technology. I would be prepared for it and find it easy, but someone else might find it harder". (Informal caregiver 3)
"I've never been asked to use technology to care for my mother. And I don't know anyone that uses it". (Informal caregiver 4)
"I don't think I need more camera or monitoring kinds of tools. I feel it's more a responsibility for the family members of the person I take care of. I believe I only have responsibilities during working hours. It could be mentioned to family members, who are those who might need them, but it's not part of my duties". (Formal caregiver 1)
"I'm not sure about what the repercussions may be in terms of my CV or recruitment". (Formal caregiver 5)
"There's a need for economic resources, everything is very expensive". (Informal caregiver 3)

3.2 Requirements and Formative Needs for the Improvement of Tasks

The caregivers interviewed were interested in the possibility of training associated with their caregiving work and the use of technology, although they found it difficult to make specific content-related suggestions. Where there was agreement was in a preference for face-to-face training, given by a teacher or guide. Although some mention was made of the possibilities of videoconferencing or online training, they mentioned that this was only feasible for young people and not older people, or in any case for more advanced training levels, rather than initial training.

There was also agreement on a "practical" focus for training (applicable to their everyday work) and a degree of organization into levels or modules. Some proposals and suggestions referred to adapting these levels based on one's experience as a caregiver or the complexity of the conditions to be dealt with, or modules with content tackling the available technologies and how to use them in each given case, psychological aspects associated with the person cared for (not imposing, making them feel valued, etc.) and specific training on caregiving in certain situations or for certain conditions (wounds, catheters, finding veins, etc.).

Neither external recognition nor the validity of the training appeared to be aspects of concern to any of the interviewees, and only one mentioned that they would be important to take into account for carrying out the training.

Table 5 shows some quotes to support those ideas.

Table 5. Quotes on requirements and training needs for improving caregiving

"A face-to-face course. Going to class with a teacher explaining how to use it". (Informal caregiver 1)
"The first choice would be face-to-face, a second option maybe online, but with a teacher, because if you had to read it on your own, nobody would do it". (Formal caregiver 2)
"Ideally face-to-face. Maybe, the odd Skype if someone can't but I think that caregivers may well be older people and they wouldn't do it online. I also think it has to be really practical". (Informal caregiver 3)
"Training should be face-to-face and in a group, as it's important to share things with other caregivers and learn from their experiences". (Informal caregiver 4)
"Its content could be modular, with different levels, initial or with a different degree of depth so you don't get bored. Advanced-level content could be online and without a teacher". (Formal caregiver 3).

4   Discussion

The UTAUT2 model is a theory widely employed in research on the acceptance of new information technologies in the workplace. More particularly, the model provides a robust explanation for variability with regard to ICT usage intentions and behavior in line with an individual's perception of technology. The proposed model suggests two types of elements: specific acceptance factors and the subjects' conditions, which modify the intensity with which the specific factors act.

None of the interviewees showed either apprehension or fear regarding the use of technologies on a personal level. Clearly, cultural and social reasons [8], together with other socio-demographic variables, such as age and gender, and circumstantial ones, such as experience and education [9] play a role in defining a person's level of usage of technology. Nevertheless, despite this personal usage, it is not translated into the professional sphere of caregiving, and therefore the use of these tools is not extensive, but rather single and contextualized [10, 11].

The role played by caregivers is crucial in understanding not so much the relationship they establish with technology as the type of technology they will employ in the performance of their activities and the value they will attach to it. The fact of whether it is formal or informal care does not seem as important as the type of work carried out. In all cases, whether the care is formal or informal, at home or in a care facility, care entails, fundamentally, physical work [12]: washing, dressing, moving, feeding, providing company, etc. So, assistive technologies are, essentially, technologies that facilitate this physical work or free them from it, in that they allow the person cared for to do it for themselves [13]. Digital technologies, which might involve the use of sensors, apps and cameras, are regarded as features of a hypothetical future, but far removed from present-day realities. However, caregivers showed different degrees of interest depending upon their previous experience of technology and the social value of its usage in everyday contexts (mainly family and professional). Those sharing the notion of social progress through technology and who adopt (more or less proactively) new digital technologies appear more in favor of its usage in caregiving tasks as well.

According to other authors [14], what the caregivers interviewed seek is technologies that make their work easier, not necessarily transforming it. None of the interviewees had contemplated, for example, the possibility of caregivers being able to delegate the work they do to some kind of more or less autonomous technology [15, 16]. They do not regard said technologies as tools for delegating the emotional and supervisory work they perform, nor even physical care work, but rather as support for work that is in itself significant, which coincides with the regard in which technology is held by those who they care for: the elderly [17].

In this regard, they believe that a caregiver should be judged on their ability to provide good care, and not for their skills in using technology [7]. This statement is supported by some works on the perception of the elderly, who do not believe that the use of technology will significantly improve their quality of life [18].

Regarding technology as a means of support for caregiving, caregivers view technologies as tools providing a response to a present need, rather than devices linked to risk prevention or detection [17, 19]. Caregivers disassociate themselves from taking decisions on introducing technology into their caregiving tasks, although they state that they are committed to its effective use if deemed necessary.

These results are clearly linked with those obtained on possible training on the matter. So, they associate possible training with practical aspects associated with a specific technology in specific caregiving situations, provided on a face-to-face, guided basis and adapted into line with their experience and the types of care they provide. In other words, they do not view it as the possibility of gaining an understanding of a catalogue of tools, usages and benefits, or ethical problems arising therefrom. We believe that these results are in line with the work of Yu et al. [7], in which the purpose of training is regarded as increasing caregivers' performance expectancy (perception of benefits) with regard to the usage of technology. Indeed, training of this type promoted by managers at long-term care facilities or by the family members responsible for the persons receiving the care would impact, not only on performance expectancy, but also on effort expectancy (ease of use), social influence (importance for others) and facilitating conditions (support for use), which are the four key elements in the adoption of technology, according to the UTAUT2 model.

Lastly, these results reveal the importance of carrying out studies prior to the use of ICT and attempting to reveal which predictors have an influence and how, especially when they are aimed at a variety of end users. Research faces the challenge of producing this evidence. In this regard, and above and beyond these initial preliminary results, future lines of research are to be found in two fields: firstly, by means of the comparison of results with other samples of caregivers from other EU countries, particularly a, inter-country comparison; and, secondly, analysis of how the determinants of the usage of the ICT by caregivers impacts upon the outcome of their work.

5 Conclusions

The concept of technology is unclear to the caregivers interviewed. In turn, despite their personal usage of ICT, they do not apply them in their caregiving tasks, be these formal or informal, or at least the caregivers do not perceive themselves as consciously using them.

Turning to the basic variables of the UTAUT2 model for the adoption of technology (performance expectancy, effort expectancy, social influence, and facilitating conditions), it has clearly been seen that there is a long way to go in the introduction of technology into caregiving, particularly because, even when its potential benefits are clearly appreciated, there is no perception of any organizational or family context to promote or facilitate it.

Given this, we believe that the recipient of any possible training should be reconsidered: so, we identify an initial need for training aimed at decision-makers (care center staff or the elderly and/or family members) associated with enhancing understanding of the tools and of their potential benefits and, subsequently, training for caregivers linked with learning and support for their effective usage.

6 Appendix. Interview Script

Demographic profile (profile)

- Gender: m/w
- Age:
- Educational level:
- Economic status (income intervals according to each country)
- Experience
- Care.
  - Training for care: yes/no (specify which one)
  - Persons you attend: health conditions and age of the persons you have experience in attending: (specify)
  - Years of experience in caring practices:
- Use of Technology (UTAUT: experience).
  - Devices you use in your personal life: (specify)
  - Devices you use for care activities: (specify)
  - Devices you use in your personal life and for care activities

Package 1: The practical parameters that determine the patient's acceptability of ALTs (anxiety for technology, privacy versus autonomy, social stigma, cultural differences, etc.).

- Have you ever thought of using any ALTs to carry out your care tasks? If yes, which one? Which was the specific problem you expected to solve or the situation you expected to improve? (UTAUT: voluntariness of use, experience)
- Do you believe that using any kind of ALTs will help you in your caring tasks? In what way? (UTAUT: performance expectancy)
- What do you think influences the acceptance of ALTs? Could it be determined by something particular that affects you personally? (UTAUT: performance expectancy)
- Do you consider yourself a person who, once you have learned something, introduces it into your daily routine as a habit? (i.e. if you have learned a new caring practise, from that moment on you always do it that way).
- Do you think this could also be applied to the use of technology (a certain program, a device, an app, etc.)? (UTAUT: habit)
- In which way can the use of ALT enable you to improve the care tasks? Can you give a few examples? (UTAUT: performance expectancy)
- Has anybody asked you to use ALTs (for carrying out caring tasks)? Who? e.g., the institution you work for, the family of the person you are caring for, the person you are caring for, yourself? (UTAUT: social influence) (UTAUT: voluntariness of use)
- Do you know anyone who is using ALTs at home? If yes, is he/she a person who is close to you, who you trust? Has his or her opinion exerted a clout on your decision to use ALTs? (UTAUT: social influence).
- Do you think that using ALT will enhance your professional standing/recognition? In which way/why not? (UTAUT: social influence) (UTAUT: voluntariness of use)
- To what extent would you be willing to use technology in your care work? (from 0 to 5) (UTAUT: voluntariness of use)
- Do you think that the benefits of using ALT are greater than their monetary cost? (UTAUT: Price Value)

Package 2: The role of the caregiver in this new environment and the smooth cooperation between the caregiver and the ALT's.

- Do you expect interaction between you and ALTs to be smooth and easy? If yes, please describe why? If not, what do you think is necessary to make it easier and smoother? (UTAUT: effort expectancy)
- Do you think it will be easy for you to learn how to operate new ALTs? Which tools would be helpful or what kind of support would you need? (UTAUT: effort expectancy)
- Which resources are necessary to implement and use the ALTs? Do you think that you have them available? (UTAUT: facilitating conditions)
- Do you have the necessary knowledge to use them? (UTAUT: facilitating conditions)
- Do you think it will be necessary to appoint a person with the expertise to assist you or solve technical problems with ALTs? (UTAUT: facilitating conditions)

- Do you know:
  - Which are the ALTs available in the market?
  - How to identify which ALT you need to meet your needs in each situation?
  - Where and How to look for the ALT you need?
  - How to appraise the quality and utility of the ALT regarding your needs?
  - How to use the chosen ALT to address your needs?

Package 3: The impact assisted living technologies have on the ethical and social sphere of the beneficiaries, namely: privacy, autonomy, obtrusiveness, passivity, reliance on automation, reduction of social interaction.

- Do you feel apprehensive about ALTs? Do you have any particular fear about using ALTs?
- Do you feel fun or pleasure when you use any technological device? And when you use ALTs? (UTAUT: hedonic motivation)
- Do you think it is important that people continue to perform daily activities in their homes for as long as possible, and with as little assistance as possible?
- If, to achieve this, you had to put a surveillance camera at the dining room, or a bracelet on the person's wrist, a sensor in the bed or WC, or a sensor in the refrigerator:
  - What do you think the benefits of this would be?
  - What are the conditions (legal, social, psychological, ethical...) that you would have to reckon with before introducing these technologies?
  - What would you want to consider personally?
- In your opinion, what would be the main contribution or the main impact of ALTs on the patients?
  - Protective (ALTs give more security to the patient)
  - Automation (ALTs automation leads to passivity)
  - Controlling (ALTs take your responsibilities)
  - Enabling/empowering (ALTs enhance patient's autonomy)
  - Isolating (ALTs decrease social contact)
  - Which adjective describes more accurately your view on ALTs?
- As we told you, we are planning to design an online training course on ALTs for caregivers.
  - Which are the contents/curricula do you think it should include?
  - In what format would you like it to have?

- Totally online/Blended
- Closed-content/Modular
- Totally self-paced/With a facilitator
- With different levels
- Any other...?

Acknowledgements. We would like to acknowledge all the caregivers who shared their doubts, insights and experiences. This work is based on a larger research project supported by the Erasmus+ program under Grant No. 2017-1-DE02-KA202-004212. TechCare project.

References

1. Chiarini, G., Ray, P., Akter, S., Masella, C., Ganz, A.: MHealth technologies for chronic diseases and elders: a systematic review. IEEE J. Sel. Areas Commun. **9**, 6 (2013). https://doi.org/10.1109/JSAC.2013.SUP.0513001
2. Mostaghel, R.: Innovation and technology for the elderly: systematic literature review. J. Bus. Res. **69**, 4896–4900 (2016). https://doi.org/10.1016/j.jbusres.2016.04.049
3. Venkatesh, V., Morris, M.G., Davis, G.B., Davis, F.D.: User acceptance of information technology: toward a unified view. Source MIS Q. **27**(3), 425–478 (2003). https://doi.org/10.2307/30036540
4. Venkatesh, V., Thong, J.Y.L., Xu, X.: Consumer acceptance and use of information technology: extending the unified theory. MIS Q. **36**(1), 157–178 (2012). https://doi.org/10.1017/CBO9781107415324.004
5. Brown, S.A., Venkatesh, V.: A model of adoption of technology in the household: a baseline model test and extension incorporating household life cycle. MIS Q. **29**(4), 399–426 (2005). https://doi.org/10.1080/01972240600791333
6. Limayem, M., Hirt, S.G., Cheung, C.M.K.: How habit limits the predictive power of intention: the case of information systems continuance. MIS Q. **31**(4), 705–737 (2007). https://doi.org/10.2307/25148817
7. Yu, P., Li, H., Gagnon, M.-P.: Health IT acceptance factors in long-term care facilities: a cross-sectional survey. Int. J. Med. Inform. **78**, 229 (2009). https://doi.org/10.1016/j.ijmedinf.2008.07.006
8. Axelsson, S.W., Wikman, A.M., Näslund, A., Nyberg, L.: Older people's health-related ICT-use in Sweden. Gerontechnology (2013). https://doi.org/10.4017/gt.2013.12.1.010.00
9. Quintiliani, L.M., Reddy, S., Goodman, R., Bowen, D.J.: Information and communication technology use by female residents of public housing. mHealth (2016). https://doi.org/10.21037/mhealth.2016.10.01
10. Selwyn, N.: The information aged: a qualitative study of older adults' use of information and communications technology. J. Aging Stud. **18**, 369–384 (2004). https://doi.org/10.1016/j.jaging.2004.06.008
11. Turner, P., Turner, S., Van De Walle, G.: How older people account for their experiences with interactive technology. Behav. Inf. Technol. **26**(4), 287–296 (2007). https://doi.org/10.1080/01449290601173499
12. Twigg, J.: Carework as a form of bodywork. Ageing Soc. **20**(4), 389–411 (2000). https://doi.org/10.1017/S0144686X99007801
13. Elwick, A., Liabo, K., Nutt, J., Simon, A.: Beyond the digital divide: young people and ICT. Read CfBT Educ Trust SSRU Inst Educ (2013)
14. Pols, J.: Review of Care at a distance: on the closeness of technology (2012)
15. Roberts, C., Mort, M., Milligan, C.: Calling for care: "disembodied" work, teleoperators and older people living at home. Sociology **46**(3), 490–506 (2012). https://doi.org/10.1177/0038038511422551
16. López, D., Sánchez-Criado, T.: Analysing hands-on-tech care work in telecare installations. In: Prendergast, D., Garattini, C. (eds.) Aging and the Digital Life Course, pp. 179–197. Berghahn Books, New York (2015)

17. Hernández-Encuentra, E., Pousada, M., Gómez-Zúniga, B.: ICT and older people: beyond usability. Educ. Gerontol. **35**(3), 226–245 (2009). https://doi.org/10.1080/0360127080 2466934
18. Skymne, C., Dahlin-Ivanoff, S., Claesson, L., Eklund, K.: Getting used to assistive devices: ambivalent experiences by frail elderly persons. Scand. J. Occup. Ther. **19**(2), 194–203 (2012). https://doi.org/10.3109/11038128.2011.569757
19. Demiris, G., Hensel, B.K., Skubic, M., Rantz, M.: Senior residents' perceived need of and preferences for "smart home" sensor technologies. Int. J. Technol. Assess. Health Care **1**, 120–125 (2008). https://doi.org/10.1017/S0266462307080154

What Technologies Can the Nurse Use to Increase the Quality of Life of the Elderly Population with Leg Ulcers? – Systematic Literature Review

Ana Ripado[1]([⊠]), Ruben Pires[1], Rita Morais[1], Pedro Parreira[2],
César Fonseca[3] ⓘ, Manuel Lopes[3] ⓘ, and Céu Marques[3]

[1] Évora University, Évora, Portugal
1.36404@alunos.uevora.pt
[2] College of Nursing of Coimbra, Coimbra, Portugal
[3] Évora University, Investigator POCTEP 0445_4IE_4_P, Évora, Portugal

Abstract. The purpose of this study was to identify the new technologies that nurses could use to increase the quality of life on an elderly person with leg ulcer. Methods: it was made a systematic revision of literature with qualitative synthesis and meta-analysis. Results: Elderly persons with chronic leg ulcers frequently experience multiple disabling symptoms and these symptoms are highly related with impairment of quality of life. Nowadays, the technology is prepared to improve diagnosis and treatment of illness. For the leg ulcer, one of the newest technologies is electrical stimulation on skin with two types: electrical stimulation therapy and electroceutical treatment. These therapies consist on the application of microcurrents of electric energy to replace the current of injury which has become disrupted in chronic wounds. The therapy reduces the wound size, pain and exudate levels. Conclusion: With this recent investigation and with the enforcement of new technologies in association with the usual therapies it is possible to improve the quality of life of the patient, however, it is extremely important to continue the investigation on this area.

Keywords: Leg ulcer · Quality of life · Technology

1 Introduction

A leg ulcer is defined as an ulceration below the knee and it is inserted on the group of chronic wounds [1]. These wounds can be classified as venous, arterials or mixed, on accord of its etiology [3].

Studies consider this pathology became a problem of public health because it affects 1% of the adult population and increases for a 3 to 5% of the elder population [5]. In Portugal, it is verified in past few years an increase of average life expectancy, with a media of 80,62 years [7]. As a consequence of this factor and in association with the increasing of the risk factors (diabetes, obesity, smoking habits, venous stasis, use of contraceptives, among others), the morbidity of the subject with leg ulcer as a

© Springer Nature Switzerland AG 2019
J. García-Alonso and C. Fonseca (Eds.): IWoG 2018, CCIS 1016, pp. 62–69, 2019.
https://doi.org/10.1007/978-3-030-16028-9_6

tendency to grow [5]. Is estimated that in Portugal close to 1,42% of individual per 1000 habitants suffers this problem [1].

This type of wounds causes physical, psychological and social repercussions to the patient, and causes a series of changes on the patient quotidian and on family life [2]. Because of the ulcer, the person can have pain, unpleasant odor on the wound lay, negative emotional reactions, changes on body image, depression, sleep problems e consequently social withdrawal [3]. This situation becomes extremely lowering and causes a negative impact on patient quality of life.

The quality of life is defined as an individual sensation of life satisfaction and well-being [3], being that this term involves all the components of the human condition: physics, physiologic, social, cultural and spiritual [2]. When this concept is related with health it become to be influenced by the impact of the disease and treatment [2].

In the health area, the technology innovation brings the appliance market and techniques more sophisticated, that help on a quick and beneficial diagnoses and treatment of illness. With this, the men can solve problems that doesn't have remedy in last few years and consequently develop better life conditions [6]. The modern technology has the purpose of increasingly the human activity and in a direct and indirect way, are associated with health care services [4].

It's important to detach that the technology can be a humanization facto rand can become an agent and an object of the human touch, even on the environments technologically intense of care. In nursing, if it exists a balance between the application of recent scientific knowledge and the role played by the nurse, it is possible to best suit the needs of the person and enable them to a better quality of life [4].

2   Methodology

A Systematic Review of Literature has been developed, and the following PICO [8] starting point has been defined: "What technologies can the nurse (I) use to increase the quality of life (O) of the elderly population with leg ulcers? (P)".

Carried out research in the EBSCO search engine: CINAHL (Plus with Full Text), MEDLINE (Plus with Full Text) and Academic Search Complete sought full text article, It is considered that the systematic reviews should take into account the scientific evidence of the last 5 years [8], for that reason, the articles searched for writing the systematic review were published between 01/01/2013 and 09/31/2018 with the following key words (Nursing OR Nurse) AND (Leg Ulcers) AND (Quality of Live) AND (TX Technology) AND (TX Aged OR Elderly OR Senior OR Older People).

We obtained a total of 25 articles: 7 articles in CINAHL, 13 articles in MEDLINE and 5 articles in Academic Search Complete, 5 of which were repeated. For the elaboration of the discussion and respective conclusions, 7 articles were filtered.

As inclusion criteria, articles focusing on the problematic where the results are sensitive to the use of technology in the improvement of the quality of life of the elderly, using quantitative, qualitative methodologies and systematic review of the literature, were favored. The exclusion criteria included all the clinical articles with no relation to the object of study, repeated in the two databases, with an unclear methodology with a date lower than 2013.

3   Results

To make visible and transparent the methodology used to explicit listing of 7 filtered articles, which were the substrate for the preparation of the discussion and respective conclusions.

In order to know the different types of knowledge production patent in the filtered articles, three levels of evidence were used: Level A – Data derived from multiple randomized clinical trials or meta-analyses; Level B – Date derived from a single randomized clinical trial or large non-randomized studies; Level C – Consensus of opinion of the experts and/or small studies, retrospective studies, registries (Table 1).

Table 1. Analysis of the articles included in the systematic review

Title	Author	Year	Participants	Methodology	Results
Electrical stimulation therapy and electroceutical treatment for the management of venous leg ulcers	Ovens, L. et al.	2017	1 man with 80 years	Case study Evidence Level B	Significant improvement of chronic inflammation in leg ulcers when electrical therapies are used compared to standard therapies. These technologies allow patient involvement, improving the quality of life
Factors associated with health-related quality of life in chronic leg ulceration	Hopman, W. et al.	2014	407 individuals	Quantitative Approach Evidence Level A	Individuals with leg ulcers have a lower quality of life compared to others. The most significant risk factors for this reduction are: age, sex, presence of pain, ulcer duration and size, and mobility restrictions
The results of a clinical evaluation of Accel-Heal® electroceutical treatment in a large NHS Trust	Turner, N. & Ovens, L.	2017	17 patients with leg ulcers with mean age of 66 years	Quantitative Approach Evidence Level B	The use of Accel-Heal® can improve patients' clinical outcomes when used as a complement to standard therapy

(*continued*)

Table 1. (*continued*)

Title	Author	Year	Participants	Methodology	Results
Distinct Wound Healing and Quality-of-Life Outcomes in Subgroups of Patients With Venous Leg Ulcers With Different Symptom Cluster Experiences	Finlayson, K. et al.	2017	247 patients with venous ulcer	Quantitative Approach Evidence Level A	There is a relationship between late ulcer healing and the quality of life. It indicates that the comprehensive assessment of symptoms is needed to identify patients at higher risk of adverse outcomes and enable early intervention
Identifying relationships between symptom clusters and quality of life in adults with chronic mixed venous and arterial leg ulcers	Hien, D. et al.	2015	110 people with chronic leg ulcer	Quantitative Approach Evidence Level B	Both the systemic symptoms (pain, fatigue and depressive symptom) and localized symptoms in the leg (pain, fatigue, exudate, inflammation and edema) are related to quality of life. Therefore, health professionals should analyze these symptoms and then alleviate the symptoms and improve the quality of life of the patients
Identification of Symptom Clusters in Patients with chronic venous leg ulcers	Edwards, H. et al.	2014	318 patients with venous ulcer	Quantitative Approach Evidence Level A	The identified 2 groups of symptoms: pain, depression, sleep disorder, fatigue and inflammation, exudate, edema of the lower limbs. These symptoms have an influence on the quality of life

(*continued*)

Table 1. (*continued*)

Title	Author	Year	Participants	Methodology	Results
The effectiveness of afour-layer compression bandage system in comparison with Class3 compression hosiery on healing and quality of life in patients with venous leg ulcers: a randomised controlled trial	Finlayson K. J. et al.	2014	103 participants	Randomized Controlled Trial Evidence Level A	This study provides a better understanding of wound healing and in this way, it is to improve ulcer healing rates, quality of life and reduce the costs of health care

4 Discussion of Results

Chronic leg ulcers affect 1% of the adult population and 3.6% of people older than 65 years [10], they are a significant cause of decreased functional ability and quality of life (QOL) [11]. The etiology of leg ulceration is usually multifactorial, with venous disease accounting for approximately 70%, mixed etiology for 15% [10].

Between 60% and 70% of leg ulcers [9] are caused by failure of venous return mechanisms in the lower limbs, [3] they are due to underlying structural damage in the circulatory system of the affected leg [9], which results in chronic venous insufficiency [11].

For venous leg ulcers, wear and tear or trauma in both the valves and vessels of veins hinders the flow of blood up the affected leg, which results in the accumulation of blood within the leg veins [9]. Increased pressure where the blood pools causes further vessel damage. In addition, a continuous leakage of blood outside the veins leads to a build-up of biologic material in that area of the leg [9].

On average, each ulcer remains an open wound for about 12 months. Unfortunately, when healing occurs, a high probability (i.e., 60% and 70%) exists that another ulcer will develop in its place [9]. This process causes chronic inflammation and leads to the formation of an open wound that is intrinsically impaired from healing [9]. Because many ulcers take years to heal, followed by recurrence shortly after, the long-term chronicity of the disease can lead to uncertainty, disappointment, loss of hope, or despair [11]. Seniors with chronic leg ulcers frequently experience multiple disabling symptoms, including pain, depression, sleep disturbance, fatigue, lower limb swelling, and symptoms associated with lower limb inflammation (e.g., pruritus, discomfort from high levels of exudate, localized heat, and redness) [9]. In addition, Edwards E, in her article refers that patients reported "tightness" or aching from lower leg edema [11]. The excess fluid in edematous legs often results in large amounts of wound exudate, causing further discomfort or excoriation or both from wet dressings and bandages and embarrassment associated with leakage and odor [11]. Many of these physical symptoms contribute to psychological symptoms. The nature of the condition can result in problems with body image and embarrassment [11].

Pain in patients with chronic leg ulcers is often inadequately managed and is associated with significant decrements in QOL [11]. In addition to pain, venous leg ulcers are associated with a number of symptoms that occur as a result of chronic venous insufficiency [11]. Previous studies found that certain symptoms, such as pain or depressive symptoms, are associated with poorer quality-of-life (QOL) and/or wound-healing outcomes [9].

Importantly, chronic leg ulcers significantly decrease QOL and cause a loss of independence [10]. This condition has a negative impact on activities of daily living, with 50% of patients reporting severe restrictions in mobility, 40% reporting social isolation, and 27%–68% reporting negative psychological impacts, such as depression, anxiety, and poor body image [10].

In a study conducted in 2015, with the aim of identifying relationships between symptom clusters and quality of life in adults with chronic mixed venous and arterial leg ulcers it was concluded that, both the systemic symptom cluster (pain, fatigue and depressive symptom) and the localized-leg symptom cluster (pain, fatigue, exudate, inflammation and edema) were highly correlated with physical QOL. Another particularly strong relationship was observed between the systemic symptom cluster and mental health QOL [10].

Leg ulcers have a difficult healing process and that results in an intensive use of resources to the treatment. Around 70% of chronic leg ulcers are caused by venous disease and evidence shows that compression therapy is an effective treatment [15]. Despite that in the past few years, technology is more used to diagnoses and treatment of some pathologies. Chronic leg ulcers are not an exception.

One of does new technology is using electric stimulation on skin with two types of therapy: electric stimulation therapy and electroceutical treatment. Human physiology is electrochemical in nature and within the skin a stream of electrical current, known as "skin battery", is created by the difference in voltage between the surface of the epidermis and the deeper layers, and produces a low amperage current, called "skin current". With the presence of a wound the skin current is discontinued at the wound site and the flow of the current flows outwards, establishing a "current of injury". This last current is important to orchestrate tissue repair, to stimulate cell proliferation and to collagen synthesis. However, it can disrupt when adverse events of the wound occur, such as the presence of foreign bodies, slough, necrotic tissue or following the development of biofilms and/or infection. With this information comes the therapies named above. Electrical stimulation therapy and electroceutical treatment is the application of microcurrents of electrical energy to replace the current of injury [12].

Firstly, appeared electrical stimulation therapy. This device used an electro-stimulation impulse generator, adapting the intensity according the patient tolerance, and applying the current twice daily for 30 min for up 12 weeks. Studies prove that this treatment reduce the wound size, encourage granulation and change the wound from an inflammatory phase to the repair phase. Until now studies don't prove the existence of side effects. The size of the device and need for such regular application could cause challenges for its use in the community [12].

Secondarily appeared electroceutical treatment that delivers a sub-sensory level of electrical energy to cause a physiological change to the impaired biological functions in the wound. With a push of button, the treatment provides a precise dose of electro-ceutical treatment over a fixed period of 12 days [12]. The dose is delivered by two portable electrodes, applied opposite each other avoiding any macerated skin [14]. The treatment doesn't heal the wound within the 12-day treatment but kick-starts the wound healing physiological process. The treatment reduces the wound size (and applied to leg ulcers with a mean age of 1 year can cause full wound closure within 2,5 months), reduces the pain and the exudate levels. In opposite of electrical stimulation therapy, this treatment is smaller and allows health professionals to use alongside standard treatment, including compression bandage [12].

Like any therapy/treatment, these therapies have contraindications include: active cancer and pregnancy, use should be avoided near the head for patients with epilepsy and near the chest for patients with pacemakers. It is important to ensure the devices do not get wet and should be removed prior to electrical investigations such as echocar-diograms, electroencephalograms and magnetic resonance imaging [12].

Research shows that the use of this therapies brings benefits to the patient with chronic wounds. Studies recommend that advanced therapies, like these, should be used in clinical practice to reduce alongside standard treatment to reduce chronic inflammation, pain and other symptoms common to this type of wounds, and even-tually improves quality of life [12].

5 Conclusion

The evidence shows that and consequently shows a huge impact on quality of life. However, if we consider the technological evolution of the past few years, especially in medical area, and the number of patients with leg ulcers is increasing, health profes-sionals can create a balance between this too vectors. From the clinical point of view, these advanced technologies using electrical stimulation are effective, without side effects and with staff and economic benefits, but the application in Portugal becomes a challenge, perhaps because the lack of investigation on this area or perhaps because the lack of "will" of Portugal government to provide this technology.

We approached just this type of new therapy, with recent investigation and with good results, results not just on the healing process or on the kick-start of wound healing physiological process, but also results on increasing quality of life of patients with this type of pathology.

It is extremely important to continue the investigation on this area. We have to remind that these therapies, in a certain way, increases the quality of life of the people that, as health professionals, we swear to take care.

References

1. Furtado, K.: Úlceras de perna – Tratamento baseado na evidência. Nursing (176), 35–42 (2015)
2. Saraiva, D., Bandarra, A., Agostinho, E., Pereira, N., Lopes, T.: Qualidade de vida do utente com úlcera venosa crónica. Referência (10), 109–118 (2013)
3. Alves, D., Nunes, I., Marques, M., Novas, M.: Qualidade de vida na pessoa com úlcera de perna, revisão integrativa. RIASE 2(1), 454–467 (2016)
4. Pereira, C., Pinto, D., Tourinho, F., Santos, V.: Tecnologias em Enfermagem e o Impacto na Prática Assitencial. Revista Brasileira de Inovação Tecnológica em Saúde 2(4), 29–37 (2013)
5. Cruz, M., Baudried, T., Azevedo, F.: Causas infrequentes de úlceras de perna e a sua abordagem. Revista da SPDV 69(3), 383–394 (2011)
6. Lorenzetti, J., Trindade, L., Pires, D., Ramos, F.: Tecnologia, inovação tecnológica e saúde; uma reflexão necessária. Texto Contexto Enfermagem 21(2), 432–439 (2012)
7. PORDATA Base de Dados Portugal Contemporâneo. https://www.pordata.pt/Europa/ Esperan%C3%A7a+de+vida+%C3%A0+nascen%C3%A7a+total+e+por+sexo-1260. Accessed 08 Oct 2018
8. Melnyk, B., Fineout-Overholt, E., Stetler, C., Allan, J.: Outcomes and implementation strategies from the first U.S. evidence-based practice leadership summit. Worldviews Evid. Based Nurs. 2(3), 113–121 (2005)
9. Finlayson, K., et al.: Distinct wound healing and quality-of-life outcomes in subgroups os patients with venous leg ulcers with different symptom cluster experiences. J. Pain Symptom Manage. 53(5), 871–879 (2017)
10. Do, H., Edwards, H., Finlayson, K.: Identifying relationships between symptom clusters and quality of life in adults with chronic mixed venous and arterial leg ulcers. Int. Wound J. 13(5), 903–911 (2016)
11. Edwards, H., Finlayson, K., Skerman, H., Alexander, K., Miaskowski, C., Aouizerat, B., Gibb, M.: Identification of symptom clusters in patients with chronic venous leg ulcers. J. Pain Symptom Manage. 47(5), 867–875 (2014)
12. Ovens, L.: Electrical stimulation therapy and electroceutical treatment for management of venous leg ulcers. Br. J. Commun. Nurs. 22, S28–S36 (2017)
13. Hopman, W., VanDenKerkhof, E., Kuhnke, J., Harrison, M.: Factors associated with health-related quality of life in chronic leg ulceration. Qual. Life Res. 23(6), 1833–1840 (2014)
14. Turner, N., Ovens, L.: The results of a clinical evaluation of Accel-Heal electroceutical treatment in a large NHS Trust. Wounds UK 13(4), 92–99 (2017)
15. Finlayson, K., Courtney, M., Gibb, M., O'Brien, J., Parker, C., Edwards, H.: The effectiveness of a four-layer compression bandage system in comparison with Class 3 compression hosiery on healing and quality of life in patients with venous leg ulcers: a randomized controlled trial. Int. Wound J. 11(1), 21–27 (2014)

Loneliness and Aging. Do Public Policies Dream of Technological Solutions?

Borja Rivero Jiménez(✉)⬤, David Conde Caballero⬤,
Beatriz Muñoz González, Nuria García Perales, Julián F. Calderón García⬤,
and Lorenzo Mariano Juárez⬤

University of Extremadura, Cáceres, Spain
{brivero,dcondecab,bmunoz,nuria,jfcalgar,lorenmariano}@unex.es

Abstract. The aging of population entails a series of phenomena, among which is the reality of loneliness experienced by many elderly people. Different publications point out the relationship between loneliness and health problems, something that is translating into a lower quality of life for these people during their last years. With this paper we intend to point out some important ideas about the problem of loneliness in elderly people in rural areas. For this objective, we believe it is essential that more works be developed that investigates the subjectivity of the emotional world of those who live in loneliness and that public policies develop effective actions based on this works, including technological solutions that help to alleviate this problem.

Keywords: Aging · Anthropology · Loneliness · Social isolation · Technology

1 Introduction

In one of our first incursions to the fieldwork, we held a meeting with the mayor of a rural locality. Our research is carried out in rural areas with a high rate of aging and depopulation. Among other topics, a story appeared that we believe can point to the importance of the topic we are going to deal with in this article. The mayor told us how a few years ago they discovered the lifeless body of an old man who had died during the night, on the balcony of the house where he lived alone, in a central street of the village. Neighbors discovered it after various hours, in the morning. This story may mark the most extreme side of some older people's loneliness, but it serves as a metaphor for what this sometimes means in our time: dying alone, in a space where they are seen, but without anyone in the last moments.

We believe that the growing aging population should live their last years of life with the best quality of life possible, and this significantly influences their mood and personal relationships. Our older people are generally active people, concerned about their families, interested in acquiring new knowledge, who demand a role in decision-making. The literature on active aging gives an

© Springer Nature Switzerland AG 2019
J. García-Alonso and C. Fonseca (Eds.): IWoG 2018, CCIS 1016, pp. 70–79, 2019.
https://doi.org/10.1007/978-3-030-16028-9_7

account of this reality. But they are also increasingly lonely people. Loneliness is not a exclusive problem of the elderly. Studies have already shown that more than one in three people in Western countries feels alone, regardless of age [5]. It is important, however, to point out the fact that certain factors, such as the death of the partner or the disappearance of the social network, make this especially evident in older people and, therefore, we can more easily establish the relationship between loneliness and old age in terms of socio-cultural constructs.

This article aims to pose, from a theoretical approach, the reality of loneliness of elderly people in rural contexts with a high index of aging and depopulation. To do this, we will approach the figures of the phenomenon, we will try to situate the conceptualization of the terms, the incidence of loneliness within health and, finally, the relationship between public policies and technological solutions that appear to the problem.

2 Objectives and Research

The project "International Institute for Research and Innovation on Aging" (4IE) aims to analyse the biomedical, functional and psychological aspects of aging in the context of the regions of Extremadura (Spain) and Alentejo (Portugal) through a multidisciplinary team including technologists, health researchers, anthropologists and sociologists. Among our lines of work is the development of knowledge on the aging process and care of the elderly, proposing a new model of care for the elderly to adapt the context of their lives to their needs and validate and implement various technological solutions that allow the application of innovations and new models of care developed. For these objectives, from anthropology and sociology we try to pose the structural situations and contextualize them to adapt them to the technological solutions proposed. One of the problems that most affects the elderly in this geographical context is loneliness. The main objective of this article is an approach to the situation of loneliness that older people live in rural contexts. We will analyze:

1. The official data that we have about loneliness and aging.
2. The conceptualization of the term and the different scales at which it is objectively measured.
3. The relationship between loneliness and health.
4. The public policies and actions that from the administration are being carried out to propose technological solutions to the loneliness of the elderly.

3 The Loneliness of the Elderly in Rural Contexts

3.1 The Official Data of Loneliness

The narrative of the numbers seems to leaves no doubt: loneliness is already a big problem in modern societies, with prospects of worsening in the future. The world's population is aging and virtually every country in the world is experiencing an increase in the number and percentage of elderly people in its population [20]. The demographic dependency ratio of older people (people aged 65 or over in relation to those aged 15–64) is expected to increase significantly across the EU in the coming decades [10]. Average life expectancy in Spain increased by more than 40 years between 1910 and 2010, especially from 1970 onwards due to the decrease in mortality in older ages [13]. At the beginning of the last century in Spain it was rare to reach the age of 35; today, it is normal to exceed 80. At the end of 2017 [17], people over 65 and over already represented 19.07% (8,905,738 people) of the total population, 20.44% if we look at the figure for Extremadura. The trend is increasing according to the projections: the percentage of elderly population would reach 25.6% in 2031 and 34.6% in 2066. There is no discussion, therefore, about the fact that the aging of the population is one of the central issues on the political agenda of the 21st century. The context is complex and different processes are interrelated, including the depopulation of rural areas in favour of migrations to large city centres [24]. In Extremadura, the population flows from rural zones to the cities can be seen in a reality of depopulation of the villages, which is increasingly aging. Already in 2014, according to the INE, in the municipalities of less than 2,000 inhabitants the elderly represented 30.6% of the total population, and the data reaches a 40% in some towns in Extremadura, a spectacularly high percentage with respect to the national average. And this situation looks like it is going to increase over the next few years.

In this context of very aging rural areas, the problem of loneliness has broken out with force. According to the 2017 Continuous Household Survey, in Spain 25.4% of households were unipersonal, with a fairly even distribution between the sexes (46.6% of these households were occupied by men, 53.4% by women). Of the total number of one-person households, 41.8 per cent are occupied by persons aged 65 or over. In gross, the translation is that 1,960,900 people over the age of 65 live alone, 71.9% of whom are women. The data in Extremadura show a total of 111,100 one-person households, of which 51,600 are occupied by people aged 65 or over, 71.8% of whom are women in this age group. Extremadura's demographic dynamics, therefore, are inexorably heading towards an increasingly aging population, which lives mainly in a rural environment, with little intergenerational contact and living more and more frequently with loneliness as their age advances.

3.2   The Problem of Conceptualizing the Concept

In any case and with all this evidence, the data do not reveal the whole landscape, they hardly allow to trace a part of the complete map. The definition of loneliness, its cultural construction in different populations or its impact on people's lives are today awaiting detailed analysis. Thus, the definition of the concept of loneliness generates problems from the moment we accept that it is not only equivalent to social isolation, but that it is something much more complex, which is why some authors refer to it not as a one-dimensional construct, but rather as a multidimensional fact. The feeling of loneliness is the product of a cognitive elaboration that is crossed by learned social and cultural norms that influence the behavior of subjects [4] and that, therefore, presents different patterns depending on the individuals, that make the concept of loneliness have little relation with the reductionism of assimilating it to the lack of company. At the same time, as Herrera [15] indicates, this is a concept that has undergone an important transformation in recent years, given that only 50 years ago loneliness referred to people without clear family groups who were on the margins of society; little or nothing to do with current reality.

The concept of loneliness has been interpreted in different forms, and is often seen as that subjective feeling that corresponds to the objective measure of social isolation. There is no single or universal definition of the term and in the literature it has been described in different ways: as the perceived lack of social contact, the lack of people or availability to share experiences or relationships, a state in which in spite of being able to interact with other people it is not done or the discrepancy between the reality of interaction with other people and what would be desired [28, 32]. From different theoretical perspectives (such as existentialism, cognitive theory, interactionism or psychoanalysis) there have been approaches to the phenomenon of loneliness, something that is evidenced by this variety of definitions. The concept of social isolation, however, is related to the integration of individuals within their nearby social networks [1, 28].

Social isolation has been defined as a lack of significant and sustained communication over time or also as the lack of habitual contact with family members and social networks. When we speak of social isolation, therefore, we are referring to a more objective concept, which, although it would have an important relationship with feelings of loneliness, allows it to be measured with quantitative methodological tools in a more evident way, which, as we will see later, has resulted in different scales that make it difficult, at times, to standardize the concept. On the other hand, when we talk about living alone, we only refer to a measure of the type of household in which the person lives. In the case of Spain, this would be the concept relating to "one-person household" used by the INE. Living exclusively in a household does not have to be directly related to having feelings of loneliness or living in social isolation, although sometimes it has a direct relationship. The high percentage of elderly people living alone reflects the trends in the way they live and which are often the result of the death of the partner (or their institutionalisation) and also of certain tendencies among individuals in families to live independently. With this situation and the expected increase, it is likely that future older people will have even higher rates of living alone.

There are different methodological tools to measure loneliness although two standardized instruments are generally used. On the one hand, the UCLA solitude scale, a 20 item scale designed to measure subjective feelings of loneliness and social isolation. Participants rate each element as O ("I often feel that way"), S ("I sometimes feel that way"), R ("I rarely feel that way"), N ("I never feel that way"). The measure has been revised several times since its first publication to create inverse punctuation items or to simplify the wording. On the other hand, we found the Jong Gierveld solitude scale, which, although it can be applied as a one-dimensional solitude scale, is composed of items that were developed to distinguish between social and perceived solitude. For use in large surveys, a shorter version of the scale was constructed so that the triple application of the original scale (a scale of general solitude and emotional and social subscales) was guaranteed. The UCLA scale has a greater use in research work in the United States and the Jong Gierveld scale of loneliness is more widespread in European countries. This situation has caused the difficulty to define loneliness, to categorize it and to quantify it, which very probably has distorted to a great extent the approach from which the problem has been looked at. For Gajardo [12], solitude has been approached from an epidemiological perspective whose final consequence has been the medicalisation of the process that has become a syndrome that can be prevented, detected and treated [27], and for which there are specific scales that leave no room for doubt. However, after what has been said, it seems clear that this is an insufficient approach to an extremely complex problem. Therefore, we need to go deeper into reality beyond numbers, to know the process, to describe its complexities, to understand it by entering into the worlds of intersubjective construction.

3.3   Loneliness as a Public Health Problem

Loneliness has been discovered as an important factor that has a notable influence on health. Different papers [2,12,15,22,27] point out how the decrease in family relations, social isolation and a lower participation in pleasant activities is directly linked to a worsening of the population's health and quality of life, to the point that some authors have gone so far as to define loneliness as the most devastating "disease" affecting old age [15]. Some concerns that arise as a consequence of the aging process of the population [29] highlight the increase in the proportion of people who will age with dependency and, consequently, who will need more care, and the increase in those who will live and feel lonely and alone. In this way, current figures make it possible to speak of an "epidemic" of loneliness (which some have already called a "silent epidemic"), since research has shown increasingly conclusive evidence linking loneliness, in whatever form, with disease.

A number of studies suggest that loneliness is associated with negative physical and mental health outcomes, including heart disease, depression, suicide [18] and dementia [33]. Mortality rates are significantly higher among those who are isolated or who have significant feelings of loneliness than among those who are accompanied [21]. Loneliness is also associated with a number of physiological parameters such as stress hormones [14]. Social isolation has a negative impact on the maintenance of independence, with consequent implications for the use of social and health services [9]. Lack of social contact and unelected loneliness have a significant influence on increased mortality [30]. For a person who feels lonely, scientific evidence argues, cortisol levels are elevated, resistance to blood circulation is increased, and even some aspects of immune competition are diminished. Holt-Lunstand et al., through a meta-analysis [16] of different research in the field of social psychology tried to give surnames to this relationship and pointed out an increased risk of death in those people who have little contact with other people. Furthermore, this risk was maintained regardless of the number of actual interactions with others and the time spent. Along the same lines, a recent study [26] carried out in three European countries (Finland, Poland and Spain) on older adults indicated that loneliness has a stronger association with health than the other components of the social networks of the subjects studied. This association was similar in the three countries studied, with different socioeconomic levels and different health characteristics and welfare systems. The study also highlighted the importance of evaluating and monitoring loneliness in individuals with health problems and the importance of continuing research along these lines.

Gender differences also influence the health and illness processes of those living alone. For example, there is evidence that suggests that retired men report significantly better health than housewives [25]. Perceived health status is closely related to physical, mental and functional health and leisure activities. Being a woman with total dedication to domestic work is associated with a perceived worse state of health. The social construction of gender, therefore, would make certain emotional, relational, family and public aspects of men lives vulnerable to loneliness and incapable of solving it in a simple way [11]. On the other hand, clear gender differences have been identified in the way people relate to each other, which could contribute to increasing the likelihood that men will feel more alone. While women tend to have more diverse social networks that include close relationships with family members, friends and community members, men tend to focus more on intimate relationships with their partners.

It should be stressed that, as Bazo Royo [2] points out, the explanation for this obvious relationship between health and loneliness could be that the perception one has of the state of health is influenced when there are feelings related to loneliness. In this way, those who feel more alone are those who also feel sicker, so that, although many times it does not really correspond with the physical problems they suffer, they can affect the mood of older people and even their psychological well-being. Feeling alone and being alone do not have the same meaning nor are they infallibly united [19].

3.4 Public Policies, Technology and Loneliness

In this context, from the political sphere there does not seem to have been a growing interest in tackling the fight against loneliness and social isolation as a key element in improving the quality of life of the elderly population. In January 2018, the United Kingdom Prime Minister [31] announced that public policies against loneliness would become a fundamental part of the now new Ministry for Sport, Civil Society and Loneliness. It was committed to developing a strategy at all levels of government to identify the different options for tackling loneliness and building more integrated and resilient communities. At European level, while both the 2009 Lisbon Treaty and the EU Charter of Fundamental Rights agree on the importance of non-discrimination and the active integration and participation of older people in society, there is as yet no relevant document that sets out common solutions to the loneliness and social isolation of older people. For example, none of the latest relevant communications from the European Union on aging [6–8] makes express reference to loneliness and social isolation as challenges to be faced at this stage of life. Few public policies address loneliness as a fundamental problem for the elderly and legislate to solve or alleviate this situation. The answers are usually given by organisations that work with older people and are concerned with tackling the problem. In Spain, there are few solutions proposed by public bodies, with the exception of some initiatives at the level of mayoralties such as that of Madrid, which, through the "Madrid, City of Care" space, is articulating pilot programmes that focus their attention on detecting situations of unelected loneliness that may occur in some neighbourhoods in the centre of the city.

In the document "The EU's contribution to active aging and intergenerational solidarity", it is pointed out that "information and communication technologies (ICT) play an increasingly important role in promoting active aging. The Internet and new technologies often provide cost-effective and easy access to information, goods and services, to social interaction, and to democratic and civil processes" [8]. The European Union has made efforts in recent years to make the learning and use of ICT in older people a vehicle for their full integration into society. Since 2007, when a European action plan on information and communication technologies and aging was launched, called "Ageing well in the information society", with the aim of taking advantage of new and more accessible products and services for older people, various solutions have followed this approach. For example, the EU's Digital Agenda 2020, which aims to harness the potential of ICTs to foster innovation, economic growth and progress, focuses on the potential use of ICTs to meet the needs of an aging population through digital literacy and knowledge, e-health and telemedicine services and systems. Several EU research and innovation programmes aim to follow these lines. In Spain, the Institute for the Elderly and Social Services (IMSERSO) published a document in 2015 in which the relationship between the elderly and technology was discussed. In this document, the importance of technology as a vehicle between different generations and how it could serve to reduce marginalisation and loneliness was upheld, for which measures would have to be adopted for access, participation and adaptation to technological changes for older people. The use of telecare or devices such as mobile phones or tablets (through, for example, the "Enred@te" programme) are presented as reliable technological solutions to compensate for the loneliness of the elderly.

For years, technologists have been trying to work to reduce loneliness in elderly people through interventions with a diversity of technologies to combat it. Through different proposals such as "on-line activities", what has been called "Internet-supported therapeutic interventions" [3] and the use of robots and videogames, attempts are being made to innovate in order to offer technological solutions that extend the independent life of elderly people and discuss solutions to cases of unelected loneliness. However, some authors point out that these interventions are not yet as effective as could be expected and do not gather enough evidence, with evaluations that do not fit objective evaluation criteria in many occasions [23]. Organisms that work to promote active aging and do not socially isolate the person suggest that the best context for aging is that of the home itself: it is a safer place, a friendlier environment and there is less likelihood of suffering loneliness or social isolation. The Ambient Assisted Living Joint Programme (AAL) [25] is an example of how ICT-based projects can be developed to enable adults to stay at home as long as possible autonomously and independently. It is necessary for international institutions to consider lines of action and evaluation so that technology is put at the service of older people who need it most, in an effective manner and based on evidence and evaluation of results that are sufficiently founded.

4   Conclusions

We have pointed out the importance of the phenomenon of loneliness for the elderly in rural areas. It seems to us fundamental to have a broader knowledge on this subject and with an empirical approach, to carry out a significant conceptualization for the people in question who suffer from loneliness, but from their subjectivity and the world of emotions it contains. To this end, the tools of ethnographic fieldwork can offer us an important guide for research.

Although it is clear that loneliness can lead to a public health problem in a context of growing aging, we believe that this problem is not being addressed sufficiently by public policies to be able to offer effective solutions to alleviate the problems arising from loneliness. For this purpose, we believe that it is essential to integrate technologies that are effective in tackling the problem, for which there is a great need to focus efforts on developing effective evaluation systems for these technological responses. The quality of life during the aging process depends to a large extent on the combined efforts of the protagonists involved resulting in responses that reduce the experience of loneliness of elderly people.

Acknowledgment. This work was supported by the 4IE project (0045-4IE-4-P) funded by the Interreg V-A España-Portugal (POCTEP) 2014–2020 program.

References

1. Andersson, L.: Loneliness research and interventions: a review of the literature. Aging Ment. Health **2**(4), 264–274 (1998). https://doi.org/10.1080/13607869856506
2. Bazo Royo, M.T.: Personas ancianas. Salud y soledad. Reis: Revista española de investigaciones sociológicas (47), pp. 193–223 (1989)
3. Bornemann, R.: The impact of information and communication technology (ICT) usage on social isolation including loneliness in older adults. A systematic review. Ph.D. thesis (2014)

4. Buz Delgado, J.: Envejecimiento y soledad. La importancia de los factores sociales. In: Cubillo, M., Quintanar, F. (eds.) Por una cultura del envejecimiento, México, pp. 271–281 (2013)
5. Cacioppo, J.T., et al.: The cultural context of loneliness: risk factors in active duty soldiers. J. Soc. Clin. Psychol. **35**(10), 865–882 (2016). https://doi.org/10.1521/jscp.2016.35.10.865
6. Comisión Europea: Hacia una Europa para todas las edades (1999)
7. Comisión Europea: El futuro demográfico de Europa: transformar un reto en una oportunidad, pp. 1–14 (2007)
8. Comision Europea: La aportación de la UE al envejecimiento activo y a la solidaridad entre las generaciones. Comisión Europea, p. 20 (2012). https://doi.org/10.2767/67663
9. Concannon, L.: Developing inclusive health and social care policies for older LGBT citizens. Br. J. Soc. Work **39**(3), 403–417 (2009). https://doi.org/10.1093/bjsw/bcm131
10. European Commission Directorate-General for Economic and Financial Affairs: The 2015 Ageing Report Economic and budgetary projections for the 28 EU Member States (2013–2060). Technical report (2015). https://doi.org/10.27658/77631
11. Franklin, A., Barbosa Neves, B., Hookway, N., Patulny, R., Tranter, B., Jaworski, K.: Towards an understanding of loneliness among Australian men: gender cultures, embodied expression and the social bases of belonging. J. Sociol. (2018). https://doi.org/10.1177/1440783318777309
12. Gajardo Jauregui, J.: Vejez y soledad: Implicancias a partir de la construcción de la noción de riesgo. Acta Bioethica **21**(2), 199–205 (2015). https://doi.org/10.4067/S1726-569X2015000200006
13. García González, J.M.: Por qué vivimos más? Descomposición por causa de la esperanza de vida española de 1980 a 2009 / Why Do we Live Longer? Decomposition by Cause of Life Expectancy in Spain between 1980 and 2009. Revista Española de Investigaciones Sociológicas, pp. 39–60 (2014). https://doi.org/10.5477/cis/reis.148.39
14. Hawkley, L.C., Cacioppo, J.T.: Loneliness matters: a theoretical and empirical review of consequences and mechanisms. Ann. Behav. Med. **40**(2), 218–227 (2010). https://doi.org/10.1007/s12160-010-9210-8
15. Herrera, R.R.: La soledad en las personas mayores españolas. Portal Mayores Inmerso, pp. 1–21 (2004)
16. Holt-Lunstad, J., Smith, T.B., Layton, J.B.: Social relationships and mortality risk: a meta-analytic review (2010). https://doi.org/10.1371/journal.pmed.1000316
17. Instituto Nacional de Estadística: Estadística del Padrón continuo (2018)
18. Luanaigh, C.Ó., Lawlor, B.A.: Loneliness and the health of older peopleInt. J. Geriatr. Psychiatry **23**(12), 1213–1221 (2008). https://doi.org/10.1002/gps.2054
19. Muchinik, E., Seidmann, S., Acrich de Guttman, L.: Soledad y aislamiento. Un enfoque cualitativo. Anuario de Investigaciones de la Facultad de Psicologia de la Universidad de Buenos Aires **6**, 301–312 (1998)
20. ONU: Suggested citation: United Nations, Department of Economic and Social Affairs, Population Division. World Population Ageing (2015)
21. Patterson, A.C., Veenstra, G.: Loneliness and risk of mortality: a longitudinal investigation in Alameda County, California. Soc. Sci. Med. **71**(1), 181–186 (2010). https://doi.org/10.1016/j.socscimed.2010.03.024
22. Pikhartova, J., Bowling, A., Victor, C.: Is loneliness in later life a self-fulfilling prophecy? Aging Ment. Health **20**(5), 543–549 (2016). https://doi.org/10.1080/13607863.2015.1023767

23. Pinazo-Hernandis, S., Puente, R.P.: Innovación para el envejecimiento activo en la unión europea. Análisis del programa ambient assisted living joint programme (AAL) en el periodo 2008–2015. Búsqueda (15), pp. 38–50 (2015). https://doi.org/10.21892/01239813.95

24. Pinilla, V., Sáez, L.A.: La Despoblación Rural En España: Génesis De Un Problema Y Políticas Innovadoras. Centro de Estuios sobre Despoblación y Desarrollo de Áreas Rurales p. 24 (2016)

25. Pino-Domínguez, L., et al.: Self-perceived health status, gender, and work status. J. Women Aging 28(5), 386–394 (2016). https://doi.org/10.1080/08952841.2015.1018030

26. Rico-Uribe, L.A., et al.: Loneliness, social networks, and health: a cross-sectional study in three countries. PLoS ONE 11(1), e0145264 (2016). https://doi.org/10.1371/journal.pone.0145264

27. Rodríguez Martín, M.: La soledad en el anciano. Gerokomos 20(4), 159–166 (2009). https://doi.org/10.4321/S1134-928X2009000400003

28. Scharf, T., De Jong Gierveld, J.: Loneliness in urban neighbourhoods: an Anglo-Dutch comparison. Eur. J. Ageing 5(2), 103–115 (2008). https://doi.org/10.1007/s10433-008-0080-x

29. Serrano, J.P., Latorre, J.M., Gatz, M.: Spain: promoting the welfare of older adults in the context of population aging. Gerontologist 54(5), 733–740 (2014). https://doi.org/10.1093/geront/gnu010

30. Steptoe, A., Shankar, A., Demakakos, P., Wardle, J.: Social isolation, loneliness, and all-cause mortality in older men and women. Proc. Natl. Acad. Sci. U.S.A. 110(15), 5797–801 (2013). https://doi.org/10.1073/pnas.1219686110

31. UK GOB: PM commits to government-wide drive to tackle loneliness

32. Victor, C., Scambler, S., Bond, J., Bowling, A.: Being alone in later life: Loneliness, social isolation and living alone (2000). doi: https://doi.org/10.1017/S0959259800104101

33. Wilson, R.S., Boyle, P.A., James, B.D., Leurgans, S.E., Buchman, A.S., Bennett, D.A.: Negative social interactions and risk of mild cognitive impairment in old age. Neuropsychology 29(4), 561–570 (2015). https://doi.org/10.1037/neu0000154

Internet of Things (IoT)

Interconnecting IoT Devices to Improve the QoL of Elderly People

Daniel Flores-Martin[1]([⊠])(iD), Alejandro Pérez-Vereda[2], Javier Berrocal[1](iD), Carlos Canal[2](iD), and Juan M. Murillo[1](iD)

[1] Universidad de Extremadura, Badajoz, Spain
{dfloresm,jberolm,juanmamu}@unex.es
[2] Universidad de Málaga, Málaga, Spain
apvereda@uma.es, canal@lcc.uma.es

Abstract. The number of internet-connected devices (Internet of Things, IoT) is growing at an unstoppable rate. Many manufacturers have developed specific protocols that are usually closed and do not follow any standard, hindering the interconnection and coordination of devices from different manufactures. This entails a greater effort from users to coordinate some devices and the loss of the benefits provided by this paradigm. Some works are proposing different techniques to reduce this barrier and avoid the vendor lock-in issue. Nevertheless, this interconnection should also depends on the context. IoT devices must adapt their behavior according to the people's preferences around them. In this paper, we propose a system that allows to identify a dynamic interconnection of IoT devices arising from changing situations to help elderly people with their daily tasks and improve their quality of life. Our work allows us to make this interconnection context dependent, creating a collaborative environment between people and devices. Further, in a world with an accelerated population aging, there is an increasing interest on developing solutions for the elderly living assistance through IoT systems.

Keywords: Internet of Things · Context · Interconnection · Elderly people

1 Introduction

The relevance of the Internet of Things (IoT) is increasing as more and more internet-connected devices are developed. Recent estimates state that in the next few years we will have about 30 billion smart devices connected to the Internet [13]. One of the general purposes of these devices is to make people's lives easier by simplifying tasks or helping them get things done. IoT is being applied in many domains: smart home, automotive, smart cities, healthcare, etc. [8]. Concretely, in healthcare, the IoT paradigm allows more personalized, preventive and collaborative care, where patients monitor and manage their

© Springer Nature Switzerland AG 2019
J. García-Alonso and C. Fonseca (Eds.): IWoG 2018, CCIS 1016, pp. 83–93, 2019.
https://doi.org/10.1007/978-3-030-16028-9_8

own health, and the responsibility for healthcare is shared between patients and medical staff [12]. Such solutions are particularly interesting in rural areas, where due to depopulation, the number and availability of adequately emergency equipment is limited.

IoT devices can be used to perform simple tasks, such as blood pressure monitoring, emergency situations notification, or periodic reminders, but the real potential comes when they interconnect with each other, to perform more complex tasks. This interconnection is not easy, as we find a great heterogeneity of IoT devices in the market. To achieve this interconnection each manufacturer defines its own communication protocols. Nevertheless, there is no standard to interconnect IoT devices from different manufacturers. This increases the risk of *vendor lock-in*, as we are conditioned to purchase devices from the same manufacturer if we want to achieve a full compatibility [16], or setting manually each device, something that is unbearable for people with low technical knowledge.

To mitigate this drawback, different works have promoted alternative methods to make IoT devices work with each other, such as specific *frameworks*, e.g. [17], where a framework is developed to integrate specific domain applications into IoT, or [9], which presents interfaces and interconnection procedures based on oneM2M [18]. The use of ontologies and the Semantic Web are also becoming very important to solve these interconnection problems [19]. These works help to solve the problem of device interconnection, but it is not an easy task, because technological diversity of smart devices must be taken into account, as well as the correct handling of the context, which is not always considered. The development of context-sensitive software has proved successful [14].

IoT devices are becoming intelligent thanks to the information gathered about the context in which they are located, from near people or other devices. To minimize people interaction with devices, this interconnection must be adapted to the context. These drawbacks can be addressed by developing software capable of adapting its behavior to people's needs [14,20]. Several research areas can contribute to provide this adaptation, namely Context Oriented Programming (COP), Ambient Intelligent (AmI), Semantic Web, and Machine Learning (ML). Most of these paradigms allow us to define behaviors for different scenarios at design time, so the adaptation of the devices is limited to situations that developers have been able to identify, making it impossible to adapt them to other situations that may arise from the context.

The authors of this work have proposed the Situational-Context paradigm [3], where the context is treated as a way of analyzing the conditions that exist at a particular time and place identifying people's needs. This work presents an architecture that models the Situational-Context focused on healtcare for the elderly people domain, although it can be used for other domain. In addition, it allows to obtain data from users' profile, stored in their smartphones, to use them so that IoT devices can adapt their behavior to people's needs. This happens dynamically and at runtime, because the possibilities that can occur in a context are innumerable. This makes it possible for IoT devices to adapt their behavior to situations not previously predefined. Thanks to this, it is possible for IoT devices to adapt their behavior to situations not previously predefined.

The rest of the document is structured as follows. Section 2 describes the motivations of our work. Next, Sect. 3 introduces the concept of Situational-Context. In Sect. 4 we show the used architecture. Section 5 details the devices interconnection. Then, in Sect. 6 we describe some related work. Finally, in Sect. 7 some conclusions are detailed.

2 Motivations

Nowadays, the interconnection of IoT devices to achieve a coordinated work is still a problem that prevents to exploit the full potential of IoT paradigm.

To show the impact of this problem, we are going to use a scenario based on ageing and rurality. In the rest of this article the proposed scenario will be used to show the benefits of our work.

Juan is a 74 years old man who lives in La Calera in the southeast of Cáceres, in the Las Villuercas Mountains. This morning, Juan went for a walk with his friend Emilio. They both have their mobile phones with them. Since the village is running out of inhabitants and they are getting older, their sons and daughters always ask them not to go out without their mobile phones in case something happens to them. Juan and Emilio are not aware of this, but their mobile phones can do much more than receive calls from their children. In addition, these devices are recording where they walk, where are them, with whom they are and are detecting each other so that their phones now know they are in company (Fig. 1a).

Juan has returned home and it's time to take his medicine. It is notified by the electronic pill dispenser that was given to him last month. This pill dispenser has also detected that there are no pills left for the next day (Fig. 1b). It is very important that Juan does not stop his heart treatment. Although his smartphone made the electronic prescription request, they were unable to bring his medication. There seems to have been a mistake at the pharmacy in Guadalupe. Fortunately, Emilio takes the same medication as Juan and received it last week. Juan and Emilio have received a message telling them that tomorrow Emilio must give Juan two doses (Fig. 1c).

The Semantic Web techniques and frameworks that have been seen before are not enough to solve this problem, since context information is needed.

This use case shows the need to interconnect different devices. In addition, this interconnection depends on the contextual information that surrounds the devices, so that all possible data can be had to carry out the interconnection in the best possible way. Therefore, we want to test the capacity of the Situational-Context to promote the generation of complex strategies that involve the orchestration of services of several devices.

3 Situational-Context

Situational-Context is a way of analyzing the conditions that exist at a particular time and place in order to predict, at runtime, the expected IoT

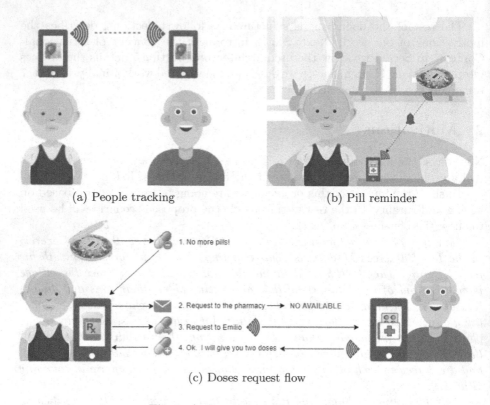

(a) People tracking   (b) Pill reminder

1. No more pills!

2. Request to the pharmacy ⟶ NO AVAILABLE

3. Request to Emilio

4. Ok. I will give you two doses

(c) Doses request flow

Fig. 1. Ageing and rurality use case

systems behavior. It is composed of entities. These entities can be both IoT devices and people represented through their smartphones, indistinctly. In addition, they have two fundamental properties: *skills* and *goals*.

This model exploits the capabilities of smart devices to collect, store and calculate locally contextual information to build their virtual profile and the virtual profile of their owner. Therefore, the devices around it can reuse it to meet the user's preferences. Situational-Context defines that the virtual profile of an entity (IoT device or a person) must contain at least the following information:

- A *Basic Profile* that contains the raw contextual information dated with the status of the entity, the relationships with other devices and its history.
- A *Social Profile*. This profile contains the results of high-level inferences made on the Basic Profile.
- The *Goals* that details the state of the environment desired by the entity. These goals are deduced from the Basic and Social Profiles at runtime.
- The *Skills* that an entity has to make decisions and take actions capable of modifying the environment and aimed at achieving the goals.

Considering environments in which there are different entities and each of them has a virtual profile, Situational-Context can be defined as the composition of the virtual profiles of all entities involved in a particular situation.

Thanks to Situational-Context it is possible to analyze the context surrounding Juan and detect nearby entities, such as Emilio, or his smart pill dispenser, which can use its skill to make the electronic prescription when it detects that it is running out of doses of some type of pill, and thus be able to continue to provide Juan with his medication. In the same way, this could be applied to other entities such as Emilio (represented by his smartphone), Emilio's pill dispenser, or another IoT devices that they can have at home. Situational-Context aims, among others, to improve the QoL of people by avoiding having to invest so much time in configuring smart devices.

This paradigm has obtained previous results of interconnection of devices at the network level [5]. We assume, therefore, that the connection through the network of IoT devices in a Situational-Context environment is feasible.

4 Entity Representation Architecture

Due to the detected need, we use the Situational-Context paradigm with which we intend to achieve a better interconnection of IoT devices, and get the maximum benefit by adapting their behavior to people's preferences at runtime. This favors the interaction of entities and allows them to be dependent on the context in which they are, at runtime. Its components are detailed in Fig. 2.

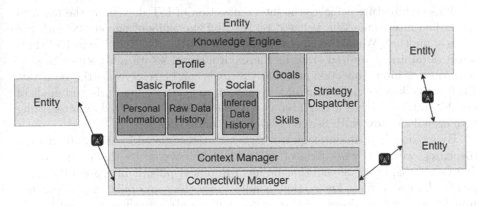

Fig. 2. Entity architecture

- **Connectivity Manager.** Establishes the physical connection between entities. It sends and receives information related to skills, goals, personal information, etc.
- **Context Manager.** Responsible for creating and updating contextual information. It contains the information of the entities belonging to the same situation in a given instant of time.
- **Profile.** Union of the *Basic* and the *Social Profile* of the entity.

- **Basic Profile.** Basic information that identifies the entity, such as the identifier, manufacturer, model, date of manufacture, etc. (Personal Information). It also contains raw data about the history of interactions with other entities (Raw Data History).
- **Social Profile.** Stores all inferred data from the basic profile (Inferred Data History). Thanks to this data, Juan's smartphone can know where Juan is moving or who he's accompanied by.

- **Skills.** Entity features. They produce a change in the context. For example, the pill dispenser can order pills from the pharmacy.
- **Goals.** They arise when one wants to obtain a state in a property of the environment that with the own capacities is not possible. For example, due to the situation that Juan's pill dispenser is empty, he must make the electronic prescription and also request some doses from his friend Emilio.
- **Strategy Dispatcher.** Devices can detect what goals there are in the environment, and which ones can be solved with their skills. A strategy is identified when it is detected how to coordinate the devices in the environment to solve the given goals. The complexity of strategies lies in the collaboration of entities to identify and solve needs. Returning to the example of Juan and Emilio, Emilio's pill dispenser must establish a strategy to give a few doses to Juan, but only if Emilio has plenty of pills.
- **Knowledge Engine.** Analyzes the history of the entity's activities to detect patterns and learn from them, with the goal of automating tasks in the future or detect routines.

This architecture achieves the interconnection of IoT devices at the features level. The interconnection is based on relating the skills of one entity with the goals of another. We know that the goals in an entity arise from the lack of skills when obtaining a desired state in the environment, so we must know how to perform this interconnection and that the goals can be resolved in the best way. Each entity has its own vision of the context, and knows the skills and goals of nearby entities, so that it can interact with them. This is achieved by integrating Situational-Context with Semantic Web and ontologies.

By looking that an ontology can represent the skills and goals of Juan's pill dispenser, we know what kind of goals could be covered by this entity. When Juan's pill dispenser detects that he has run out of pills, it interprets its social profile data and, as it knows that Emilio takes the same pills, and it can ask him for a couple of doses. In this way it will be able to automatically use its ability to cover the person need. Semantic Web will be responsible for providing knowledge to this information, making the relationships between skills and goals are defined in a more human language, and also interpretable by machines.

To better explain the composition of the entities used in our scenario, some of their components are specified in Tables 1 and 2, where we can see Juan's pill dispenser and Juan, represented through his smartphone. Apart from the personal information, we observe that Juan's pill dispenser has a series of skills with which it can solve Juan's needs.

Table 1. Juan's pill dispenser

Personal info	Skills
Manufacturer	**Pills management**
- PDOne	- Reminder doses
Model	- Distribute
- One	- Recommendations
Family	- ...
- HealthCare	Pharmacy
Device	- Request pills
- Pill dispenser	- Electronic receipt
...	- ...

Table 2. Juan

Personal info	Goals
Manufacturer	**Pills management**
- Huawei	- Reminder doses
Model	- Check dose amount
- P20 Lite	- ...
Family	**Security**
- Smartphone	- Family notify
...	- ...

In our example, Juan needs to take his daily dose according to the medical prescription that his smartphone stores, but due to the lack of dose in the pill dispenser he can not do it. In this case, thanks to the virtual profiles generated through Situational-Context, Juan knows that Emilio is taking the same medication and he can request him to send several doses. In addition, the interconnection of these entities, people and devices, is done in a totally dynamic way at runtime, so no previous configuration or manual action is necessary, which allows us to improve the people QoL by not having to be aware of the devices or having to invest our valuable time in configure them manually.

Virtual profiles are developed following the PeaaS (People as a Service) paradigm [6] and using the novel tool developed by Tim Berners-Lee's team: Solid (Social Linked Data) [11]. Solid proposes a decentralized platform for social web applications, where user data is managed independently of the applications that consume this data, a proposal that is quite aligned with our work. Solid is a framework that can be used to implement the basic pillars of PeaaS, obtaining the following benefits [2]: (1) *True data ownership*, where users should have the freedom to choose where their data resides and who is allowed to access it; (2) *Modular design*, because applications are decoupled from the data they produce, users will be able to avoid vendor lock-in, seamlessly switching between apps and personal data storage servers; and (3) *Reusing existing data*, developers will be able to easily innovate by creating new apps or improving current apps, all while reusing existing data that was created by other apps. This could be a good approach to build part of Situational-Context paradigm and could come in handful of benefits.

5   Interconnection Flow

The devices interconnection in Situational-Context has a clear objective: the needs resolution. As we mentioned in Sect. 3, an entity has a need when its skills cannot achieve the desired state in the environment and it must draw on the skills of another one.

Through the *Connectivity Manager*, entities can connect to each other, and exchange information. For example, Juan's pill dispenser and Juan's smartphone can connect each other through bluetooth.

This information is interpreted and updated by the *Context Manager*. At this point, the entity knows its own skills and goals, as well as those of the other entities in the context, and will know if it can solve any determined goal. Juan's pill dispenser knows that Juan does not have pills and that there are other elements in the environment with the skill to provide them, such as the pharmacy or Emilio's pill dispenser.

Then, Juan's smartphone will detect the information coming from the *Profile*, which contains the entity history and preferences that has a goal. Thanks to this information, Juan is reminded to have his doses by his pill dispenser every day.

Once the change to be made is detected, for example, to give a couple of doses to Juan, the *Strategy Dispatcher* will formulate a strategy and propose a change over the context. This strategy will consider the skills of the entity and also those of others that could contribute to solving the goal. Using an ontology, the strategy knows which skills and goals are related to each other. Once the strategy has been formulated it is carried out. Besides, it is stored in the profile in order to be able to infer on it and detect possible patterns, to facilitate the strategy development in the future. For the specific case of the strategy of pills in the context of Juan, the pill dispenser takes into account the preferences of Juan and Emilio to distribute the pills so that Juan can receive his doses and Emilio has enough pills for the rest of the days.

This whole process is carried out at runtime, without predefining the previous behavior of the entities, as the solutions to be explored would be innumerable.

Figure 3 shows the interconnection diagram between the entities in the scenario.

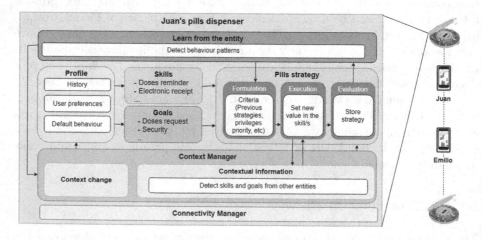

Fig. 3. Interconnection between entities

6 Related Work

As we discussed at the beginning of this research in [4], we can use different paradigms such as AmI, COP, SW and ML, to automate interactions between users and IoT systems according to user preferences. In addition, solutions to improve integration between people and IoT systems through the use of smartphones such as People as a Service (PeasS) and Internet of People (IoP) were also discussed.

When we delve into Semantic Web aspects within the scope of IoT, we find several works that follow an objective similar to ours. SocioTal [1] is a project focused mainly on issues of security and data sharing, whose aim is to create a configurable and secure IoT environment that encourages people to contribute with their devices and information, providing appropriate tools and mechanisms that simplify complexity and encourage citizen participation. Gyrard et al. also address issues related to IoT and Semantic Web, and they even have developed their own framework to facilitate interaction between IoT devices from a template generator for different IoT domains [7], based on Semantic Web technologies to explicitly describe the meaning of sensor measurements.

As mentioned in Sect. 1, healthcare domain is gaining great importance within the IoT. We can find works focused on the care or treatment of the elderly. In [15], we find We-care, a system for the assistance of elderly people that is able to monitor and record the vital information of these people, as well as provide mechanisms to activate alarms in emergency situations. Along the same lines, Mainetti et al. have designed an Ambient System Living (AAL) system to create better living conditions for older people, capable of constantly monitoring their state of health through data from heterogeneous sources [10].

In addition, if we combine Semantic Web with elderly care, we find an interesting project, SOPRANO [21], an extensible and open AAL platform for elderly people that aims to lead a more independent life in their family environment through a new generation of intelligent home with ambient intelligence.

We are aware that there are many proposals for the development of software whose behavior adapts to the context, but that, to the best of our knowledge, do not cover in many cases the problems mentioned above, such as those related to the adaptation of devices to the conditions of the context at runtime. Therefore, the research challenges we address are several. First, the lack of a unified model of human-IoT interaction. IoT devices are produced by several manufacturers, each with its own interaction model. Secondly, the lack of an automatic negotiation model for the interaction between people and IoT devices according to people's preferences. Some of the works mentioned above pursue a similar goal to ours, in terms of achieving an adaptive context in IoT, but we want to make the interconnection of these IoT devices emerge from the situation itself. If these problems could be solved, there would be a better integration of people in IoT environments in terms of interoperability.

7   Conclusions

As the health care domain is becoming increasingly important, we are concerned about the idea of being able to connect as many smart devices as possible to make the lives of older people easier. However, the problem of interconnection in the IoT world is still present today due to the heterogeneity of devices on the market. The interaction between IoT devices is crucial for the resolution of strategies to support people daily tasks, and must allow them to adapt their behaviors to people's needs, which often depends on the collaboration of several smart devices.

This work is another step towards achieving this interconnection in a dynamic way, thanks to technologies such as Situational-Context. Thus we can adapt the behavior of the devices to the needs of people in real time, without the need to attend to previous configurations in design time.

In future work we will focus on how to define the strategies that meet the goals. We know what skills and goals are going to be involved in the strategy, but we must continue along this path to determine how they should act, and refine the criteria to be taken into account. In addition, we will also continue to work on the Semantic Web line and ontologies, to make the association of skills and goals as precise as possible, by using semantic reasoners for the detection and resolution of interconnection strategies between entities.

Acknowledgments. This work was supported by the Spanish Ministry of Science and Innovation through projects TIN2015-69957-R, TIN2014-53986-REDT, and TIN2015-67083-R (MINECO/FEDER, UE), by the Department of Economy and Infrastructure of the Government of Extremadura (GR15098), by the European Regional Development Fund (ERDF) and by 4IE project (0045-4IE-4-P) funded by the Interreg V-A España-Portugal (POCTEP) 2014–2020 program.

References

1. Bernal Bernabé, J., et al.: Sociotal-the development and architecture of a social IoT framework (2017)
2. Berners-Lee, T.: Solid vision. https://solid.mit.edu/. Accessed 9 Oct 2018
3. Berrocal, J., Garcia-Alonso, J., Canal, C., Murillo, J.M.: Situational-context: a unified view of everything involved at a particular situation. In: Bozzon, A., Cudre-Maroux, P., Pautasso, C. (eds.) ICWE 2016. LNCS, vol. 9671, pp. 476–483. Springer, Cham (2016). https://doi.org/10.1007/978-3-319-38791-8_34
4. Flores-Martin, D.: Meeting IoT users' preferences by emerging behavior at runtime. In: Braubach, L., et al. (eds.) ICSOC 2017. LNCS, vol. 10797, pp. 333–338. Springer, Cham (2018). https://doi.org/10.1007/978-3-319-91764-1_27
5. Galán-Jiménez, J., Berrocal, J., Garcia-Alonso, J., Canal, C., Murillo, J.M.: Coordinating heterogeneous IoT devices by means of the centralized vision of the SDN controller (2017)
6. Guillen, J., Miranda, J., Berrocal, J., Garcia-Alonso, J., Murillo, J.M., Canal, C.: People as a service: a mobile-centric model for providing collective sociological profiles. IEEE Softw. **31**(2), 48–53 (2014)

7. Gyrard, A., Datta, S.K., Bonnet, C., Boudaoud, K.: Cross-domain Internet of Things application development: M3 framework and evaluation. In: 2015 3rd International Conference on Future Internet of Things and Cloud, pp. 9–16, August 2015. https://doi.org/10.1109/FiCloud.2015.10

8. Haluza, D., Jungwirth, D.: ICT and the future of health care: aspects of health promotion. Int. J. Med. Inform. **84**(1), 48–57 (2015)

9. Kim, J., et al.: Standard-based IoT platforms interworking: implementation, experiences, and lessons learned. IEEE Commun. Mag. **54**(7), 48–54 (2016)

10. Mainetti, L., Patrono, L., Secco, A., Sergi, I.: An IoT-aware AAL system for elderly people. In: International Multidisciplinary Conference on Computer and Energy Science (SpliTech), pp. 1–6. IEEE (2016)

11. Mansour, E., et al.: A demonstration of the solid platform for social web applications. In: Proceedings of the 25th International Conference Companion on World Wide Web, pp. 223–226. International World Wide Web Conferences Steering Committee (2016)

12. Metcalf, D., Milliard, S.T., Gomez, M., Schwartz, M.: Wearables and the Internet of Things for health: wearable, interconnected devices promise more efficient and comprehensive health care. IEEE Pulse **7**(5), 35–39 (2016)

13. Nordrum, A.: The internet of fewer things [news]. IEEE Spectr. **53**(10), 12–13 (2016)

14. Perera, C., Zaslavsky, A., Christen, P., Georgakopoulos, D.: Context aware computing for the Internet of Things: a survey. IEEE Commun. Surv. Tutor. **16**(1), 414–454 (2014)

15. Pinto, S., Cabral, J., Gomes, T.: We-care: An IoT-based health care system for elderly people. In: 2017 IEEE International Conference on Industrial Technology (ICIT), pp. 1378–1383. IEEE (2017)

16. Roman, R., Zhou, J., Lopez, J.: On the features and challenges of security and privacy in distributed Internet of Things. Comput. Netw. **57**(10), 2266–2279 (2013)

17. Shrestha, N., Kubler, S., Främling, K.: Standardized framework for integrating domain-specific applications into the IoT. In: 2014 International Conference on Future Internet of Things and Cloud (FiCloud), pp. 124–131. IEEE (2014)

18. Swetina, J., Lu, G., Jacobs, P., Ennesser, F., Song, J.: Toward a standardized common M2M service layer platform: introduction to oneM2M. IEEE Wirel. Commun. **21**(3), 20–26 (2014)

19. Szilagyi, I., Wira, P.: Ontologies and semantic web for the Internet of Things-a survey. In: 42nd Annual Conference of the IEEE Industrial Electronics Society, IECON 2016, pp. 6949–6954. IEEE (2016)

20. Taivalsaari, A., Mikkonen, T.: A roadmap to the programmable world: software challenges in the IoT era. IEEE Softw. **34**(1), 72–80 (2017)

21. Wolf, P., Schmidt, A., Klein, M.: SOPRANO-an extensible, open AAL platform for elderly people based on semantical contracts. In: 3rd Workshop on Artificial Intelligence Techniques for Ambient Intelligence (AITAmI 2008), 18th European Conference on Artificial Intelligence (ECAI 2008), Patras, Greece (2008)

A New WSN Mesh Protocol for More Transparent IoT Devices

Marino Linaje$^{(\boxtimes)}$ ⓘ and Enrique Carlos Mesías

School of Technology, Universidad de Extremadura, 10003 Caceres, Spain
mlinaje@unex.es

Abstract. We are experimenting great advances in the last years towards Weiser's Ubiquitous Computing vision. To complete his transparent computing vision, we must unnoticed the presence of computing hardware around us. Currently, we are deploying smart devices in our houses to detect e.g., smoke in the kitchen, the state of a window (open or close) and so on. However, these devices require at least an initial configuration to be able to e.g., connect to the Internet through the router and sometimes also to set up some basic parameters. This paper focuses on the way IoT devices are interconnected to be able to interact with other connected devices as well as with people (e.g. to configure them), proposing a solution closer to the Weiser's vision that is specially necessary for people not able to configure these devices for several reasons, such as elderly people that e.g., do not have the smartphone or PC to do it or are not able to do it due to functional diversity (e.g., problems with their hands for fine-grain control). More specifically, our specific target is people living in rural areas where the technical assistance is also not available and where houses tend to be big with wide stone walls that obstruct radio signals. Trying to solve this situation we propose a new IoT protocol to deal with this situation where people can throw IoT devices to a place with typically several of them already deployed and the nodes will autoconfigure themselves.

Keywords: IoT (Internet of Things) · Wireless Sensor Network (WSN) · Mesh · Elderly users · Rural houses

1 Introduction

Population living in rural areas is getting older. Nowadays, migration of young and medium age population from rural areas to bigger cities is a fact in many countries. This reality is building megapolis growing all around the world while this depopulation in rural areas is making elderly people to face more problems, such as shops closing due to low population in many areas. These problems are not only direct implications of depopulation such as a decrease in social interactions or difficulty to buy groceries, but also indirect implications such as technology related problems. Technology is evolving fast around us, a four years old smartphone is not able to run current apps and we expect this evolution also for home connected devices. Many of them include "smart" capabilities and some of them can be especially relevant for people leaving alone, such as gas or smoke detector connected to somewhere outside in the cloud to

© Springer Nature Switzerland AG 2019

J. García-Alonso and C. Fonseca (Eds.): IWoG 2018, CCIS 1016, pp. 94–106, 2019.
https://doi.org/10.1007/978-3-030-16028-9_9

notify someone when something goes wrong. Many appliances in the kitchen come just interconnected and connected to the vendors' clouds and presumably, it will become harder in the future to buy not connected devices.

These devices are a fundamental piece of what so-called Internet of Things and communications play a pivotal role inside these devices [5]. Thus, traditional home appliances complexity is growing due to their new functionalities and communication capacities. Mark Weiser's vision of ubiquitous computing could bring elderly people, especially in rural areas, with the facilities to install and operate with these devices by themselves in a more transparent way, avoiding initial communication configuration. This transparency is a necessity for elderly people in rural areas to take advantage of available and incoming IoT devices that could facilitate their livings. Examples are already available in the market or under research, such as devices to monitor their health remotely [10] avoiding unnecessary trips to the hospital in a remote city or to a central town e.g., once per week. Other researchers [12] have already stated that IoT can help increasing the quality of life for the elderly. But this is not the only service that could improve elderly life quality and we could include any kind of alert, security or safety IoT systems among others.

The main problem with elderly people and IoT devices is interaction [1]. We split this configuration into two groups: initial setup of the device and regular functions. Many researchers have worked proposing new approaches primary for the latter because many of these devices, like health-related ones among others, require technical skills to be configured [9]. In rural areas, this is a relevant issue because in big cities elderly people can ask someone else with more technical skill of going to a professional shop to solve the problem. While regular function interactions have been largely addressed by the research community, the initial communication configuration required by many IoT devices has not been so widely developed. Therefore, we can see IoT devices of big companies such a Google that require a smartphone or a PC to be properly configured for the very first time, at least specifying router connection credentials to be able to connect the device with other devices of the network as well as with other services in the cloud when required.

In rural areas, we have detected two additional problems being one of the communication issues when applying common star Wi-Fi topology connecting all the devices to a central one. Due to the wide stone walls that rural houses have in our area (Extremadura in Spain and Alentejo in Portugal) and house size, this communication technology has deployment problems regarding coverage range. A sensor out of router's range is an easy to solve problem for people with the necessary technical skills and just adding one or more Wi-Fi repeaters could solve the range problem but, how an elderly is going to figure out what is happening when he deploys the sensor and no connection is established, how is (s)he going to configure the new required repeater device... and this leads us to the second problem: cost. Advances in electronic devices have also brought the decrease of their cost but, including not just a microcontroller, but the required radio communication module, the sensor for the required operation as well as the power system. So, adding additional hardware just to increase the network range without adding new capabilities makes less sense.

Merging all the stated problems, an ideal solution requires a network which should be able to allow zero configuration during the deployment phase while also able to interconnect devices without requiring extra dedicated hardware, such as repeaters. Even when the new IoT device that we want to deploy is out of the router (also known as sink in the telecommunication field) range. These necessities perfectly match the idea of mesh networks and there have been several attempts, from the research community as well as from the industry, to implement a communication protocol able to use this topology while maintaining a low power consumption of the devices. The power consumption is important because to simplify the deployment, many devices are battery-operated ones. But also, because losing battery power faster will lead to increase the time devoted to device maintainability, avoiding the Weiser's vision of transparent devices.

Being the first publication of this work, the objective of this paper is discussing the design decisions as well as presenting an overview of the proposal. Furthermore, the repository with the open source implementation is available at https://github.com/enriquecml/SnorlaxMesh for others to contribute for greater improvements. Our work does not deal with very specific devices such as cameras, that require large bandwidth and continuous operation, but sensing/acting sensors that require low bandwidth and where the information/sampling of just one reading is not critical. So, if one sensor sampling is lost while transmitting, there are so many of them that it is a minor incident.

2 Requirements

R1 - No Configuration. The user must be able to "throw"/deploy the new IoT device into an ambient where at least the router with a preconfigured connection device (called sink) is available. Ideally, the sink and the router could be integrated into a single multiprotocol router. According to the IoT forecasts [7] dozens of these devices should be already deployed in the close future. Thus, no range problem at all should appear being always one device (called sensor node or just node) near to another one. So, being able to use multihopping from one node to another until arriving the sink should not be a problem.

R2 - No Extra Hardware to Extend Coverage. The development must not require specific devices to extend network configuration range, such as repeaters. The network nodes must be able to send communications from one to another to increase its communication range. So, only homogenous nodes are expected.

R3 - Low Cost. The development must run on very low-cost devices. On the one hand, this would ideally increase the price of the IoT devices as lower as possible (e.g., an oxygen meter with or without connection capabilities should increase its value just a couple of euros, making the price different irrelevant even for most cheap electronic devices). On the other hand, low cost implies low memory and processor capabilities as well as constrained connection ones. Therefore, the protocol must be lightweight, easy to compute and must not require large RAM to store communication-related issues (such as queues and so on). The cost of something is always relative but, we think 1–2€ is a reasonable price for a microcontroller and the communications capabilities.

R4 - Respect Device Main Operation Interval. The users must not notice the added communication layer when compared to a device already doing the same operation without this layer. That is, if the sensor registers the temperature of the room each minute, it must maintain this behavior even when new functionality is added e.g., registering also the data in the cloud. To deal with this requisite, the solution must respect the originally intended sensor node interval to read and process its attached sensors, supposed to be its primary contribution. The nodes in a WSN, like those in houses, can sense a great variety of situations to help to build a more realistic digital context to identify to envision the situations going on. Due to these different necessities, not all the nodes read their sensor values with the same periodicity. On the one hand, e.g. a temperature sensor in the living room is not going to change drastically every second, so we can just wake-up the microcontroller read the sensor and transmit this value every couple of minutes. But e.g., a smoke detection sensor in the kitchen cannot be waiting a couple of minutes between readings for safety reasons. On the other hand, e.g. a presence sensor is sensing all the time its environment and only inform the microcontroller (typically waking it up) when something is moving. Thus, node sensing operations may be time-triggered or event-triggered and the solution should cover both.

R5 - Minimize Maintenance. This requisite could be stated has low power, but all the requirements have been elicited from the user's point of view. Some IoT devices cannot be battery operated because they require e.g., real-time continuous sensing or they do not need it because they are connected to a continues power source. However, other ones can be or must be battery operated. This is especially relevant when there is no previous deployment planning. Hence, the sensor node can be deployed anywhere without cable dependencies. Battery-operated nodes require battery maintenance, charging or replacing the batteries from time to time. When this is the case, the battery life should be maximized avoiding unnecessary battery drain. The communication is typically the most relevant issue when dealing with battery life in IoT devices, consuming more battery than the sensing or processing operations in most of the cases. On the one hand, to save energy, microcontrollers follow a sleep and awake cycle as part of their operation, that also includes the communications switching on-off. Typically, microcontrollers and communications consume in the order of μA while sleeping, in the order of mA when they are awake, and dozens or few hundreds of mA when using communications (there is a great variability depending on the chosen communications).

3 Related Work

As explained in the introduction, these requirements guide us to a specific set of WSNs called mesh networks or multi-hop networks, where a message goes from one node to another goes hopping from one node to its neighbors until the destination (the sink node) is reached. Not all the mesh communication proposals analyzed have been designed to consider all the requirements previously stated and we will discuss it now on.

On the one hand, there have been several attempts to create mesh networks from the research community e.g., [8] as well as from the industry. Maybe the most notable one has been ZigBee, based on IEEE 802.15.4, and just very recently Bluetooth, based on IEEE 802.15.1. ZigBee mesh capabilities have been discussed widely in the literature due to the great difference between its theoretical and practical power consumption. Also, ZigBee have coordinator, router and regular node roles that must be configured (and programmed) before being deployed.

On the other hand, all the proposal named above increase the price of the product to a point where it is not viable for cheap objects, being the communication module more expensive than the not connected product itself. E.g., a sensor to emit a "bip" when a door or a window is open can be purchased for 2€ or less but, just a ZigBee communication module is over 20€. Some solutions (e.g., [8]) just increase the price of the IoT device requiring one processor as microcontroller and another for communication.

Regarding the mesh capabilities of Bluetooth (version 5), maybe due to its very recent appearance or due to the low amount of development boards related with the latest Bluetooth 5 standard, it has not been intensively tested. Anyway, we have not found a Bluetooth module in the price range stated by the requirement R3, and not even for older Bluetooth standard versions including the low energy ones from Bluetooth 4.

Some other researchers are trying to provide Wi-Fi, based on 802.11, with mesh topology. On top of the 802.11 standard, many communication protocols have arisen at different OSI layer levels, such a CoAP for constrained environments, TCP or HTTP to build what we know as Web of Thing (WoT) to name a few. However, none of them include mesh capabilities natively. Furthermore, some of them like HTTP were not conceived for small packets (e.g. info of a sensor measure) and low power consumption, being its power consumption in most microcontroller using Wi-Fi around or above 100 mA when transmitting.

Regarding Wi-Fi, some works trying to create a mesh network protocol related to the selected microcontroller have been implemented. We can classify them between related work just using or based on the Arduino IDE ESP8266 mesh example (trivial and just a proof of concept), and abandoned, incomplete implementations (e.g., [2]) or not formalized ones. Finally, other code repositories mixing MQTT (a trending publish/subscribe telemetry communication protocol) and mesh for ESP8266 (e.g., [3]) just do not cope with the requirements stated in Sect. 2.

4   Our Approach: A Low Cost Effective Mesh Protocol

It was easy for us to find a microcontroller within the price range stated as R3, due to our integration inside the Smart Open Lab, a FabLab, in Cáceres. We selected one of the *makers* favorite products for IoT devices, the ESP8266 microcontroller [4]. This microcontroller was originally conceived as a Wi-Fi communication module, but due to its hardware capabilities, it can be programmed integrating the microcontroller and the communication functionalities into a single integrated circuit. It has not been created to measure many sensors at the same time having just an analog input pin, but it is quite capable to use many digital sensors at the same time. The price of the microcontroller is in the range of 1,20–1,50€ depending on the quantity planned to buy. One of the constraints of ESP266 is its poor communication support, that is our case is especially relevant since this microcontroller and other similar microcontrollers do not support full duplex communications. Thus, we will need to deal with separated transmission and reception time frames.

While there is a new microcontroller from the same company named ESP32 including Wi-Fi and Bluetooth communications, doubling the microcontroller clock speed and the number of microprocessors as well as the General Purpose Input and Outputs (GPIO) capabilities. However, also its price is over 2,50€–2,95€, just above our requirements. Anyway, we have also tested this microcontroller and its power consumption is a little bit higher than the ESP8266 one because microcontroller is also more capable, but this affects requirement R5. Currently, there are few research papers about these microcontrollers being both quite new and very recently adopted by the research community [11]. We would have preferred sub-GHz communications (the ESP8266 only includes 2,4 GHz Wi-Fi) that expose better wall penetration, but we did not find a microcontroller including communication in the price range required.

Once selected the microcontroller, we deal with the rest of the requirements. There are many standards related to IoT communications and we detailed some of them in Sect. 3. In communications, there is not one rule to solve any situation. Enterprises developing IoT devices are typically using these standards plus other ad-hoc solutions to fill the gap of standardization between them. Summarizing Sect. 3, no current protocol in our knowledge can be directly applied to cope with the Sect. 2 requirements. So, we have developed a new Wi-Fi mesh communication protocol taking special care of sleep intervals and making all the nodes in the network homogeneous from the communications point of view. Without specific roles, we avoid complex configurations that could eventually affect some requirements such as R1 and R3. Thus, nodes will configure themselves during all its life. Selected mesh topology avoids repeaters and related additional hardware to achieve requirement R2 (also contributing to minimize costs stated as requisite R3) while configuration autonomy is required to achieve requirement R1.

There are several design decisions that we have taken during the mesh protocol development and all of them have been carefully evaluated and some of them even implemented totally or partially to be tested with real hardware before taking a decision.

Regarding the wake-up schema, several options have been proposed by other authors regarding communication. It can be synchronous (periodic just with the neighbors, with the communication path or the whole network or just no periodic), asynchronous (initiated by the transmitter, the receiver, random or combined) or mixed. Full synchronous schemas can be eliminated due to the requisite R5. ESP8266 is monocore, so multitasking is virtual and not real, being only one functionality executed by the processor at any moment (e.g. receiving, sensing or processing data). So, when multitasking in monocore microcontrollers while the microcontroller is processing data, some data transmissions from other nodes could be missed. To solve it some traditional protocols implements ACKs that are simple to implement. However, they require an additional transmission (the ACK itself plus the original data one) as well as retransmitting when required. This functionality has been avoided here because while the node is sensing an ACK and a potential retransmission, the sender and the receiver cannot be sleeping and must have the radio links switched on. So, this solution would drain the battery damaging the achievement of requisite R5. We started implementing a fully asynchronous approach, but we had problems with the different nodes waking up schemas and the number of messages in the queues with some of the tested solutions that we will cover in this section. So, the implementation evolved into a mixed communication schema, periodic but asynchronous where the nodes do not share a common clock, one of the problems that some mesh protocols show. It is asynchronous to reduce power consumption, maximizing the time the node can be in sleep mode, and synchronous because each node has his own wake-up/sleep periods that can be different from the rest of the nodes. It is synchronous because each node knows the reception interval of each of its neighbors, so it synchronizes its transmission interval with the reception interval of its neighbors. For sake of simplicity, we include the period duration codified as part of its unique network name. Hence, while receiving data, the node is also announcing its existence to its neighbors, a way to connect with it (exposing its SSID) and the node period. So, its neighbors are then able to calculate the next reception intervals to minimize unsuccessful transmission attempts while draining the battery.

Regarding the routing protocols for this specific WSN, we avoided evaluating pure flooding due to the selected microcontroller memory restrictions, but we evaluated and combined other techniques such as gossiping (i.e., controlled flooding), spin and direct broadcast as following discussed.

The regular communication operations that have been designed for the WSN nodes are: *announce and receive* messages (the protocol calculates its maximum sleeping time support for any node to calculate the next reception time), *scan* the neighbors (to search for neighbors when the neighbors list is empty), *send* a message to a neighbor (there are different type of messages as we will specify bellow into this Section) and *sleep* (to save battery until the next interval or if there are messages in the sending queue to be sent). Announce and receive functionality is performed simultaneously by means of the node period codified as part of the SSID as stated above.

We have also defined a set of user and maintenance operations that are mostly used internally by the protocol that are the following ones. *Duplicate messages check*, to avoid messages already send or that already are in the sending queue. *Sending queue message deletion*, to eliminate all the messages already sent to the neighbor list. *Select next node to send it a message*, that considers which neighbors have received messages more recently to avoid their memory overflow but, also establishes a random probability of each node to be selected or not for the same reason. All this user and maintenance level operations are available for other researchers as methods so, anyone could test different approaches to improve the mesh network.

When creating the state transition diagram for the communication protocol (depicted in Fig. 1) we gave priority to *sense/process* functionality that stands typically for sensor reading and its (pre)processing and/or actuator executions. Regarding the communication operations, the state machine give priority to *announce and receive* (because we don't know if other nodes are still waiting for a node to wake-up to send it a message) and *send* (because the sensing data must arrive at its destination) functionality, while the rest of the functionality is only addressed when these two ones have been completed.

By agreement with the mixed approach adoption that we made for this mesh WSN protocol, time intervals become now necessary not only for the node to complete their normal operations, but also to communicate with other nodes. Typically, a microcontroller taking care of power consumption and with no communication capabilities has two states/intervals, the sensing/process one and the sleeping one that repeats periodically when no event-based sensors are used in the node. Because both intervals cannot be active at the same time (i.e., the microcontroller is awake or sleeping) for an entity other than the node to know when the node is going to be awake is just necessary to know a moment when the node was awaked and the node period. From now on, this entity could always find the sensor awake when necessary. The same principle has been adopted in our approach in order to know when a node is ready to receive data transmissions (i.c., reception interval) because is the same that the announcement interval that also exposes it period to all its neighbors. For a regular IoT device, only one more state should be required for transmission, that it is performed typically after the sensing/processing state and before going back to sleep.

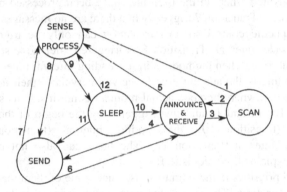

Fig. 1. State machine for the sensor nodes including communication, processing and sleeping capabilities

However, our case is more complex as detailed in Fig. 1, and other states become necessary to receive from other nodes that the node must previously discover autonomously within its surroundings. The time intervals devoted to each node state inside the whole node period are dynamic according to the node transmission, retransmission, reception, announcement and sensing/processing necessities at any wake-up time. Our nodes just need to maintain his own clock to calculate when a neighbor is ready to receive data with a simple operation (Eq. 1), maximizing sleeping interval in the node until the next neighbor will be ready.

$$next\_sending\_time\_to\_a\_neighbor = \frac{node\_actual\_time - neighbor\_discovery\_time}{neighbor\_period} \quad (1)$$

Even when not detected in the deployment tests, the only problem we envisioned with the previous solution is quite strange and only occurs when two neighbors that want to communicate have the same *announce and reception* interval time and period. Thus, both nodes overlap their *announce and reception* state making impossible them to communicate. To solve it, the communication protocol randomly doubles the announce and reception interval duration in the receiver or just keep it when this situation is detected. So, even while this problem may occur, the communication will eventually work in one of the next intervals after the first failed attempt.

The state machine can go from one state to another due to time-based or operation-based conditions (usually when the state main operation has finished) as follows. Transition 1 (from scan to process state), 5 and 7 are activated when the sensing/processing time is event or time-triggered. Transition 2 is triggered when the announce and receive interval starts. Transition 3 is activated when there is remaining operation time after completing the announce and reception of messages operations. Transition 4 is triggered when there are pending messages to be sent. Transition 5 is only triggered when no scan or sending operations must be performed at that moment. Transition 6 is activated when all the messages have been processed or the announce operation is necessary. Transition 7 triggers when there are no messages to be sent, here there is also a specific control so, this transition can only be triggered once per microcontroller awake interval. Transition 8 is triggered after node sensing and processing is done but, only when the node is in its sending interval time (autoconfigured by the node according to the announce and receive intervals of their neighbors) while transition 9 is initiated when the node actual moment is not inside its sending interval time. Transitions 10, 11 and 12 are time-triggered by the begin of the announce and receive interval (transition 10), the sending interval (transition 11) or the sensing/processing interval (transition 12). The latter can also not be triggered by sensor events as explained for requisite R4.

We also added priorities to these transitions, since some of them may be potentially triggered at the same time. The transitions with higher priority in the protocol have more possibilities to be executed during the current awake interval. Transitions 1, 5, 7, 9 and 12 have the higher priority while transitions 4 and 11 has a medium priority and finally transitions 2, 3, 6, 8 and 10 have the lower priority. The designed state machine is not preemptive so, the priorities only affect the tasks/states ordering and it is not able to stop a state task to go to another state until it will be finished. According to our tests, the microcontroller is quite capable at 80 MHz (80.000 instruction cycles per second) and communication operations have been kept as simple as possible while the node period is measured in seconds to ensure the nodes sleeping most of the time.

Regarding the types of message, the solution needs some different ones. One of the most interesting ones is control messages to avoid memory overflows in the reception nodes. Thus, prior to a data transmission, this type of message is always sent. This short message includes ID to identify the sender, CHANNEL fixed to _RATE for this type of message and a RATE field for the node to specify the difficulty to send it data in the next periods until the node will change this parameter. This control messages are read by the receiver while performing communication maintenance tasks. Due to the previously unknown number of nodes and their locations is impossible to previously know the number of neighbor nodes and some of them could be saturated with messages maybe throwing away some of them. So, RATE is used by the sender node to express its potential to receive data in the close future. It is calculated by the sender node using the number of received messages divided by the number of eliminated messages and just zero if no messages were eliminated. So, when a node must send information, it does a multicast to no all its neighbors, but just some of them (while at least one). Then, the new sender node randomly establishes the possibility to send information to each of its neighbors with a possibility from 0 to the inverse of the _RATE when _RATE is different to zero and only sending the data if the result of this operation is zero.

Another type of messages is data messages, that are used to send the sampling data as well as the required retransmission of data from its neighbors. This message type includes fields to specify CHANNEL, as a native extension mechanism for the communication protocol to include e.g., _STATS or _DEBUG channels among others that any node could be aware of; DATA that contains the data itself, that may include the sensed data and other relevant information such as timestamp among others); SEQUENCE to order data messages from the same sender because due to the multi-hopping behavior of the protocol, a message send before another one could arrive later to the destination; IDs that contains an ordered list with the nodes unique identifiers that have retransmit the message as well as the node that send the original message (so if a particular message has already arrived at the node for retransmission, it can just be eliminated to save memory) and NUMBER_IDs that is just a number indicating the number of IDs in the previous list to be able to decode them.

The UML class diagram for the main pieces of the communication protocol is depicted in Fig. 2 where the main classes go as follows. AP manage the neighbors list of the node. BROADCASTNODE manage the Wi-Fi radio of the node, that is based on TCP server using the native ESP8266 communication capabilities including for example the Extended SSID (ESSID) that include the announce and receive interval time of the node coded with the SSID. MESSAGEBROKER to manage the message queues. Finally, SCHEDULERNODE that is quite complex because control the state machine detailed in Fig. 1 including all the intervals to throw the transitions also according to their priorities.

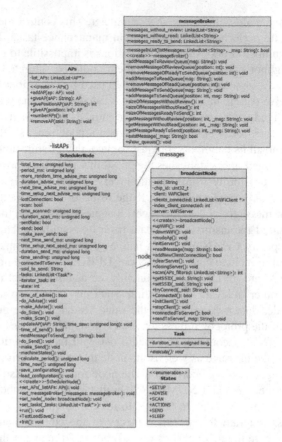

Fig. 2. Left: UML class diagram for the mesh node specification.

5 Conclusions

Nowadays, the IoT communication future is still undefined but, as researchers, we cannot leave all the work to the enterprises. Their focus is business, not people and they create for the masses, usually with a typical set of *personas* and contexts in their minds while designing solutions. This situation may leave the elders to their fate, living into large houses with wide walls and no enough technical skills or technicians around to solve the communication problems with their devices. Therefore, the research community must use its tools to include them all proposing new approaches.

The proposed solution achieve all the requirements in Sect. 2, but even when we have guessed many potential scenarios while designing the solution and we have performed deployments using real hardware up to 10 nodes working for days while manually switching randomly one or more on and off to monitoring network behavior, the proposal should be deployed in a real scenario with daily usage and real elderly users in rural areas. We hope to be able to complete this work as part of 4IE+ (see acknowledgments). So, this is a work in progress shared with the community as an open source project that we expect to continue developing in the future.

For multihopping mesh WSNs, like the one proposed here, it is debatable how to measure many common and easy to calculate times to check network performance, such as the time for a message to arrive at its destination. This occurs because many common network time measures depend on each of the nodes sleep-awake intervals, neighbors discovery moment and network saturation to name a few. Therefore, more complex measures and explanations are required. That work was done to achieve the current level of refinement in the protocol design (and implementation) but that work explanation would exceed the current paper length.

Some other questions remain still in the air, maybe being security one of the most relevant ones and many optimizations could be achieved by the research and open source communities. For the later we plan to simulate complex situations with the One following the work carry out be [6].

Acknowledgements. Instituto Internacional de INvestighación e Innovación del Envejecimiento (4IE), Ref. 0445_4IE_4_P. Proyecto cofinanciado por el Fondo Europeo de Desarrollo Regional (FEDER) a través del Programa Interreg V-A España Portugal (POCTEP) 2014–2020.

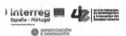

References

1. Das, R., Tuna, A., Demirel, S., Yurdakul, M.K.: A survey on the internet of things solutions for the elderly and disabled: applications, prospects, and challenges. Int. J. Comput. Networks Appl. **4**(3), 1–9 (2017)
2. EasyMesh code repository. https://github.com/Coopdis/easyMesh. Accessed 15 Sept 2018
3. ESP8266MQTTMesh code repository. https://github.com/PhracturedBlue/ESP8266MQTTMesh. Accessed 15 Sept 2018
4. Expressif. ESP8266 specifications. https://www.espressif.com/en/products/hardware/esp8266ex/resources. Accessed 12 Oct 2018
5. Ezechina, M.A., Okwara, K.K., Ugboaja, C.A.U.: The Internet of Things (Iot): a scalable approach to connecting everything. Int. J. Eng. Sci. **4**(1), 09–12 (2015)
6. Galán-Jiménez, J., Berrocal, J., García-Alonso, J. Canal, C., Murillo, J.M.: Situational and adaptive context-aware routing for opportunistic IoT networks. In: 28th International Telecommunication Networks and Applications Conference (2018)
7. Gubbia, J., Buyyab, R., Marusic, S., Palaniswami, M.: Internet of Things (IoT): a vision, architectural elements, and future directions. Future Gener. Comput. Syst. **29**(7), 1645–1660 (2013)
8. Kim, H.S., Lee, J., Wook, J.: Blemesh: a wireless mesh network protocol for bluetooth low energy devices. In: 3rd International Conference on Future Internet of Things and Cloud (FiCloud). IEEE (2015)
9. Memon, M., Wagner, S.R., Pedersen, C.F., Beevi, F.H.A., Hansen, F.O.: Ambient assisted living healthcare frameworks, platforms, standards, and quality attributes. Sensors **14**(3), 4312–4341 (2014)

10. Ray, P.P.: Home Health Hub Internet of Things (H^3IoT): an architectural framework for monitoring health of elderly people. In: International Conference on Science Engineering and Management Research. IEEE (2014)
11. Singh, K.J., Kapoor, D.S.: Create your own Internet of Things: a survey of IoT platforms. IEEE Consum. Electron. Mag. **6**(2), 57–68 (2017)
12. Suraki, M.Y., Jahanshahi, M.: Internet of Things and its benefits to improve service delivery in public health approach. In: 7th International Conference on Application of Information and Communication Technologies. IEEE (2013)

Health Gains of Telephone Follow-up Nursing Intervention to Patient with Heart Disease

Sara Correia[1(✉)], Ana Correia[1], Isabel Videira[1], Paula Abrunhosa[1],
Célia Cuco[1], Raquel Bolas[1], Dilar Costa[1], and César Fonseca[2]

[1] Centro Hospitalar Universitário de Lisboa Norte,
Av. Prof Egas Moniz, 1649-035 Lisbon, Portugal
sara.fr.correia@gmail.com
[2] Universidade de Évora, Évora, Portugal

Abstract. Aim: To identify the health gains related to nursing interventions in the telephone follow-up of adult patients with heart disease.

Methodology: Systematic literature review by research in EBSCO, (CINAHL and MEDLINE) in the publication time interval between January 2012 and October 2017, using the PICO method. Elected 8 articles for analysis.

Results: By the using of a telephone nursing intervention with heart disease patient's health gains were identified related to: symptomatic control, management of the therapeutic regimen, use of health services, safety/adverse events and quality of life.

Conclusions: The telephone nursing intervention contributes to optimize the follow-up to the patient, translating into health gains sensitive to nursing care.

Implication to professional practice: In the contexts of nursing practice for adult patients with heart disease, telephone follow-up proves to be an intervention to be considered, translating into gains in health, promoting patient follow-up and improving training in disease management.

Keywords: Tele-nursing · Counseling · Nursing · Cardiac patient

1 Introduction

Heart failure (HF) is a syndrome with high prevalence, morbidity and mortality, which represents a great economic and social overload [1]. In Portugal, it affects about 400,000 people and is increasing, constituting a high cost to the National Health Service, by the consumption of medication, exams and medical devices. As consequences it's well know the physical and psychological limitations, with related loss of quality of life [2].

The current challenge lies in the identification of nursing interventions that translate health gains sensitive to nursing care [3]. These gains are directed to the needs of individuals or groups, in their health and life context, and are based on organizational factors, experience and level of knowledge, with a direct impact on functional status, selfcare, symptom control, management of disease, safety/adverse events, use of health services and quality of life [4]. Nursing care-sensitive outcomes can be defined as all

© Springer Nature Switzerland AG 2019
J. García-Alonso and C. Fonseca (Eds.): IWoG 2018, CCIS 1016, pp. 107–113, 2019.
https://doi.org/10.1007/978-3-030-16028-9_10

those relevant, based on nursing domain and intervention, for which there is empirical evidence linking the nurse's input and the outcome of the intervention [4].

The use of the interactive means of communication via telephone has main advantages, as the rapidity of response, greater accessibility of the individual to healthcare and the nurse to the individual, greater equity in access to healthcare and potential of health gains in good time [5].

This systematic review of the literature aims to identify the health gains of nursing interventions using interactive means of communication via telephone in follow-up of adult patients with heart disease (HD).

2 Methods

Systematic literature review using the PICO method (What are the health gains (O) of telephone follow-up nursing intervention (I) to the adult patient with heart disease (P)?) was performed.

The electronic database used for search was EBSCO (MEDLINE with Full Text, CINAHL, Plus with Full Text), retrospectively from January 2012 to October 2017. The descriptors were validated in the MeSH (Medical Subject Headings) and searched by the following order: ["nursing" OR "nursing care" OR "nursing intervention"] AND ["heart failure" OR "coronary disease" OR "heart diseases" OR "heart"] AND ["telenursing" OR "after care" OR "counselling"]. From this search process strategy resulted 117 articles in total. To assess the levels of evidence of the articles the contributes of Melnyk and Fineout-Overholt [6] were used. The search and articles selection process it's represented in the following Table 1.

Table 1. Articles search and selection process

Identification:
• N° of identified articles on database (MEDLINE & CINAHL) - 727
Selection:
• N° of excluded articles - 392
• Full text articles – 335
• Temporal limit (2012–2017) – 117
• Excluded articles repeated – 104
Eligibility (by integral reading):
• Articles without inclusion criteria – 96
• Articles with inclusion criteria – 8
Inclusion:
• Included articles to analysis – 8
• Level II – 1; Level III – 3; Level V – 1; Level VI - 2; Level VII – 1.

3   Results

See Table 2.

Table 2. Results

Article	Aim	Results	Level of evidence
Author: Arredondo-Holguín et al. [7]. **Methods:** Experimental study. **Participants:** 29 users >30 years old with HF. **Aim:** To evaluate the improvement in nursing care in self-care (pharmacological and non-pharmacological adherence, adaptation to the illness and request for help), after educational nursing intervention in patients with HF. **Results:** Nursing educational intervention had beneficial effects in most of the evaluated self-care behaviors. Since several intervention strategies (group educational sessions, home visits and telephone follow-up, and supporting documentation) have been evaluated, it is not possible to indicate which is more efficient, which makes it necessary to do other studies to compare specific strategies. **Level of evidence:** V			
Author: Rojas et al. [8]. **Methods:** Quasi-experimental study. **Participants:** 21 users, average age 67 years. **Aim:** To determine if motivational interview as a nursing intervention is a promoter of self-care (therapeutical compliance, ability to adapt to the disease and seek help before the exacerbation of the symptoms), in patients with HF. **Results:** The nursing intervention that uses as a strategy the telephone follow-up as a support to the motivational interview contributes to improve the self-care of the patient with HF. **Level of evidence:** III			
Author: Hobbs et al. [9]. **Methods:** Systematic literature review. **Articles:** 7 **Aim:** To determine if the intervention performed (telephonic follow-up, telemonitoring, interprofessional interventions) to the patient with HF, through telephone contact reduces their re-hospitalization within 30 days after discharge, compared to those who are not submitted to this intervention. **Results:** Multidisciplinary programs are effective in reducing hospital rehospitalization in the period studied in patients with HF. **Level of evidence:** VI			
Author: Arredondo-Holguín et al. [10]. **Methods:** Descriptive research. **Participants:** 31 users with HF **Aim:** To describe the difficulties encountered in telephone follow-up related to the self-reported (adherence to non-pharmacological treatment) in patients with HF. **Results:** Nursing education programs, through telephone follow-up, to HF users, have been effective in improving adherence to therapy, resulting in better control of disease. **Level of evidence:** VI			
Author: Rodríguez-Gázquez et al. [11]. **Methods:** Controlled, randomized, non-blinding clinical trial. **Participants:** 33 users in the study group and 30 in the control group. **Aim:** Evaluate the efficiency of an educational nursing program for the improvement of self-care behaviors (pharmacological and non-pharmacological			

(continued)

Table 2. (*continued*)

Article	Aim	Results	Level of evidence

adherence, adaptation to the disease, request for help and empowerment) in patients with HF.

Results: The educational nursing intervention studied has a beneficial effect on self-care behaviors of people with HF.

Level of evidence: II

Author: Kim et al. [12]. **Methods:** Quasi-experimental and longitudinal design. **Participants:** 61 patients with cardiac disease.

Aim: To develop a comprehensive program (teaching, documentation, support, telephone follow-up) for cardiac rehabilitation that considers the learning needs of cardiac patients in their cultural context in Korea. Check the effects of the program on physiological and psychosocial factors and recurrent symptoms or cardiac events

Results: The results showed that participants in the program had decreased body mass index and abdominal perimeter, as well as improved left ventricular diastolic function and improved quality of life related to heart disease.

Level of evidence: III

Author: McCarthy et al. [13]. **Methods:** descriptive study pilot. **Participants:** 20 participants.

Aim: To describe the results of an evaluation process of exercise counseling and symptom management using the motivational interview.

Results: There are beneficial behavioral changes with motivational interviews.

Level of evidence: VII

Author: Dunbar et al. [14]. **Methods:** Clinical randomized trial. **Participants:** 134 man.

Aim: To test an integrated intervention of self-care (functional capacity, physical activity and quality of life), in patients concomitantly with HF and diabetes mellitus.

Results: Improvement of functional capacity and quality of life in patients with HF.

Level of Evidence: III

4 Discussion

The information resulting from the critical analysis of the selected articles contributed to answer the initial question, since, explicitly or implicitly, they address the telephone follow-up to the patient with HD.

Through the analysis of the results it is possible to identify that the educational intervention of nursing has a beneficial effect on the self-care behaviors of people with HD. It should be noted that educational activities included educational group sessions, information leaflets, home visits and telephone follow-up [11]. An increased knowledge and higher adherence in the management of the non-pharmacological therapeutic regimen, regarding salt intake, weight control, urine measurement, fluid restriction, lower limb elevation, influenza prevention, physical activity, adequacy of daily life activities to the effort and reduction of alcohol and tobacco consumption were identified.

Telephone intervention is a good strategy in patient education and continuity of care in assessing adherence to self-care behaviors. During the telephone sessions conducted in a study, improvement was observed in the patients' interest in knowing more about the disease and altering inappropriate behaviors [10]. In other studies, the health gains obtained from the teaching were improved, namely, improved weight control and fluid intake, elevation of the lower limbs in the seated position, physical exercise performance [7] and reduction of salt intake in the diet [8].

It was verified that nursing education programs carried out through telephone follow-up, to patients with HD, contribute to increase the knowledge about the therapeutic regime by the patient/family [11]. The active participation of the patient in the therapeutic plan is essential for effective adherence to the management of the therapeutic regimen [8]. Strategies such as the implementation of the list of medicines have contributed to maintain or improve the therapeutic compliance of the individual [7]. In fact, motivational interviews over the phone reinforce the received information in face-to-face sessions [13].

Regarding to symptom control and based on the studies analyzed, the use of strategies, such as distributing activities throughout the day in order to manage the effort, decrease fatigue [7] and to adjust the activities to the effort [10], contribute to the improvement of daily physical activity tolerance [12, 14]. Other gains have been identified for the individual, such as a decrease in body mass index and abdominal perimeter [12].

One of the analyzed papers indicates that the management of multidisciplinary programs are effective in reducing the rehospitalization of patients with HD, namely the intervention of specialist nurse in HD and the intervention through phone follow-up [9]. The use of health services was described by three authors regarding the search for healthcare and the search for healthcare assistance in the phase of exacerbation of the disease [7, 8, 11].

Regarding safety/adverse events, the analyzed articles found improvement in the ability to adapt to the disease [7, 11], improving the perception of health status, namely the modification of self-concept and self-acceptance, learning to live with HD and the effects of treatment [11], and a reduction in complications at the HD disease [14]. To prevent and avoid the occurrence of adverse events, strategies have been developed namely stay away from people who are cold [7] and adoption of measures to prevent influenza [10].

Health is not the only factor that influences the quality of life, however, it has a central importance. In the analysis of the studied articles, it was verified that two authors identified health gains related to the improvement of quality of life [12, 13]. The follow-up consultation via telephone and the daily record made by the patient increase the knowledge about the disease and its management [9, 13, 14].

The authors argue that the support network and the family favor the promotion of self-care [8], which may contribute to improve the quality of life of the patient.

5 Conclusion

The nursing intervention that uses as a strategy the telephone follow-up as a support to the motivational interview contributes to improve the selfcare of the patient with HD.

It is fundamental that the nurse uses the motivational interview complemented with the telephone follow-up as a tool to promote self-care in patients with HD and simultaneously use a work of articulation with other healthcare professionals.

Multidisciplinary programs are effective in reducing hospital readmissions in patients with HD. It is recommended that health education programs for HD patients include telephone follow-up as a strategy to improve adherence to treatment.

The telephone follow-up associated with other nursing interventions, contribute to optimize patient follow-up (knowledge about the disease, behavior change, motivation, symptom management, complication prevention, health service utilization management, therapeutic regime management and quality of life improvement), translating into health gains sensitive to nursing care.

Due to the health gains found, telephone follow-up should be considered in the care of patients with heart disease in different contexts, promoting follow-up of the patient and improving their capacity to manage the disease.

References

1. Fundação Portuguesa de Cardiologia: Insuficiência Cardíaca cuide da sua máquina (2017). http://www.fpcardiologia.pt/insuficiencia-cardiaca-cuide-da-sua-maquina/
2. Fonseca, C., et al.: Pela melhoria do tratamento da IC em Portugal – documento consenso. Rev. Port. Cardiol. 36(1), 1–8 (2017)
3. Doran, D.M.: Nursing Sensitive Outcomes: State of the Science. Jones Bartlett Publishers, London (2003)
4. Doran, D.M., Pringle, D.: Patient outcomes as accountability. In: Doran, D. (ed.) Nursing Outcomes: The State of the Science, 2nd edn, pp. 1–27. Jones and Bartlett, Sudbury (2011)
5. Ordem dos Enfermeiros: Conselho Jurisdicional. Parecer CJ 102, Consulta de Enfermagem por via telefónica (2009). http://www.ordemenfermeiros.pt/documentos/CJ_Documentos/Parecer102_2009_consulta_enfermagem_telefone.pdf. Accessed 21 Jan 2018
6. Melnyk, B.M., Fineout-Overholt, E.: Evidence-Based Practice in Nursing & Healthcare: A Guide to Best Practice. Lippincott Williams & Wilkins, Philadelphia (2011)
7. Arredondo-Holguín, E., Rodríguez-Gázquez, M., Higuita-Urrego, L.: Improvement of self-care behaviors after a nursing educational intervention with patients with heart failure. Investigación & Educación en Enfermería 30(2), 188–197 (2012)
8. Rojas, C.M., Rojas, D.N., Reyes, A.M.: Motivational interviews as a nursing intervention to promote self-care in patients with heart failure in a Fourth-Level Institution in Bogotá, Colombia. Investigación en Enfermería: Imagen y Desarrollo 15(1), 31–49 (2013)
9. Hobbs, J.K., Escutia, D., Harrison, H., Moore, A., Sarpong, E.: Reducing hospital readmission rates in patients with heart failure. Medsurg Nurs. 25(3), 145–152 (2016)
10. Arredondo-Holguín, E., Rodríguez-Gázquez, M., Higuita-Urrego, L.: Difficulties with adherence to non-pharmacological treatment of patients with heart failure detected through telephone follow-up. Investigación en Enfermería: Imagen y Desarrollo 16(2), 133–147 (2014)

11. Rodríguez-Gázquez, M., Arredondo-Holguín, E., Herrera-Cortés, R.: Effectiveness of an educational program in nursing in the self-care of patients with heart failure: randomized controlled trial. Revista Latino-Americana de Enfermagem **20**(2), 296–306 (2012)
12. Kim, S., Lee, S., Kim, G., Kang, S., Ahn, J.: Effects of a comprehensive cardiac rehabilitation program in patients with coronary heart disease in Korea. Nurs. Health Sci. **16**(4), 476–482 (2014)
13. McCarthy, M., Dickson, V., Katz, S., Sciacca, K., Chyun, D.: Process evaluation of an exercise counseling intervention using motivational interviewing. Appl. Nurs. Res. **28**(2), 156–162 (2015)
14. Dunbar, S.B., et al.: Randomized clinical trial of an integrated self-care intervention for persons with heart failure and diabetes: quality of life and physical functioning outcomes. J. Cardiac Fail. **21**(9), 719–729 (2015)

Supporting Active Ageing Interventions with Web and Mobile/Wearable Technologies and Using Microservice Oriented Architectures

Francisco Carranza-García[1] , Francisco M. García-Moreno[1] ,
Carlos Rodriguez-Dominguez[1] , José Luis Garrido[1] ,
María Bermúdez Edo[1] , María José Rodriguez-Fortiz[1] ,
and José Manuel Pérez-Mármol[2(✉)]

[1] Dpt. Lenguajes y Sistemas Informáticos, CITIT-UGR,
University of Granada, Granada, Spain
{carranzafr, fmgarmor, carlosrodriguez, jgarrido,
mbe, mjfortiz}@ugr.es
[2] Dpt. of Physiotherapy, Faculty of Health Sciences,
University of Granada, Granada, Spain
josemapm@ugr.es

Abstract. New solutions in the e-Health domain are been applied to address problems such as monitoring, user adaptation and context influence, particularly if the patients are older people. The social and economic burdens associated with age decline can be decreased by providing more holistic technological solutions. Our aim is to contribute to the integration of different aspects in the active ageing process (cognitive, physical and social) to achieve more complete evaluations and by performing more effective interventions in the elderly. To this end, in this research work we propose a technological solution based on microservices architectures, which has been validated in two different projects: cognitive training and frailty prevention. The solution involves a system of systems engineering, thus improving reusability, extensibility, and performance in the e-Health domain.

Keywords: Microservices architecture · e-Health · Active ageing ·
VIRTRAEL · PREFRA

1 Introduction

Active ageing focuses on the recognition and reinforcement of the human rights of older people. Although some of them remain active and participate in their community and in family matters, many others face isolation and a lack of adequate health or social care [5]. Despite cultural and political influences, cognitive and health decline related to ageing is the main reason for elderly people to feel that they are a social burden.

To decrease that social burden and empower the elderly, new policies that imply the involvement of older people are arising in Europe, with projects and solutions to provide access to culture, long life learning, home healthcare services, physical activity for seniors, leisure and welfare activities, etc.

© Springer Nature Switzerland AG 2019
J. García-Alonso and C. Fonseca (Eds.): IWoG 2018, CCIS 1016, pp. 114–123, 2019.
https://doi.org/10.1007/978-3-030-16028-9_11

ICTs are involved in most of these projects as a tool to monitor, train, intervene or help the elderly to improve their quality of life and state, keeping them active and healthy, physically and cognitively. For these reasons, the domain of active ageing requires the design of complex systems addressing these key aspects.

The objective of "systems of systems" engineering is the integration of systems, creating a system with more functionality than the sum of its parts [13]. The microservices architecture is aligned with the building of "systems of systems" because of their main principles such as reusability, extensibility, interoperability and composition.

In this paper, we show how a microservices architecture is also a useful software design solution to develop complex systems that make use of different technologies (web and mobile) in the health application domain. In particular, we present two examples for active ageing intervention in elderly people. The first one, VIRTRAEL, is a web-based system oriented towards cognitive assessment and training, and the second one, PREFRA, is a mobile/wearable-based system devised for the prevention of the frailty status. Both systems are designed and implemented based on a microservices architecture as a means to fulfil certain quality properties.

Initially these systems were designed independently, although several microservices can be reused as shared resources and even integrated in other future applications.

The paper introduces in Sect. 2 the microservices architecture. Sections 3 and 4 describe two systems that are focused on active ageing research, in which microservice-oriented architectural design has been applied despite requiring the use of different technologies, that is, web-based technologies in a cognitive assessment and training program (VIRTRAEL), and mobile/wearable ones in prevention of frailty (PREFRA). The final section summarizes conclusions and future work.

2 Microservices Architecture

Microservices architectures are inspired by service-oriented computing. Moreover, this architecture enables the continuous delivery/deployment of large, complex applications [9].

Additionally, it is an approach to the development of software that consists of building an application as a set of small services (i.e., that offer a single, very specific functionality), which are executed in their own process and communicate through lightweight mechanisms (usually an HTTP resource API). Each service is responsible for implementing the complete business functionality considering three layers of models: reference model, implementation model and deployment model.

Thus, microservices oriented architectures are a relevant design proposal to fulfil requirements for systems to be designed to support any kind of intervention in the health application domain, especially when these systems have to be extended and/or integrated in the future.

There are several proposals that describe the advantages of using microservices architectures in the literature. We highlight the following ones in the Health field. In [14] a microservice-oriented software architecture provides enough flexibility to facilitate the integration of heterogeneous devices and dynamic reconfigurations into systems for an assisted living of the elderly in their natural environment (AAL - Ambient Assisted

Living). A large number of data can be collected in IoT systems through data-driven microservices thus providing better care to patients, while reducing time and cost [7]. IoT models of microservices have been proposed to assist people with depressive crisis and it especially works in certain situations and emotional states of users [1].

The design and development of the two research studies presented in this paper are based on the principles of this architecture as will be described in detail in the following sections.

3   VIRTRAEL: Cognitive Assessment and Training

This section presents the VIRTRAEL system by describing its main characteristics and architecture.

3.1   VIRTRAEL Project

VIRTRAEL is a web-based system developed with funding from the Andalusia Regional Government (Junta de Andalucía) [15]. It supports a computer-based cognitive training program and a set of assistance tools to allow the management of the different user profiles (therapists, informal careers and older people) and access privileges, supervision and assessment of the users' performance.

VIRTRAEL provides 18 types of serious games to evaluate and train the main cognitive skills: memory, attention, planning and reasoning. We have demonstrated the concurrent validity of these activities and performed a previous pilot study to analyse the users' responses. Some of these activities include 3D virtual-reality environments. VIRTRAEL carries out three key functionalities organized on 3 main concerns/tools: configuration, communication, and performing games.

The configuration tool allows the administrator and the therapists to match end-users (patients) and supervising therapists. It also allows supervisors to know which games have been carried out by the patient and the scores that were achieved. Each therapist can configure which games will be carried out and in which order, for each patient. The supervisor can track, in real time, the progress of each patient while performing each exercise, and decide if the next planned game should be skipped or not.

The communication tool provides both a forum to exchange messages between the stakeholders in the cognitive assessment and training, and a chat to allow real-time collaboration between end-users and therapists. This tool is intended to improve user engagement, decrease the sense of isolation, and increase the sense of collaboration with other people.

The games area includes the serious games distributed in pre-defined work sessions. A session at the beginning and another one at the end evaluate the cognitive skills of the user before performing the exercises, and after completing them. The aim of the intermediate sessions is to train the cognitive abilities of the user to improve them. Each game trains at least one or two of the following skills: memory, planning, reasoning, and attention. A customized avatar (intended to improve user engagement) guides the elder to play the games in each session, and occasionally provides positive reinforcements. The games require the user to read instructions and, based on them, to give an answer by selecting between a set of items (text or images) or writing in some specific cases. During the performance of a game, several measures are taken to evaluate the success, play time, number of fails, omissions and hits.

VIRTRAEL has been tested in a pilot study in which its usability for elderly people was checked and also the concurrent validity of tests for cognitive assessment and the effectiveness of the cognitive stimulation exercises [12].

3.2 VIRTRAEL Architecture

Regarding the development of the system, it is designed as a set of services, which provide core functionalities: exercise management, user administration, collaboration and adaptation.

The architecture consists of four main concern-oriented services that interoperate which each other: ExerciseCollection, Administration, Adaptation and Collaboration (Fig. 1). The services consist of a set of microservices. The following subsections will describe them.

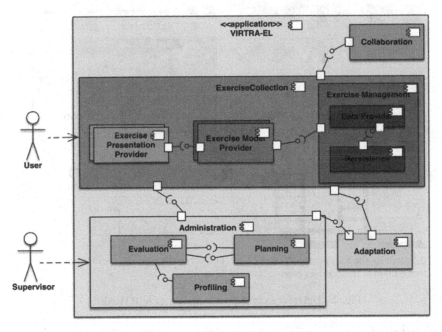

Fig. 1. Service-based architecture of VIRTRAEL.

ExerciseCollection

This service provides the foundations for managing exercises and their presentation to the end user. Internally, it is composed of three microservices:

- **Exercise Model Provider:** Given a type of exercise, it provides a model (XML) for that exercise. Figure 2 shows the interface of some types of exercises. This model includes a set of rules to accomplish and evaluate the exercise, a set of elements to be presented to the user (questions, places, images, puzzles, instructions, etc.), an ordering in the overall set of exercises, a repetition scheme (the times to be presented to the user, the rules to show it again, etc.), aspects to be measured, etc.

- **Exercise Presentation Provider:** Given an exercise model, it provides the graphical user interface (front-end) for it, considering the user device and the web browser to adapt the presentation: specific contents, selected widgets, etc.
- **Exercise Management:** Any given exercise model makes use of this microservice to retrieve its ordering from a database, according to how it has been configured by the supervisors for each end-user. Consequently, this microservice behaves as a back-end for each exercise model. Moreover, the exercise model uses this microservice to make persistent its internal status (information about number of fails, omissions and successes, time between interactions, number of helps required, etc.).

Previous microservices make use of the adaptation service to adapt the exercise models to the previous results obtained by the user, the way he/she interacts, etc.

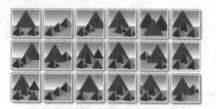

A. Choose the pictures with two pyramids facing the sun

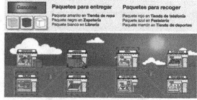

B. Plan the delivery of a set of packages

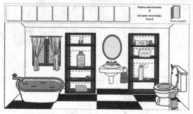

C. Search for the missing objects and move them to their correct place

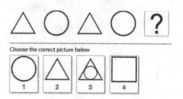

D. Choose the next picture in the series

Fig. 2. Different examples of exercises of VIRTRAEL

Administration

This service provides functionalities to manage the users (therapists and patients) and control their access permissions and privileges. It is internally composed of three main microservices:

- Assessment: Given any exercise model, it can evaluate the users' scoring and provide a result in the form of a "medal". as a positive reinforcement to the end user. Moreover, this microservice provides more advanced information to the therapists, allowing them to see the scoring progress for each user, group statistics, etc.

- Planning: This microservice provides tools to plan the ordering of the exercises and establish "sessions" of exercises, that is, an ordered set of exercises to be accomplished by the user at a specific period.
- Profiling: The profile of each user is provided by this microservice. Some information is manually provided by the users, such as personal information, while other information is automatically calculated. Moreover, this microservice provides tools to control their access permissions and privileges.

Collaboration

This service is used by the Exercises service to support collaboration and supervision. It provides functionality for managing the users of a work group and determining if they are performing the exercises in a collaborative or competitive way. It also maintains the awareness of the patients, showing the results of the interaction of a user to his peers or to a supervising therapist. Consequently, the service must exchange and share information between different instances of an exercise model and presentation, each instance running on different devices and with different users.

The key internal mechanism to support exercise sharing is a middleware that provides a high-level API to facilitate information exchange between peer users, and separate low-level communication management from exercise logics. The middleware is called BlueRose [10, 11], and it includes a publish-subscribe communication model to make more effective event distributions among different VIRTRAEL instances. Currently, only the middleware is integrated in the system, but nevertheless, different ways of collaborating will be provided by this service in future extensions of the system.

Adaptation

This service consists of two microservices to customize the system. The first one performs adaptations according to the user's devices and the web browsers of each user. The second one contains a set of rules to automatically adapt the exercises according to the results obtained by the users and their profiles. It is related to the ExerciseCollection service since it needs the data collected by the Exercise Management model to decide, using an "if-then" rule system, if the characteristics of the exercise models or exercise presentations must change.

The adaptation involves modifying the presentation of the exercise, its contents, level of difficulty, and the number of repetitions in each session.

4 PREFRA: Prevention of Frailty

This section presents the PREFRA project, the aim of which is the collection of data to identify older people with frailty and the analysis of these data to perform a clinical intervention based on the prevention of frailty.

4.1 Frailty Definition

The frailty syndrome is "a state of increased vulnerability of the deficit resolution of homeostasis after a stressful event due to the accumulation of age-related problems in the physiological systems" [16]. A more multidimensional explanation of it is: "dynamic state that affects an individual who experiences losses in one or more domains of human functioning (physical, psychological and social), which is caused by the influence of a range of variables and which increases the risk of adverse outcomes" [4]. Examples of these outcomes are deterioration of balance, falls, hospitalization, and even causation of death.

A person with frailty suffers a progressive loss of functionality until reaching a state of dependence in performing daily-life activities. It is important that frailty is assessed by professionals to measure some factors to identify when it is present in an older person [3, 6, 8]. Prevention is the key point to avoid future complications and dependence because the intervention can reduce the frailty status. In order to improve and enhance preventive actions, a holistic and ecological model to assess frailty is required.

With that aim, we propose the creation of an elder-centered model, obtained with a traditional assessment test and adapted technological support. ICT can contribute to collect more data, with more precision, transparently and ecologically, while the elderly is performing basic, instrumental and advanced daily life activities.

Up to now, some research has been done on the use of wearables to identify the physical state of users, gathering patterns, movement or detection of stress situations [2]. However, they do not consider all the factors influencing frailty, and there are few studies that perform the assessment in the environment of the user, as opposed to in health care centers.

4.2 User Model

Our proposal identifies variables, related to functional capacity in an ecological way, by providing a structured and comprehensive assessment of the health status and independence of the elderly according to the activities of daily life (ADL) performance, and considering the dimensions present in frailty (clinical, physical, psychological and social). We propose nine categories with the following variables:

- Sociodemographic: age, sex, educational level, number of children.
- Clinical: pluripathology, drug adherence, height, metabolic syndrome, hand dominance, foot dominance, blood pressure changes.
- Healthy and toxic habits/life styles: physical exercise, sleeping, smoking habit, alcohol habit.
- Sensory perception components: vision, hearing, tactile sensing.
- Musculoskeletal components: hand-grip strength, pinch strength.
- Motor components: walking aids, fall risk, balance, ambulation (walking function), upper-limb coordination, velocity of movement.
- Cognitive components: orientation, language, memory, attention resources, emotional components, anxiety, depression.
- Social components: perceived social support.
- Context/environment components: vital accompaniment, being cared for, caregiver function/role, physical environment.

The sociodemographic, clinical and healthy/toxic habit categories of variables provide information about the quality of life and physical health of the elder, which can promote wellbeing. The sensory perception variables can give information about the existence of sensory disabilities of the individual. The other categories include variables to measure different factors that influence frailty when performing Activities of Daily Living (ADLs). Most of this information will be measured by using mobile/wearable devices with built-in sensors, allowing the collection of the data dynamically and in a non-intrusive way. Specifically, a Samsung Gear S3 smartwatch has been used for collecting data with the following sensors: accelerometer, gyroscope, heart rate, GPS, gravity, linear acceleration, light.

4.3 Software Architecture

A system based on mobile/wearable platforms and the Service Oriented Architecture (SOA 2.0) approach has been designed. The software architecture (shown in Fig. 3) consists of three types of services: basic microservices, infrastructure services and pub/sub services.

- **Basic microservices** implement basic functions, also in relation to the resources present in the device, e.g. there exists a microservice that is responsible for communication with the accelerometer sensor for collecting the data this can provide. The following list briefly describes the basic microservices that are currently implemented:
  - Accelerometer: it is responsible for collecting the activity of the accelerometer sensor.
  - Gyroscope: responsible for collecting gyroscope sensor activity.
  - Gravity: responsible for collecting the activity of the gravity sensor.
  - HeartRate: responsible for collecting the activity of the heart rate sensor.
  - LinearAcceleration: responsible for collecting the activity of the linear acceleration sensor.
  - Light: responsible for collecting the activity of the luminosity sensor.
  - Pedometer: responsible for collecting the activity of the step sensor.
  - GPS: responsible for collecting available localization data.
  - Data Register: responsible for registering the activity of a sensor in the internal storage of the device and/or the server hosted in the cloud.
- **Infrastructure services** can interact with several of the basic microservices. Currently three infrastructure services have been included:
  - Service Discoverer is used when basic microservices need to seek the functionality of other basic microservices.
  - Device Discoverer is used when services want to know which other devices are close to the device where they are deployed.
- **Pub/Sub Service** (publish/subscribe messaging, or pub/sub messaging) enables communication of facts between services/apps in event-driven architectures. It is part of the SOA 2.0 paradigm, which is required, for instance, to implement the discovery of the protocol required by the Device Discoverer.

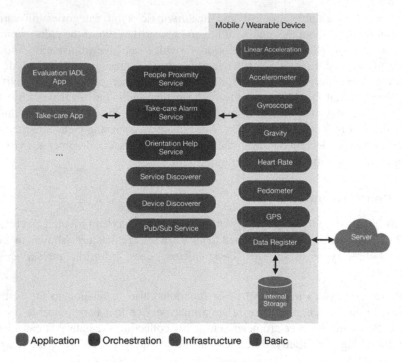

Fig. 3. Service-based architecture for assessing frailty

5 Conclusions

In the health domain, there is a need to address integration to support cases that embrace different factors (physical, cognitive, social, etc.), thus building more holistic and comprehensive models. They have to be supported by advanced computer-based systems in order to go one step further, for example, focusing on active ageing from an ecological perspective. This leads to the development of complex systems, where microservice-oriented architectures turn out to be one viable solution focused on fulfilling the required quality attributes for easy integration and extensibility. This is the case for the two different e-health projects described for elderly people, in which microservices are used: cognitive training and frailty prevention.

The software architectures in both projects have been presented. Several microservices could be reused in both projects because their basic functionality is identical. For instance, the microservice responsible for the user profile or model could be the same with the objective of complementing the data of the individuals. Another example is the Exercises Management microservice from VIRTRAEL that could also be reused in the PREFRA project in the same way, i.e. to collect measures related to the ADL performance (time, effectiveness, etc.).

Future work will focus on improving the design of the architecture to exploit the sharing, integration and composition of microservices to create systems with more capabilities and better quality. We think that both end users and developers will obtain clear benefits from this.

Acknowledgements. This research work is funded by the Spanish Ministry of Economy and Competitiveness - Agencia Estatal de Investigación - with European Regional Development Funds (AEI/FEDER, UE) through the project ref. TIN2016-79484-R and the scholarship FPU program ref. FPU16/07100 granted by the Spanish Ministry of Education, Culture and Sports.

References

1. Ali, S., Kibria, M.G., Jarwar, M.A., Kumar, S., Chong, I.: Microservices model in WoO based IoT platform for depressive disorder assistance. In: International Conference on Information and Communication Technology Convergence (ICTC), pp. 864–866. IEEE (2017)
2. Fontecha, J., Navarro, F.J., Hervas, R., Bravo, J.: A mobile and ubiquitous approach for supporting frailty assessment in elderly people. Pers. Ubiquit. Comput. **17**(6), 1073 (2013)
3. Fried, L.P., et al.: Frailty in older adults: evidence for a phenotype. J. Gerontol. Med. Sci. Am. **56**(3), 146 (2001)
4. Gobbens, R.J.J., Luijkx, K.G., Wijnen-Sponselee, M.T., Schols, J.M.G.A.: In search of an integral conceptual definition of frailty: opinions of experts. J. Am. Med. Dir. Assoc. **11**(5), 338–343 (2010)
5. Human rights of older persons. United Nations. https://www.ohchr.org/en/issues/olderpersons/pages/olderpersonsindex.aspx
6. Irlarte, E., Araya, A.X.: Criterios de fragilidad en personas mayores que viven en la comunidad: una actualización de la literatura. Rev. Med. Chile **144**, 1440 (2016)
7. Jarwar, M.A., Ali, S., Chong, I.: Exploring web objects enabled data-driven microservices for E-health service provision in IoT environment. In: 2018 International Conference on Information and Communication Technology Convergence (ICTC), pp. 112–117. IEEE (2018)
8. Pfeifer, E.: A short portable mental status questionnaire for the assessment of organic brain deficit in elderly patients. J. Am. Geriatr. Soc. **23**, 433–441 (1975)
9. Richardson, C.: Microservices: decomposing applications for deployability and scalability. InfoQ **25**, 15–16 (2014)
10. Rodriguez Dominguez, C.: https://code.google.com/archive/p/thebluerose/
11. Rodríguez-Domínguez, C., Benghazi, K., Noguera, M., Garrido, J.L., Rodríguez-Almendros, M.L., Ruiz-López, T.: A communication model to integrate the request-response and the publish-subscribe paradigms into ubiquitous systems. Sensors **12**(6), 7648–7668 (2012). Ubiquitous Computing and Ambient Intelligence
12. Rute-Pérez, S., Santiago-Ramajo, S., Hurtado-Torres, M.V., Rodriguez-Fortiz, M.J., Caracuel-Romero, A.: Challenges in software applications for the cognitive assessment and training of the elderly. J. Neuroeng. Rehabil. **11**, 88 (2014)
13. Sage, A.P.: System of Systems Engineering: Innovations for the 21st Century, vol. 58. Wiley, Hoboken (2011)
14. Schmidt, M., Obermaisser, R.: Adaptive and technology-independent architecture for fault-tolerant distributed AAL solutions. Comput. Biol. Med. **95**, 236–247 (2018)
15. Virtrael System. http://www.everyware.es/webs/virtrael/
16. Xue, Q.L.: The frailty syndrome: definition and natural history. Clin. Geriatr. Med. **27**(1), 1 (2011)

Smarts Technologies and Algorithms for Health

Automatic Learning for Improvement in Joint Mobility in the Elderly

Sara Romero Valencia[1,4], Sagrario Gomez Cantarino[2,4] (iD),
Margarida Sim-Sim[3,4] (iD), Blanca Espina[1,4] (iD),
and David Mendes[3,4(✉)] (iD)

[1] Health Service of Castilla-La Mancha (SESCAM),
Talavera de la Reina, Toledo, Spain
[2] E NDOCU Group, University School of Nursing and Physiotherapy Toledo.
(Nursing, Pain and Care), Avda. Carlos III s/n, 45071 Toledo, Spain
[3] School of Nursing S. João de Deus, University of Evora,
Largo do Senhor da Pobreza, 7000-811 Évora, Portugal
dmendes@uevora.pt
[4] Castilla-La Mancha University, Toledo,
Avda. Carlos III, s/n, 45071 Toledo, Spain

Abstract. In Europe, the elderly are the majority group, an issue that implies specific attention. On many occasions, they need to be taken care of by other people. It is essential to talk about the gait, this plays an important role and it is necessary to maintain a joint width of movement adequate in the hip, knee and ankle so that the standing and walking are functional. Among the physical factors that limit mobility in the elderly are the articular and capsular, which can produce an immobility of the person and the appearance of pain, causing a significant deterioration in the quality of life of the elderly, a question that will give rise in most cases to the appearance of depressive symptoms. It is an obvious fact that public coverage must offer health activities to promote the health of this group. The purpose of this work is to document in a bibliographic and visual way a table of physical exercises and psychological techniques for its future implantation within the Primary Health Care (PHC) and the Machine Learning tools to develop a virtual gerontology nurse to assist in deploying the exercises at home. After an adequate automatic learning and health education, with greater implication of the nursing specialist in geriatrics and gerontology (GS) and once exercised, allow the elderly to develop with a maximum of autonomy and independence at home, as well as reduce the doses of drugs, an issue that will benefit health expenditure. We are proposing a Virtual Agent based in Computer Vision, Artificial Intelligence and Natural Interfaces that can perform unattended sessions for joint mobility improvement.

Keywords: Pain · Aging · Elderly · Nursing · Care · Exercise ·
Machine learning · Deep learning · Reinforcement learning · Sensors ·
Wearables · Computer Vision · Virtual nurse

© Springer Nature Switzerland AG 2019
J. García-Alonso and C. Fonseca (Eds.): IWoG 2018, CCIS 1016, pp. 127–142, 2019.
https://doi.org/10.1007/978-3-030-16028-9_12

1   Introduction

Aging is a continuous process in which there are multisystemic changes that modify all structures and organic functions at the metabolic, psychological and bodily levels, causing postural alterations that lead to a progressive loss of mobility [1, 2]. All this causes a loss in the quality of life and a possible social isolation, with the loss of active participation in their environment.

The rate of aging increases every year as well as the consumption of drugs and it is necessary to expand the knowledge of the management of pathologies with pain [3, 4] since pain in the elderly is a health and social challenge [5].

Assistance, like the health programs that have traditionally met the demands of these elderly people, lead us to plan new models of care that respond to these growing demands, increasing their quality of life and reducing costs, as aging allows older adults to live longer with disabilities[6].

Spinal diseases with pain are one of the most common in Spain and increase every year with the aging of the population, causing a bad perception in the elderly of their health [7]. Emotional discomfort and involvement at the functional level are aspects that are of great importance among the factors of adjustment related to chronic pain in the elderly [8].

The WHO defines the quality of life as: "an individuals perception of their position in life in the context of the culture and value systems in which they live and in relation to their goals, expectations, standards and concerns". This is a very broad concept that is influenced in a complete way by the physical health of the subject, his psychological state, his level of independence, his social relations, as well as his relationship with the essential elements of his environment [9]. Aging will affect taxes to a greater or lesser extent, to transfers, to the financing of the Social Security system and, ultimately, to the entire Welfare State as it is currently conceived [10].

On the concept of functional health in old age it should be noted that, obviously, the functional status of the person depends on the state of health in other areas such as physical health, cognitive and affective status and social situation and even pain management, because some deficits of those stated by themselves are determinant.

Within the evaluation and pain management strategies, we must promote programs for the elderly population with other non-pharmacological measures to reduce the consumption of these drugs [7]. Psychological relaxation therapy reduces pain and decreases levels of anxiety, which, along with physical activity, performing stretching exercises and strengthening the spine, is a viable, inexpensive, accessible intervention and also has psychosocial benefits improving cognitive function [11–13].

As an objective, it was stated that based on the acceptance that spinal diseases with pain are one of the most common in Spain and are increasing every year with the aging of the population, the implementation of a program with non pharmacological techniques through the use of psychological techniques and physical exercise that improve the quality of life of the elderly and diminish the pharmacological burden of these.

2   Methodology

A narrative review of the available evidence was carried out about programs aimed at avoiding pain in the elderly, in a period between the years 1999 to 2017, in databases: PubMed, Dialnet, Cuiden, IME, LILACS, Cochrane Library Plus, ENFISPO, Medline, Elsevier. The descriptors used were: "aging", "autonomy", "specialist nursing", "os-teoarthrosis", "rachialgia", "joint pain", "vertebral pain", "somatization", "aging and older". Likewise, a review of the book deposits located at the University of Castilla la Mancha was carried out.

Three books were selected, two from the Toledo campus and another from the Albacete campus. Once the information was collected, a critical analysis of the content was started, establishing the importance of physical exercise and psychological relaxation techniques as a non-pharmacological measure of functionality and improvement of the rachialgia in the elderly.

2.1   Inclusion and Exclusion Criteria

As an inclusion criterion, the following were established: (a) free full text articles and under subscription; (b) articles that include the descriptors joint pain, physical exercises and relaxation techniques; and (c) articles in Spanish and English, (these same terms were included in English, for the search in international databases). In all cases, the type of source selected was scientific journals. Free natural language was used, combined with Boolean operators ("and/and", "o/or", "no/not").

They excluded those who: (a) articles written in languages other than Spanish and English; (b) articles not found in full texts; (c) not related to the topic of study.

2.2   Sensorizing the Elderly Environment for Computer Vision (CV)

To apply CV techniques in our study an IP Camera is installed and aligned for complete vision of the elderly activities. A Sricam HD IP Camera (www.sricam.com/) that offers several possibilities like 360° pan-tilt, two way audio, motion detection and night vision is used to interact naturally with the patient.

To simplify the location of the different body parts in the CV environment, several different colored stickers are positioned in an ordered way to cover the complete 16 muscle training groups presented ahead. Several body points, however, do not need to be tagged since inference can be made of the positioning according to the Foundation Model of Anatomy. Those that are used are orderly positioned, in the left shoulder, right shoulder, left wrist, right wrist, left outer knee, righty outer knee, left outer ankle, right outer ankle. With the specific colored stickers with normalized 3M pantone post-its:

The body alignment is based in the very well developed face detection algorithms that are very fast and triggers the colored stickers positioning that controls the full body location and movement.

3 Physical and Psychological Techniques in the Elderly

Physical exercises are positive both functionally and psychologically, including pain, rigidity, physical function, vitality and mental health. In addition, it balances movements, muscles and joints, thus reducing back pain, back pain, sciatica, herniated discs, neck, neck or head pain in the elderly [14].

The behavioral reorganization that the psychological relaxation techniques originate, has a pain reducing effect. Trying to normalize the life of the elderly, as much as possible and improving the situations of stress and reducing the excessive activation of our body [15].

Therefore, a program consisting of a limited number of simple exercises focused on reducing stress and excessive activation of our body, increasing the range of joint mobility and mobility of the spine. It will be important in these people the presence and help of the figure of nursing, and in particular of the nursing EG, health professional who provides nursing care and care to the elderly population, being able to teach, supervise, investigate, manage and lead the care assigned to this group in complex situations. It also acts as an advisor at all levels of the social health system [16]. It will be proposed to carry out sessions supervised by the Eir-Geriatrics every day until the learning of the respiratory techniques and the techniques of muscular relaxation concluding with physical exercises of stretching and strengthening of the spine, an issue that will improve notably the pain situation in this type of collective [17].

3.1 Applied Physical Techniques: Avoid Pain in the Elderly

In the first phase of the program, a variable duration is expected, which will depend on the learning time of the different techniques of the elderly. There are exclusion criteria in the development of the program [18], among which are: Severe high blood pressure (HBP), severe vision impairment, cardiovascular diseases, hemophilia, severe deafness, dizziness, epilepsies. uncontrolled, cardiac insufficiency with rhythm disorders and chronic renal failure [18].

In the development of the second phase, some exercises will be carried out to evaluate the physical conditions of the older adult. It will be necessary to initiate them with a warm-up and theoretical-practical knowledge and support related to health in relation to the activities to be developed, with this function being carried out by the EG Nursing [17], and once the elderly has been instructed, such movements should be carried out for 5 min. How to walk, go up and down stairs, turns left trunk-right and right-left [15].

After the warm-up and within this second phase, the movements established to evaluate the articulation will be strengthened, such as the mobilization of the neck, mobilization of the shoulder (in all the planes of the joint route) as well as the turns and flexion of the trunk [15–17]. Next, an evaluation of the joint flexibility will be carried out, which will lead to knowing how the physical state is in the elderly, the risk of possible injuries, interventions to be carried out and knowing the causes of a limited performance in the activities of daily life [18]. According to the reviewed articles, the elderly is safer both for mobility and stability if all the exercises are carried out on mats [15–18].

In general, the applied programs tend to imply an evaluation of the state of mind using the state anxiety scale of the State-Trait Anxiety Inventory (STAI/E) STAI/E, which evaluates the anxiety of "here" and "now". A pain assessment is also performed, for which the EVA scale is applied [13, 19].

3.2 Applied Psychological Techniques: Avoid Pain in the Elderly

In a second phase is the application among others of respiratory techniques that serve to facilitate the voluntary control of respiration by automating it to be used in situations of stress, thus controlling physiological activation. Respiratory exercises will be performed in a room without noise, where the older adult will be lying on a mat with comfortable clothes and concentrated in the exercises [13, 19, 20].

The techniques of (a) abdominal breathing will be worked on: emptying the air from the lungs by pressing the belly inwards, and inspiring and directing the air to the lower part of the lungs. The air will be retained for a few moments and the elderly will be instructed to exhale; (b) chest breathing: by emptying the air from the lungs and by breathing air into the chest cage, it will feel like the intercostal muscles dilate [20]. The breath will be held for a moment and exhaled; (c) clavicular breathing: we empty the air from the lungs and breathe carrying the air to the vertices of the lungs with the participation of the abdomen and the intercostal muscles. The air will be retained for a moment and it will breathe. In the complete breathing the three exercises are united in one only [21, 22].

In this phase are also present progressive relaxation techniques, with them is intended to achieve a state of intense relaxation learning to tense and relax different muscle groups. The older adult will concentrate on the sensations associated with the tension and relaxation of each muscle group [23].

In the application of relaxation techniques, known as the psi-coeducational phase, E-G nursing is a key point to carry out personal health education (PHS), considered essential to respond in a better way to the changes facing our country in particular to the increase in the quality of care granted to this group of people [16]. The nurse will perform sixteen tension-relaxation exercises of the different muscle groups [22–24]:

Muscle training groups:

1. Right foot.
2. Right leg.
3. Right thigh.
4. Left foot.
5. Left leg.
6. Left thigh.
7. Abdominal region.
8. Chest, shoulder and upper back.
9. Neck.
10. Mouth.

11. Eyes and nose.
12. Front.
13. Right hand and forearm.
14. Right arm.
15. Hand and left forearm.
16. Left arm.

Exercises with muscle training groups:

1. Right foot: Bend your fingers towards the floor holding them tight.
2. Right leg: Extend the toes upwards.
3. Right thigh: Squeeze the thigh against the mat.
4. Left foot: Curl your fingers towards the floor keeping them tight.
5. Right leg: Extend the toes upwards.
6. Left thigh: Squeeze the thigh against the mat.
7. Abdominal region: shrink stomach and abdomen tightening towards den-tro.
8. Shoulder chest and upper back: Pull shoulders back, trying to touch shoulder blades.
9. Neck: Push the chin toward the chest.
10. Mouth: Tighten lips, teeth and tongue against the palate.
11. Eyes and nose: Squeeze the eyelids and wrinkle the nose.
12. Front: Raise the eyebrows and wrinkle the nose.
13. Right hand and forearm: Squeeze your fist.
14. Right arm: Squeeze the elbow against the mat.
15. Hand and left forearm: Press the fist.
16. Left arm: Press your elbow against the mat.

In this sense it is very important to know the ways of performing relaxation as well as the compartment. It will be carried out in a cabin without noise, lying the elderly on a mat with comfortable clothes and concentrated in the exercises. They start by exerting a stronger tension on the toes of the right foot maintaining the 10 s, paying attention to the sensation that we have while being in tension. We release the tension of those muscles, relax them and become aware of the appreciable difference when tension is exerted and when we relax them. Repeat the same thing successively with each of the 16 muscle groups for 30 min [25–27].

It is recommended that the sessions be carried out in a sequence as indicated below [23, 24, 28]:

• First, second and third exercise the 16 muscle groups with the procedure of: tension-relaxation for 30 min.
• fourth and fifth: exercise 7 muscle groups, joining the groups (1-2), (3-4), (5-6), (7-8), (9-10), (11-12-13)) and (14-15-16) in tense-relaxation procedures with a duration of 25 min.
• Sixth and seventh sessions: using the 7 muscle groups with a duration of 15 min.
• octave and ninth sessions: 4 muscle groups will be exercised, joining the groups (1-2-3-4), (5-6-7-8), (9-10) and (11-12-13-14-15-16) with the procedure of relaxation by evocation, with a duration of 10 min.
• Tenth session: the procedure will be the recount.

Regarding relaxation through evocation distension, the memory of what we feel when having tense muscles and later when relaxing them should be evoked [25]. For this, the same 4 muscle groups used in the exercise explained above were used:

1. Foot, leg and thigh.
2. Abdomen, chest, shoulders and back.
3. Forehead, cheek, jaw and neck.
4. Hands, forearms and arms.

These elderly should have a very conducted training in such a way that they should concentrate on the sessions of tension and relaxation of these muscles during a period of 10 min [21, 23, 28].

Regarding relaxation using the counting procedure, one must have one to four in deep relaxation [22, 24]:

1. can notice how the muscles of the feet, legs and thighs are deeply relaxed.
2. are noted as the muscles of the abdomen, thorax, shoulders and back relax deeply.
3. notices as the muscles of the face and neck are deeply relaxed.
4. feels as the muscles of the hands, forearm and arms relax deeply.

3.3 Monitoring Through Deep Learning

Deep learning involves the gathering of multiple raw data signals (features) to produce a classification hypothesis (label). We gather the exercises performance by guiding the elderly through monitoring using both the camera and colored tags, smartphone, and health band. In our proposed sensorized environment, introduced in Sect. 2.2 we have a camera that can simultaneously "speak" to produce coaching for adequate completion of the set of exercises. We have developed the model of exercising for joint mobility improvement based in a set of ontological base models of anatomy namely FMA (Foundational Model of Anatomy) [29] ontology. All the features that take part of the data fusion process are automatically weighted in our model, and produce the coaching instructions that are then transmitted to the elderly in a natural way.

4 Stretching and Strengthening Phase at Home Level

The set of exercises described have a phase of stretching and another of strengthening, so they are extremely beneficial for the back, receiving a gentle massage and toning the muscle tissue and bones. We emphasize the activation and unblocking of the vertebrae of the spine, especially the lumbar area. The exercises must be well executed, paying attention to perform the effort only in the area indicated, the rest of the body will be relaxed, observing how the column is modified with the exercises. The older adult will be asked to practice at home daily at least 15–20 min [15, 25, 30].

4.1 Stretching Phase

It is recommended that the elderly lie supine and have the neck stretched, with the chin raised to the maximum without lifting the head, the shoulders offer no resistance. The chin will be lowered back to the sternum. It is recommended to repeat 10 times [14, 28, 31] (Illustration 1).

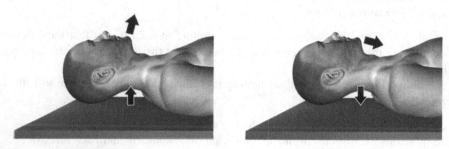

Illustration 1: Author image: David García Fernández. Creative Commons License Recognition (by)

1. Pull from the lumbar to the floor, from the groin and pubis up towards our chest. We repeat 10 times (Illustration 2).

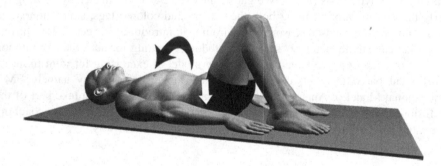

Illustration 2: Author image: David García Fernández. Creative Commons License Recognition (by)

In the standing position the elderly will place the arms hanging, the legs loose, the pelvis without inclination (neutral pelvis), the spine and neck stretched, the head high without raising the chin.

1. Opening of the shoulder blades: The shoulder blades slide smoothly towards the shoulders and arms. These are carried away without resistance. When the shoulder blades separate from the column, they lead the shoulders to an internal rotation and the dorsal vertebrae bulge, inclining the head down naturally. The curvature of the lumbar vertebrae tends to disappear, softening their movement. It will be recommended to repeat 5 times (Illustration 3).

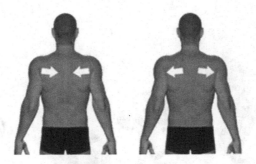

Illustration 3: Autor imagen: David García Fern Licencia Creative Commons Reconocimiento (by)

2. Closing the shoulder blades: When moving the shoulders back and down, we take the shoulder blades next to the spine towards the dorsal vertebrae inwards. This compression pushes up the nape of the neck, aligning the cervical vertebrae and moving the head backwards. It will be recommended to repeat 5 times (Illustration 3).
3. The closing of the shoulder blades favors the verticality of the dorsal vertebrae, correcting the kyphotic tendency, strengthening the musculature of the dorsal area. This better supports the rib cage, eliminating the shortening of the pectoral muscles extending the alignment of the vertebrae to the nape, stretching the neck and verticalizing the head (Illustration 4).

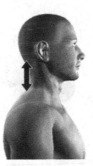

Illustration 4: Author image: David García Fernández. Creative Commons License Recognition (by)

4. Collapse of the spine: When performing a pelvic retroversion, the lumbar spine is rounded off, the spine rounded, the flexion of the knees and the head falls forward with the chin near the chest and the arms hang from the shoulders forward. From this position, the column slowly de-rises until the hands reach the floor and the head is close to the knees. We take several slow breaths to produce greater relaxation to the spine and the entire back (Illustration 5).

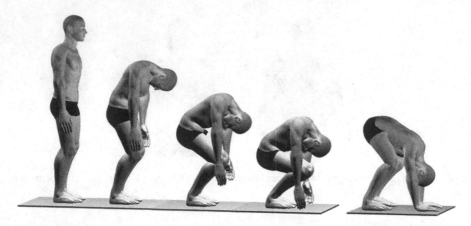

Illustration 5: Author image: David García Fernández. Creative Commons License Recognition (by)

5. Reconstruction of the spine: To return to verticality we push forward with the buttocks placing the pelvis on the shaft, bending the legs more and straightening the spine more. From this position a pelvic anteversion is made, straightening the spine while the legs are stretched (Illustration 6).

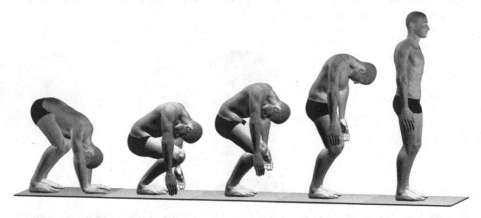

Illustration 6: Author image: David García Fernández. Creative Commons License Recognition (by)

4.2 Strengthening Phase

The spine is directly related to the pelvis, the shoulder girdle and the head. The activation of the spine stimulates these different zones and conversely through these zones the spine is activated and mobilized, preventing and correcting different dysfunctions such as lordosis, kyphosis, scoliosis, osteoporosis and eliminating the pain of the back. The exercises described below should be carried out very slowly, so the monitoring during the learning by geriatric nursing is fundamental [16]:

1. Quadruped: The arms descend vertically from the shoulders, supporting the hands on the floor, the column must be flat, the head aligned with the column. The weight of the body distributed between the knees and the hands. Being relaxed in this position for 3 breaths (Illustration 7).

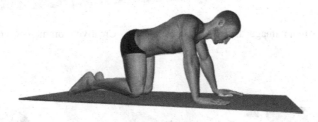

Illustration 7: Author image: David García Fernández. Creative Commons License Recognition (by)

2. Ripple of the spine by weight transfer: Once in quadruped position, we move the weight to the hands slowly until we have the feeling that we are going to fall flat on our face, we stay at that point, The thighs and the arms should remain parallel. It will be recommended to repeat the weight transfer 3 times (Illustration 8).

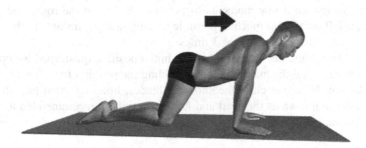

Illustration 8: Author image: David García Fernández. Creative Commons License Recognition (by)

3. Transfer weight to the knees: We carry the weight back, to the knees and feet, we repeat moving the weight from the knees to the hands and again from these to the knees very slowly, observing the breathing and the path of the movement in the column. It is recommended to repeat 3 times (Illustration 9).
4. Head movement, from top to bottom: From the initial quadruped position where the view is directed to the ground, we move looking forward and climb as much as possible, feeling the mobility of the vertebrae, we go back down our look between our feet back, as much as we can. It will be recommended to repeat the route 3 times (Illustration 10).

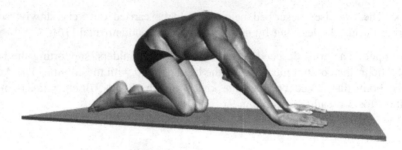

Illustration 9: Author image: David García Fernández. Creative Commons License Recognition (by)

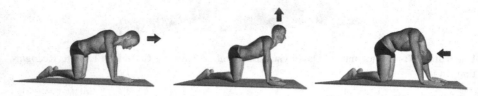

Illustration 10: Author image: David García Fernández. Creative Commons License Recognition (by)

5. Head movements from left to right: From the initial position with the gaze to the front at the height of the head, we turn the head to the right arriving as much as possible, we remain a few moments in position. We undo the route and turn the head to the left arriving as much as possible remaining a few instants in the position. It will be recommended to repeat 3 times.
6. Movement from shoulder blades: From the initial position quadruped we open both shoulder blades until the maximum, after holding the position for a few seconds we slowly loosen. Next, we close the shoulder blades, bringing them back by modifying the column towards the head and lumbar. It will be recommended to repeat 3 times (Illustration 11).

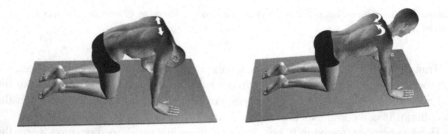

Illustration 11: Author image: David García Fernández. Creative Commons License Recognition (by)

7. From the pelvis-retroversion: From the initial position, we contract the buttocks pushing the coccyx inward, we continue to contract the ab-domen pushing up and in with the gut, slow and continuous movement. It will be recommended to repeat 3 times (Illustration 12).

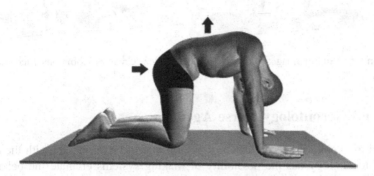

Illustration 12: Author image: David García Fernández. Creative Commons License Recognition (by)

8. From the pelvis-anteversion: From the initial position we take out and lift the buttocks without moving the thighs back, we continue pushing the waist down. The vertebral vertebrae repercussion along the spine is clear. It will be recommended to repeat 3 times (Illustration 13).
9. Integration of the legs: From the initial position, when moving the weight towards the hands when we do the anteversion, stretching the leg back and lifting it stretched and flexed (Illustration 14).

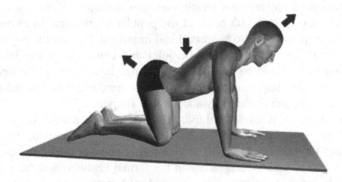

Illustration 13: Author image: David García Fernández. Creative Commons License Recognition (by)

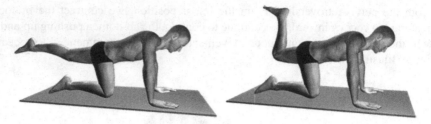

Illustration 14: Author image: David García Fernández. Creative Commons License Recognition (by)

5 Virtual Gerontology Nurse Agent

We intend to explore the recent dawn of natural interfaces to interact with the elderly. Currently technology has the possibility of making systems emulate the behavior of specialists in any given domain. The most natural way of interfacing with a person is by talking to him/her. The objective of our team is the creation of an automated bot for deliverance of the adequate training, based in the present work, by the cameras configured in the elderly environment. Having such an infrastructure installed permits the joint mobility recovery at the patient's own rhythm, on demand, without the requirement of having a personal, available on location human nurse.

6 Conclusion

Spain is one of the countries that ages faster. This question is mainly due to the decline in fertility, without forgetting that Spain has one of the highest life expectancies after 65 years in Europe, a problem that greatly increases the aging of the population. This problem greatly affects the health needs of the population, not only in its quantity, but also in the type of pathologies to be treated and improved. Among the physical factors that limit mobility in the elderly are the joint and capsular. At the joint level in connective tissues, it should be noted that the change in collagen is the first cause of resistance. It is of great importance in the elderly the need to strengthen the muscles of the lower extremities and the hip to walk without support.

The high frequency of spinal cord injuries leads to an increasing use of healthcare resources and a greater reliance on the elderly, increasing the costs of these services, which increases the pressure of health service managers to optimize the use of public services. That is why family caregivers and the formal health system have a common goal, to provide timely solutions to an existing health problem, such as caring for the elderly, providing experiences, knowledge and resources.

Knowing the benefit of therapeutic exercise in both pain and physical function and psychological benefit, improves the quality of life in this group of people. Equally, known is the therapeutic efficacy of psychological relaxation techniques, which improve pain, anxiety and depression.

For all this after this review, it is considered appropriate to indicate that the early use of both techniques would be useful in these pathologies in the elderly. It should be questioned whether life expectancy is an indicator of success in the health system.

The automatic domiciled monitoring and exercise development possible autonomously by our proposed system, improves the joint mobility in the elderly in their most favorable environment, their home.

References

1. Arce, C.I., Ayala, G.A.: Fisiología del envejecimiento. http://www.revistasbolivianas.org.bo/scielo.php?pid=S2304-37682012000200001&script=sci_arttext&tlng=es
2. Piedras-Jorge, C., Meléndez-Moral, J.C., Tomás-Miguel, J.M.: Beneficios del ejercicio físico en población mayor institucionalizada. Rev. Esp. Geriatr. Gerontol. **45**, 131–135 (2010). https://doi.org/10.1016/j.regg.2009.10.012
3. Fernández-Travieso, J.C.: Revista CENIC. Ciencias biológicas. Rev. CENIC. Ciencias Biológicas **46**, 203–221 (2015)
4. Espejo Antúnez, L., Cardero Durán, M.Á., Caro Puértolas, B., Téllez de Peralta, G.: Efectos del ejercicio físico en la funcionalidad y calidad de vida en mayores institucionalizados diagnosticados de gonartrosis. Rev. Esp. Geriatr. Gerontol. **47**, 262–265 (2012). https://doi.org/10.1016/j.regg.2011.06.011
5. Gómez Conesa, A.: Envejecimiento y dependencia. Fisioterapia **30**, 111–113 (2008). https://doi.org/10.1016/S0211-5638(08)72966-3
6. Alguacil Gómez, J.: La calidad de vida y el tercer sector: nuevas dimensiones de la complejidad. Boletín CF+S, pp. 35–48 (2014)
7. Arteaga, C.E., Santacruz, J.G., Ramírez, L.J., Bogotá, D.C.: Evaluación del dolor musculoesquelético en el anciano. Acta Medica Colomb. **36**, 30–35 (2011)
8. López, A., et al.: La experiencia de dolor crónico en personas mayores con artrosis: dimensiones cognitivo-conductuales y adaptación 1 gracias a la financiación parcial de la Sociedad Española de Geriatría y Gerontología y a la colaboración desinteresada para la selección d (2010). https://www.researchgate.net/profile/Ignacio_Montorio/publication/262829217_La_experiencia_de_dolor_cronico_en_personas_mayores_con_artrosis_dimensiones_cognitivo-conductuales_y_adaptacion/links/5a1b07150f7e9be37f9be775/La-experiencia-de-dolor-cronico-en
9. Fernandez-Ballesteros, R., Macia, A.: Calidad de Vida en la Vejez. Psychosoc. Interv. **2**, 77–94 (1993). https://doi.org/10.1063/1.121339
10. Guijarro, M., Peláez, Ó.: La longevidad globalizada: un análisis de la esperanza de vida en España (1900-2050). Scr. Nova. Rev. Electrónica Geogr. y Ciencias Soc. **12** (2008). https://doi.org/10.1344/sn2008.12.1406
11. Alonso Dosouto, H., Silva Ganso, N.: Exploración del efecto de la actividad física y su relación con distintas variables relevantes para un envejecimiento saludable en personas mayores con discapacidad intelectual. Int. J. Dev. Educ. Psychol. INFAD Rev. Psicol. No 2 **1**, 165–173 (2014)
12. Rodríguez Díaz, O.: Rehabilitación funcional del anciano the elderly functional rehabilitation. MEDISAN, vol. 13 (2009)
13. Pérez, J.A., Fernández, J.C., Fernández, B., Durán, M.: Empleo de metáforas en las sugestiones hipnóticas para manejar el dolor articular: estudio de caso = Use of metaphors in hypnotic suggestions for joint pain management: a case study. Rev. Psicopatología y Psicol. Clínica. **17**, 57 (2012). https://doi.org/10.5944/rppc.vol.17.num.1.2012.10369

14. Benito Vallejo, J.: Cuerpo en armonía: leyes naturales del movimiento. Inde (2001)
15. Ibañez, A., Torrebadella, J.: 1004 Ejercicios De Flexibilidad (2008)
16. Gómez Cantarino, S., Duque Teomiro, C., Sukkarieh Noria, S.: Otras unidades multiprofesionales en la formación sanitaria especializada desde el punto de vista de la enfermería. Principios de Educación Mé-dica. Desde el grado hasta el desarrollo profesional. Principios Educ. Médica. Desde el grado Hast. el Desarro. Prof., pp. 439–440 (2015)
17. Anrich, C.: Stretching y movilidad. PAIDOTRIBO, Badalona (2008)
18. Soares De Araújo, C.G.: FLEXITEST Un método innovador de evaluación de la flexibilidad. PAIDOTRIBO, Rio de Janeiro (2005)
19. Martín, A., Vicente, P., Vicente, E., Sánchez, M.: Depresión y calidad de vida relacionada con la salud en pacientes con artrosis: diferencias de género. Rev. Psicopatología y Psicol. Clínica. **15**, 125–132 (2010)
20. Redondo, M.M., León Mateos, L., Pérez Nieto, M.A., Jover Jover, J.A., Abasolo Alcázar, L.: El dolor en los pacientes con artriris reumatoide: variables psicológicas relacionadas e intervención. Clínica y Salud. **19**, 359–378 (2008)
21. Gónzalez, J.F.: Procedimientos de relajación. EOS, Madrid (2015)
22. Caballo Vicente, E.: Manual para el tratamiento cognitivo-conductual de los trastornos psicológicos, vol. 1. SIGLO XXI de España, Madrid (2008)
23. López, B.: Terapia ocupacional en discapacitados físicos: teoría y práctica. Editora Médica Panamericana, Madrid (2004)
24. Neira, F., Ortega, J.: Tratamiento del dolor en la artritis reumatoide fundamentado en medicina basada en la evidencia. Rev. la Soc, Española del Dolor (2006)
25. Kempf, H., Schmelcher, F., Ziegler, C.: Libro de entrenamiento para la espalda. Un programa garantizado para vencer el dolor de espalda (2007)
26. Esnault, M., Kapandji, I., Arajol, L.: Columna vertebral y stretching. PAIDOTRIBO (2009)
27. Borges, L.J., Bertoldo Benedetti, T.R., Mazo, G.Z.: Undefined: Influencia del ejercicio físico en los síntomas depresivos y en la aptitud funcional de ancianos en el sur de Brasil. Rev. Esp. Geriatr. Gerontol. **45**, 72–78 (2010)
28. Martin Rodríguez, M.: Influencia de un programa de actividad física sobre aspectos físicos y psicológicos en personas de más de 55 años en la población del Algarve (2006). https://www.tdx.cat/handle/10803/9713
29. Smith, B., Kumar, A., Ceusters, W., Rosse, C.: On carcinomas and other pathological entities. Comp. Funct. Genomics **6**, 379–387 (2005). https://doi.org/10.1002/cfg.497
30. Souchard, P.E.: RPG. Principios de la reeducación postural global, Editorial PAIDOTRIBO (2005)
31. Strahl, C., Kleinknecht, R., Dinnel, D.: The role of pain anxiety, coping, and pain self-efficacy in rheumatoid arthritis patient functioning. Behav. Res. **38**, 863–873 (2000)

Psychometric Properties of the Elderly Nursing Core Set

César Fonseca[1]([X]) (iD), Manuel Lopes[1] (iD), David Mendes[1] (iD),
Pedro Parreira[2] (iD), Lisete Mónico[1,3] (iD), and Céu Marques[1]

[1] Évora University, Investigator POCTEP 0445_4IE_4_P, Évora, Portugal
cesar.j.fonseca@gmail.com
[2] Nursing School of Coimbra, 3046-851 Coimbra, Portugal
[3] Faculty of Psychology and Educational Sciences, University of Coimbra,
Coimbra, Portugal

Abstract. Aim: To assess the psychometric properties of the Elderly Nursing Core Set.

Methods: Cross-sectional descriptive study; convenience sample composed of 427 individuals aged 65 years old or older.

Results: Factor analysis of principal components allowed extracting 4 concepts, i.e., Self-Care, Learning and Mental Functions, Communication, and Relationship with Friends and Caregivers, which explained 82.25% of the total variance. Varimax rotation indicated a very good measure of sampling adequacy (KMO = 0.947), with Bartlett's test of sphericity (X2(300) = 11131.28, p < 0.001) and an excellent Cronbach's alpha value of 0.963.

Conclusion: The Elderly Nursing Core Set exhibits excellent psychometric properties, i.e., consistency, reliability, and internal validity, for which reason it is recommended as a means of determining the nursing care needs of individuals aged 65 years old or older and assessing the outcomes of nursing interventions targeting that population.

Keywords: Ageing ·
International Classification of Functioning, Disability and Health

1 Introduction

The ageing of the population is an increasingly pressing reality [1], given that the demographic representativeness of the proportion of individuals older than 65 years of age is increasing exponentially [2]. This population group is the target of negative social perceptions associated with disability [3] and the increase in social and health costs and resources [1]. This phenomenon has several causes, among which the association between the continuous increase in life expectancy at birth and reduction in the synthetic index of fertility stand out [1]. On the global level, the life expectancy at birth shifted from 47.7 years in 1950 to 69.3 years in 2010. In some of the most aged countries (e.g., Portugal), the average life expectancy has reached 79.8 years (men: 76.7 years; women: 82.8 years), while the synthetic index of fertility is 1.37 children per women [2].

© Springer Nature Switzerland AG 2019
J. García-Alonso and C. Fonseca (Eds.): IWoG 2018, CCIS 1016, pp. 143–153, 2019.
https://doi.org/10.1007/978-3-030-16028-9_13

In Portugal, the percentage of individuals aged 65 years old or older was 19% in 2011, while it was 16% in the previous decade [3]. The ageing index of Portugal is 129 [4].

Ageing, understood as a stage of development, poses specific demands that must be properly understood. According to various biological, psychological, and social theories, ageing is a stage characterized by progressive losses. From the perspective of the health sciences, progressive ageing is associated with chronic multiple morbidity [5]. Thus, ageing presents us with a scenario characterized by the developmental demands proper to age and demands that result from deviations from the state of health. Both types of demands influence the self-care capacity, i.e., the set of activities independently performed by an individual to promote and maintain his or her personal well-being throughout life [6]. When the self-care capacity is deficient, therapeutic interventions, which might be fully or partially compensatory or supportive-educative, are needed [7].

The repercussions on the self-care capacity are largely due to functional limitations. Thus, the development of instruments to assess the functional status of older adults as an indicator of their care needs and to foresee healthcare costs and resources is highly relevant [8]. Assuming that the demands of nursing care are high among older adults, the elaboration of instruments to assess their needs to allow for the appropriate planning of the required resources is of considerable interest [9].

To classify the degree of functioning, the World Health Organization has formulated the International Classification of Functioning, Disability and Health (ICF), which has been adopted in Portugal [10] and has multiple advantages. Indicators of disability, and more particularly of limitations in activities and of limitations in the functional capacity, allow establishing healthcare needs [11]. Based on the abovementioned classification, we have developed the Elderly Nursing Core Set.

The process began with a cross-sectional, descriptive study conducted with a stratified random sample composed of 931 older adults from the Alentejo region of Portugal, with a confidence level of 95% and margin of error of 3.2%. That study, based on the ICF [9, 10], allowed developing a multi-professional instrument to assess the functioning of older adults, designated the Elderly Core Set (*Core Set dos Idosos - CSI*). The Elderly Nursing Core Set that is described here was elaborated as an instrument containing indicators sensitive to nursing care that allow assessing not only care needs but also the outcomes of nursing interventions [11].

Based on the aforementioned considerations, we understand that the nursing care of older adults is the process of care performed by nurses in connection with the rest of the health team targeting older adults within their own settings and taking their functioning, which is understood as a process of interaction or a complex relationship between the state of health and contextual factors, into consideration. The process of care aims at maintaining autonomy [12, 13] and/or promoting adjustment to eventual deficits in the self-care capacity [14–16] and in the participation in activities, considering bodily functions and structures and environmental factors.

2 Methods and Techniques

As noted above, the Elderly Nursing Core Set includes indicators that are sensitive to nursing care. These indicators were selected by means of 2 complementary paths. The first path consisted of a systematic literature review [14] performed to identify internationally described ICF codes that are sensitive to nursing care. The codes thus found were reunited with the codes included in the CSI, and a Delphi panel was established [15] with 52 nurses trained and experienced in the application of the CSI. The participants were requested to rank the codes according to their degree of sensitivity to nursing care. As a result, 31 codes that were included in the first version of Elderly Nursing Core Set were selected.

We then applied the instrument to an intentional sample comprising 427 older adults (65 years old or older) distributed across 4 different healthcare settings. We selected 2 Continuing Integrated Care teams, one from a rural area (Continuing Integrated Care Teams of Coastal Alentejo – 180 older adults) and the other from an urban area (Continuing Integrated Care Teams of Odivelas – 95 older adults). These teams are part of the National Network of Continuing Care and provide long-term care to older adults living in the community. Some of the criteria that older adults must meet to be eligible to be monitored by these teams include the following: being functionally dependent and/or meeting the criteria for frailty; exhibiting progressive chronic diseases and severe functional dependence due to progressive or permanent bodily disease and terminal illness.

The third setting corresponded to a Community Care Unit (69 older adults) that is charged with the care of a certain population group. In the present case, we chose a Community Care Unit responsible for several villages in Redondo County, where older adults living in the community predominate, with a reasonable degree of autonomy.

Finally, we also selected a nursing home for older adults (SAMS [Serviços de Assistêcia Médico Social/Medical-Social Assistance Services] Nursing Home for Older Adults – 83 older adults) affiliated with a bank in Lisbon, in which former bank employees or their relatives reside, either of their own will or because they are functionally dependent.

All the older adults in the aforementioned settings who agreed to answer the questionnaire over a defined period of time were selected for the present study.

The mean age of the participants was approximately 80 years old in all the investigated settings, ranging from 75.7 years old in the group assisted by the Community Care Unit of Redondo to 83.5 years old among the older adults residing in the SAMS Nursing Home.

Of the 31 ICF codes initially selected for the Elderly Nursing Core Set, only 25 remain in the final version of the instrument. The latter are the codes that exhibited communalities above 0.5 (Table 1), while the other 6 were eliminated [8]. The resulting instrument comprises 25 items considered to be sensitive to nursing care and is designed to assess the needs and outcomes of nursing care of individuals aged 65 years old or older. Each item is answered on a 5-point Likert scale (1. no problem: 0–4%; 2. mild problem: 5–24%; 3. moderate problem: 25–49%; 4. severe problem: 50–95%; 5. complete problem: 96–100%), as in the ICF. The instrument allows assessing

4 factors, i.e., Self-Care; Learning and Mental Functions; Communication; and Relationship with Friends and Caregivers, which were identified by means of factor analysis of principal components.

Table 1. Communalities of the Elderly Nursing Core Set, Portugal, 2017

	Initial	Extraction
Carrying out daily routine (d230)	1.000	0.871
Changing body basic position (d410)	1.000	0.768
Maintaining a body position (d415)	1.000	0.831
Hand and arm use (d445)	1.000	0.765
Walking (d450)	1.000	0.801
Moving around using equipment (d465)	1.000	0.830
Washing oneself (d510)	1.000	0.886
Caring for body parts (d520)	1.000	0.884
Using the toilet (d530)	1.000	0.777
Dressing (d540)	1.000	0.918
Eating (d550)	1.000	0.879
Drinking (d560)	1.000	0.875
Consciousness functions (b110)	1.000	0.794
Orientation functions (b114)	1.000	0.885
Attention functions (b140)	1.000	0.877
Memory functions (b144)	1.000	0.773
Emotional functions (b152)	1.000	0.865
Higher-level cognitive functions (b164)	1.000	0.616
Communicating with – receiving – spoken messages (d310)	1.000	0.887
Speaking (d330)	1.000	0.915
Conversation (d350)	1.000	0.917
Family relationships (d760)	1.000	0.643
Friends (e320)	1.000	0.541
Personal care providers and personal assistants (e340)	1.000	0.626
Health professionals (e355)	1.000	0.638

The data were collected by nurses in structured interviews based on the Elderly Nursing Core Set. These professionals previously received training in the assessment of functioning based on the ICF. They were also provided a manual for using the Elderly Nursing Core Set and the contact information of one of the investigators for clarification of eventual doubts. A total of 427 individuals aged 65 years old corresponding to the Continuing Integrated Care Teams of Coastal Alentejo and Odivelas, the Community Care Unit of Redondo, and the SAMS Nursing Home were called by the healthcare professionals to perform functional assessments. In some cases, data collection was performed at the participants' dwellings during home visits. On average, administration of the questionnaire lasted 20 min. Data collection was performed from

August to December 2012. The study complied with the required ethical norms; it was approved by the committee of ethics in health sciences of the University of Évora, and the participants signed an informed consent form. Data analysis was conducted using the IBM SPSS software and included factor analysis of principal components with varimax rotation, sensitivity analysis by means of the Kolmogorov-Smirnov (K-S) test, and reliability analysis through Cronbach's alpha [8, 17].

3 Results

In the sensitivity analysis, the normality of the distribution of the 4 factors extracted in the principal component analysis (PCA) and the Global Total were tested by means of the K-S test. The results showed that neither any of the factors nor the Global Total ($p < 0.05$) [7] exhibited normal distribution.

Analysis of the asymmetry of the distributions showed that all 4 factors and the Global Total exhibited positive skew, i.e., the distribution was concentrated on the left. Regarding kurtosis, all 4 factors and the Global Total exhibited a platykurtic distribution, as the curve was quite flat, slightly thin and with heavy tails due to the type of convenience sample we used. Table 2 summarizes the results of the sensitivity analysis.

Table 2. Results of the K-S test, skewness, kurtosis, and descriptive statistics relative to the Elderly Nursing Core Set, Portugal, 2017

Factor	K-S and P	Skewness coeff.	Kurtosis coeff.	Mean	SD	Median	Mode
Factor 1 – Self-Care	K-S = 2.327. $p = 0.000$	0.122	−1.443	2.95	1.393	2.92	5
Factor 2 – Learning and Mental Functions	K-S = 3.527. $p = 0.000$	0.797	−0.737	2.37	1.280	2.00	1
Factor 3 – Communication	K-S = 4.874. $p = 0.000$	1.153	−0.072	2.01	1.307	1.25	1
Factor 4 – Relationship with Friends and Caregivers	K-S = 2.155. $p = 0.000$	0.162	−1.009	2.25	0.875	2.33	1
Global	K-S = 1.643. $p = 0.009$	0.407	−0.984	2.59	1.076	2.44	2.24

The scale reliability was assessed by means of Cronbach's alpha [8, 17]. First, the internal consistency of the global scale was estimated and then each of its 4 factors. The Cronbach's alpha value of the global scale (25 items) was 0.963, which is indicative of excellent internal consistency. Relative to the 4 factors extracted by means of PCA (Table 3), factor 1 (Self-Care) exhibited the highest Cronbach's alpha value ($\alpha = 0.976$), which is also indicative of excellent internal consistency. The values corresponding to factors 2 and 3 ($\alpha = 0.942$ and $\alpha = 0.948$, respectively) are indicative of good internal consistency, while the value of factor 4 ($\alpha = 0.624$) is questionable. Relative to the latter, most statistics authors [8, 17] agree that a value of 0.6 is the minimum acceptable value.

Table 3. Alpha coefficients of the Elderly Nursing Core Set global scale and factors, Portugal, 2017

Factor	Number of items	Alpha
Global	25	0.963
Factor 1 – Self-Care	12	0.976
Factor 2 – Learning and Mental Functions	6	0.942
Factor 3 – Communication	4	0.948
Factor 4 – Relationship with Friends and Caregivers	3	0.624

In the analysis of the scale construct validity, we subjected the data to factor analysis by means of the principal component method with varimax rotation [8, 17]. The relational structure of the Elderly Nursing Core Set items was analyzed by means of factor analysis of principal components. This analysis resulted in the extraction of 4 concepts (or dimensions), according to the Kaiser criterion for a sample of 427 individuals, given that only the concepts with eigenvalues greater than 1 were considered, i.e., each eigenvalue quantifies the part of the variance (from the total of the variables) explained by each concept. However, the screen test (scree plot analysis) indicated that 5 concepts could be extracted, given that concepts may be extracted until the point at which the line (curve) levels off.

The 4 concepts extracted explain 80.25% of the total variance, having been constructed with a weight over 0.5 (Table 4). Assuming that a larger variance explained corresponds to greater differentiation, these 4 factors are associated with a decreasing degree of relevance relative to the functional aspects of older adults.

Table 4. Functional aspects of older adults by means of factor analysis of principal components of the Elderly Nursing Core Set, Portugal, 2017

Indicators	Components				h^2
	Self-care	Learning and mental functions	Communication	Relationship with friends and caregivers	
Washing oneself (d510)	**0.901**	0.211	0.154	0.083	0.886
Dressing (d540)	**0.894**	0.198	0.263	0.106	0.918
Caring for body parts (d520)	**0.884**	0.230	0.221	0.028	0.884
Moving around using equipment (d465)	**0.871**	0.157	0.193	0.096	0.830
Walking (d450)	**0.849**	0.195	0.187	0.088	0.801
Carrying out daily routine (d230)	**0.839**	0.240	0.296	0.146	0.871
Maintaining a body position (d415)	**0.803**	0.142	0.374	0.163	0.831
Changing body basic position (d410)	**0.779**	0.126	0.361	0.122	0.768

(*continued*)

Table 4. (*continued*)

Indicators		Components				h²
		Self-care	Learning and mental functions	Communication	Relationship with friends and caregivers	
Toileting (d530)		**0.736**	0.264	0.402	0.066	0.777
Hand and arm use (d445)		**0.685**	0.168	0.502	0.127	0.765
Drinking (d560)		**0.673**	0.270	0.591	−0.014	0.875
Eating (d550)		**0.643**	0.255	0.633	0.017	0.879
Emotional functions (b152)		0.163	**0.869**	0.285	0.039	0.865
Orientation functions (b114)		0.217	**0.861**	0.312	−0.019	0.885
Attention functions (b140)		0.243	**0.859**	0.282	0.008	0.877
Memory functions (b144)		0.185	**0.842**	0.164	0.048	0.773
Consciousness functions (b110)		0.289	**0.772**	0.337	0.017	0.794
Higher-level cognitive functions (b164)		0.125	**0.768**	0.086	0.061	0.616
Speaking (d330)		0.333	0.379	**0.812**	0.030	0.915
Conversation (d350)		0.345	0.403	**0.795**	0.052	0.917
Communicating with − receiving − spoken messages (d310)		0.354	0.428	**0.757**	0.080	0.887
Family relationships (d760)		0.213	0.246	**0.720**	0.140	0.643
Personal care providers and personal assistants (e340)		−0.085	0.063	0.021	**0.784**	0.626
Health professionals (e355)		0.195	−0.092	0.098	**0.763**	0.638
Friends (e320)		0.334	0.129	0.077	**0.638**	0.541
Cronbach's Alpha		0.976	0.942	0.948	0.624	
Kaiser-Meyer-Olkin		0.948	0.918	0.850	0.627	
Bartlett's test of sphericity	Approx. Chi-Square	6949.813	2586.864	2175.781	123.511	
	df	66	15	6	3	
	Sig.	0.000	0.000	0.000	0.000	
	Total	8.207	5.237	4.859	1.760	
	% Explained variance	32.827	20.946	19.437	7.042	

4   Discussion

The first component of the CSI is generically associated with factors that represent functional aspects related to self-care, for which reason it is designated "Self-Care". This component explains the largest percentage of the total variance (32.83%) and includes 12 indicators answered on a 5-point Likert scale (1. NO problem: 0–4%; 2. MILD problem: 5–24%; 3. MODERATE problem: 25–49%; 4. SEVERE problem: 50–95%; 5. COMPLETE problem: 96–100%).

This first component was a very good fit for factor analysis (KMO = 0.948) (Meskell et al., 2014). Given the results of Bartlett's test of sphericity ($p < 0.001$), we rejected the null hypothesis and concluded that the variables were significantly correlated. In addition, we established that the 12 indicators included in this component exhibit excellent internal consistency ($\alpha = 0.976$).

As a function of the nature of the setting proper to each of the 4 subsamples, it was assumed that their nursing care needs were different. Thus, relative to the first component, we sought to establish whether the problems detected were related to the aforementioned settings for older adult care based on the following working hypothesis: The setting in which care is provided is associated with the level of problems relative to self-care. Application of the Kruskal-Wallis test showed that, on average, the participants cared for by the Continuing Integrated Care Teams of Coastal Alentejo exhibited the most serious problems relative to self-care (231.05), followed by the participants assisted by the Continuing Integrated Care Teams of Odivelas (190.08), SAMS Nursing Home (116.40), and Community Care Unit of Redondo (49.79). Given that these differences were significant (K-W(3) = 161.415; $p = 0.000$), at least one group differed from all the others in the severity of the problems related to self-care. We further found a strong (Eta = 0.702) and significant ($p < 0.001$) association between self-care level and the care provision setting.

The second component includes elements related to orientation, attention, memory, and consciousness, for which reason we designate it "Learning and Mental Functions". This component explains 20.95% of the total variance and 53.78% in combination with the first component. It comprises 6 indicators answered on the same Likert scale as the scale described above.

Additionally, in this case, the fit of this component for factor analysis was very good (KMO = 0.918), and we were able to reject the null hypothesis to conclude that the variables are significantly correlated (Bartlett's test $p < 0.001$). The 6 indicators included in this component exhibited good internal consistency ($\alpha = 0.942$).

Furthermore, for the same reasons as in the case of the first component, we here formulated the following working hypothesis: The setting in which care is provided is associated with the level of problems relative to learning and mental functions. Application of the Kruskal-Wallis test showed that, on average, the participants cared for by the Continuing Integrated Care Teams of Coastal Alentejo exhibited the most serious problems relative to learning and mental functions (189.04), followed by the participants assisted by the Continuing Integrated Care Teams of Odivelas (178.74), SAMS Nursing Home (156.08), and Community Care Unit of Redondo (130.33). Given that these differences were significant (K-W(3) = 16.845; $p = 0.001$), at least one group differed from all the others in the severity of the problems in learning and mental functions. We further found a weak (Eta = .261) but significant (p < 0.001) association between the learning and mental functions level and the care provision setting.

The third component is generically associated with factors related to communication and relationships, including speaking and conversation, for which reason we designated it "Communication". This component explains approximately 19.44% of the total variance and 73.22% in combination with the first 2 components. It includes 4 indicators answered on the same Likert scale as the scale described above.

Because the KMO value is 0.850, the fit of this component for factor analysis was good. As a function of the results of Bartlett's test of sphericity (p < 0.001), we rejected the null hypothesis and concluded that the variables are significantly correlated. In addition, we established that the 4 indicators included in this component exhibit excellent internal consistency (α = 0.948).

Additionally, in this case, we formulated a working hypothesis associating the level of problems in this component with the care provision setting: The setting in which care is provided is associated with the level of problems relative to communication. Application of the Kruskal-Wallis test showed that, on average, the participants cared for by the Community Care Unit of Redondo exhibited the most serious problems relative to communication (195.61). This group of participants lived in the community, in this case, small villages with reasonable levels of isolation. Relative to the remainder of the groups, the level of problems related to communication were more serious in the participants assisted by the Continuing Integrated Care Teams of Coastal Alentejo (181.09), followed by SAMS Nursing Home (153.62) and Continuing Integrated Care Teams of Odivelas (149.14). Given that these differences were significant (K-W (3) = 10.685; p = 0.014), at least one group differed from all the others in the severity of problems with communication.

The fourth component includes elements related to personal care providers and friends, for which reason we designate it "Relationship with Friends and Caregivers". This component explains 7.04% of the total variance and 80.25% in combination with the other 3 components. It comprises 3 indicators answered on the same 5-point Likert scale as the scale described above.

Based on the KMO value (=0.627), the fit of the fourth component for factor analysis was reasonable. Based on the results of Bartlett's test of sphericity (p < 0.001), we rejected the null hypothesis and concluded that the variables are significantly correlated. The internal consistency of the 3 indicators was questionable (α = 0.624); however, according to some theoreticians, a Cronbach's alpha value of 0.6 is acceptable.

In this case, we also formulated the following working hypothesis: The setting in which care is provided is associated with the level of problems relative to relationships with friends and caregivers. Application of the Kruskal-Wallis test showed that, on average, the participants cared for by the Continuing Integrated Care Teams of Coastal Alentejo exhibited the most serious problems relative to their relationships with caregivers and friends (190.55), followed by the participants assisted by the Community Care Unit of Redondo (183.56), Continuing Integrated Care Teams of Odivelas (179.84), and SAMS Nursing Home (102.33). The statistical evidence allowed affirming that at least one group differed from all the others in the severity of the problems relative to the relationships with friends and caregivers (K-W(3) = 36,257; p = 0.000). We further found a weak (Eta = .311) but significant (p < 0.001) association between the level of relationships with friends and caregivers and the care provision setting.

We then analyzed the correlation matrix by means of Pearson's coefficient, which measures the linear association between variables. We assumed that correlations at the 5% significance level should have a probability of less than 0.5/300 = 0.000166; thus, we were able to establish that nearly all the variables included in the dimensions extracted using PCA exhibited significant relationships (p < 0.001), except for variable "Personal care providers and personal assistants". The variables included in the "Self-Care" component exhibited strong to very strong mutual associations, with the coefficient values varying from 0.7 to 0.9. The variables included in the "Learning and Mental Functions" and "Communication" components exhibited moderate to very strong mutual associations, with the coefficient values varying from 0.5 to 0.9. In turn, the variables included in the "Relationship with Friends and Caregivers" component exhibited weak relationships with the remaining variables, which reinforces the aforementioned weak relationships among the indicators.

This full analysis provides further evidence of the high internal and the relational consistency of the variables that compose the concepts [8, 17].

5 Conclusion

Based on the analysis of the psychometric properties of the Elderly Nursing Core Set, we conclude that the instrument as a whole exhibit's excellent consistency, reliability, and internal validity as evidenced by the content, construct, convergent, and discriminant validity. The concept designated "Self-Care" predominates in the explanation of the functioning of older adults. By contrast, the aspects related to "Relationship with Friends and Caregivers" play a less predominant role in this regard.

As a function of the results described above, we recommend the use of the Elderly Nursing Core Set to assess the nursing care needs and/or the outcomes of nursing interventions of individuals aged 65 years old or older.

References

1. Bongaarts, J.: United Nations, Department of Economic and Social Affairs, Population Division, Sex Differentials in Childhood Mortality. Popul. Dev. Rev. **40**(2), 380 (2014)
2. Burke, D., Gorman, E., Stokes, D., Lennon, O.: An evaluation of neuromuscular electrical stimulation in critical care using the ICF framework: a systematic review and meta-analysis. Clin. Respir. J. **10**, 407–420 (2014)
3. Direcção-Geral da Saúde (DGS): Translation of: World Health Organization (resolution WHA54.21). International classification of functioning, disability and health (2004)
4. European Commission (EC): Population, Key figures on Europe – 2014 edition. Luxembourg: Publications Office of the European Union (2014). ISSN 2315-201X

5. Florin, J., Ehrenberg, A., Ehnfors, M., Björvell, C.: A comparison between the VIPS model and the ICF for expressing nursing content in the health care record. Int. J. Med. Inform. **82**(2), 108–117 (2013)
6. José Lopes, M., Escoval, A., Gamito Pereira, D., Sandra Pereira, C., Carvalho, C., Fonseca, C.: Evaluation of elderly persons' functionality and care needs. Revista Latino-Americana De Enfermagem (RLAE) **21**, 52–60 (2013)
7. Maric, M., de Haan, E., Hogendoorn, S.M., Wolters, L.H., Huizenga, H.M.: Evaluating statistical and clinical significance of intervention effects in single-case experimental designs: An SPSS method to analyse univariate data. Behav. Ther. **46**(2), 230–241 (2015)
8. Marôco, J.: Análise Estatística com Utilisação do SPSS [Statistical Analysis using SPSS], 6th edn., p. 990. Edições Silabo (2014). ISBN: 9789899676343
9. Meskell, P., Murphy, K., Shaw, D.G., Casey, D.: Insights into the use and complexities of the Policy Delphi technique. Nurse Res. **21**(3), 32–39 (2014)
10. Orem, D.E.: Nursing: Concepts of Practice, 6th edn. Mosby, St. Louis (2001)
11. Pereira, C., Fonseca, C., Escoval, A., Lopes, M.: Contributo para a classificação da funcionalidade na população com mais de 65 anos, segundo a classificação internacional de funcionalidade. Revista Portuguesa de Saúde Pública **19**(1), 52–62 (2011)
12. Shen, P., Chen, C.: The WHO's international classification of functioning, disability, and health (ICF): essential knowledge for nurses. Hu Li Za Zhi (J. Nurs.) **59**(6), 92–97 (2012)
13. Sidani, S.: Effects of patient-centered care on patient outcomes: an evaluation. Res. Theory Nurs. Pract. **22**(1), 24–37 (2008)
14. So, H., Kim, H., Ju, K.: Prediction model of quality of life in elderly based on ICF model. J. Korean Acad. Nurs. **41**(4), 481–490 (2011)
15. The United Nations 2012 Population Projections (UN). Popul. Dev. Rev. **39**(3), 551–555 (2013)
16. World Bank (WB): The World Bank Annual Report 2014: Year in Review, p. 67 (2014)
17. Zhu, H.: Correctly selection methods of building up a model function of known categories in SPSS 16.0. J. Capital Inst. Phys. Educ. **26**(1), 91–96 (2014)

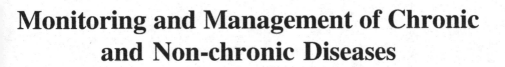

Monitoring and Management of Chronic and Non-chronic Diseases

The Communication with the Elderly Person Suffering from Auditive Deficiency: Psychomotricity and Supportive Technologies

Adriana Feijão[1], Maria Queiroga[1], Rafaela Moreira[1(✉)],
Raquel Jordão[1], and César Fonseca[2]

[1] Évora University, Évora, Portugal
138215@alunos.uevora.pt
[2] Évora University, Investigator POCTEP 0445_4IE_4_P, Évora, Portugal

Abstract. Growing old is a stage in Human development in which gains and losses can be accounted for but where, more often than not, the losses overcome the gains. Auditive deficiency can be one of those losses. Auditive deficiency is characterized by the reduction or total loss of the hearing capacity, where the communication is made in either a verbal or non verbal way.

The communication is of extreme importance in any exchange between the elderly and the health care professional, since it is the vehicle through which cognitive stimulation can be made, it being an essential factor in the acceptance of the individual and his/her capacities. For this reason, the health care professionals, willing to provide a superlative service, should be aware of a few strategies that facilitate the communication with this particular population.

It is important to optimize communication since difficulties in communicating have socio-emotional implications, including the speeding up of the ageing process. For this motive, some up-to-date technologies that facilitate the communication processes will be presented.

Last, but not least, one appeals to the investigation on how best to communicate when dealing with auditive impairments, in order to allow Psychomotor therapy to become more efficient when dealing with this population.

Keywords: Elderly · Hearing impairment · Communication · Psychomotricity · Gerontology · Quality of life

1 Introduction

Ageing is a stage in Human development during which changes occur due to the process of growing old. The Human Being develops until reaching his/her full potential. After reaching a peak, there occurs a diminishing of aptitudes and capacities. In every stage of life gains are losses are part of the scenery but, during the ageing process, losses are to be expected greater than the gains (d'Araujo 2015). The increment of losses and its evolution in a more or less gradual and progressive depends, among other factors, on the clinical condition of the individual. Therefore, two different kinds of ageing have to be considered: healthy ageing being physiological or primary and pathological or secondary ageing (Barreto 2017).

© Springer Nature Switzerland AG 2019
J. García-Alonso and C. Fonseca (Eds.): IWoG 2018, CCIS 1016, pp. 157–161, 2019.
https://doi.org/10.1007/978-3-030-16028-9_14

The auditive deficiency is characterized by the partial or total loss of hearing, thus compromising the capacity to perceive sounds and the understanding of words (Fernani et al. 2015). Presbycusis is the partial or total loss of hearing capacities due to the ageing of the auditive structures (Ribas et al. 2014).

Communication can be done in two distinct ways: verbal and non verbal. This last one includes gestures, facial expressions, body language and/or Proxemia (Paschoallin and Perensim 2016).

Further ahead, some perspectives regarding the communication between health care professionals and the elderly with hearing impairment, showing some strategies used, will be presented. Furthermore, other important factors regarding the quality of life of this population will be approached. Among other factors, up-to-date aiding technologies will be mentioned.

2 Methodology

Scientific articles were used when formulating this article. Research was done using the online data base EBSCO, Library of Knowledge Online (B-on), Science Direct and Scientific Electronic Library Online (SCIELO).

The data compilation was initiated on the 3rd of April 2018 and ended on the 7th of October 2018. In the research, the following descriptors were used: old man, hearing deficiency, communication, psychomotricity, gerontology and quality of life. The criteria for exclusion were articles published only in summary format and articles published prior to 2014.

3 Development

Communication is essential to any activity between the health care provider and the elderly, being it of extreme importance to the cognitive stimulation, which promotes acceptance of the body, of the characteristics and capacities the individual, thus avoiding the taking over by negative stereotypes (Paschoallin and Perensim 2016).

The quality assistance in health care requires communicative skills that will allow for a good understanding between the health care professional and the patient. For this motive, individuals suffering from hearing loss do prefer to be attended by health care professionals that are familiar with sign language since it allows them to be more independent and autonomous (Oliveira et al. 2015).

Still, the vast majority of health care professionals does not grasp the sign language system existing in their own country, making it necessary to employ the use of writing or lip reading. None of these methods is the ideal solution since writing can cause to constraints or frustrations to the patient, while lip reading demands great levels of attention, thus provoking mental tiredness in the patients (Oliveira et al. 2015). One other strategy that can be used to facilitate communication is to make use of an interpreter, thus having someone to mediate between the health care professional and the patient, but this technique also allows for some disadvantages: it weakens the therapeutic relation, promotes a fake integration of the person with hearing impairment and can result in the distortion of the information (Oliveira and Costa 2015) (Table 1).

Table 1. Communication strategies used by health care professionals assisting patients with hearing impairment. (adapted from Nascimento et al. 2015)

Strategies	%
Verbal communication	34
Written Portuguese Language	19
Lip reading	17
Translator/hearing companion	11
Mimic/gestures	9
Drawings	6
Figures	2
National sign language	2

In the elderly with hearing impairment communication can be compromised, thus creating difficulties in leading an active life in society (Paschoallin and Perensim 2010). The difficulty in communicating verbally is an important factor leading to the individual not feeling socially integrated. Individuals with hearing deficiency or total loss of it are commonly labeled as incapable (Oliveira et al. 2015).

The difficulty in mutual understanding generates anguish and incapability in both the health care professional and the patient (Oliveira et al. 2015).

One also has to consider that nowadays the opinions and wishes of the elderly are not taken into account, even by the family. The isolation is caused by the factors mentioned above and, subsequently, the elderly's social world becomes increasingly smaller. Obviously, social isolation can speed up the ageing process (Paschoallin and Perensim 2016). It is therefore possible that, in individuals with hearing impairment the ageing process is accelerated. This inference requires more scientific investigation in order to be validated.

Nowadays there are various technological advances that aim to facilitate the communication with the individual suffering from hearing impairment. as stated by Carneiro (2016), one should organize them in three greater groups: Tecnogestual, Tecnofacil e Tecnosw. The first includes all technologies that allow access to videos, in which the national sign language system can be integrated and one can also use to visualize facial expressions, such as Viavel, Skype and the Webcam. The second refers to systems that pertain to writing, such as the mobile phone, Facebook, Whatsapp, and even Instagram. Last, Tecnosw includes all systems that use sign writing. These three components make up the so called 'Deaf Technology' (Rangel and Stumpf 2015).

Lets now explain in what constitutes the Brasil Viavel System. Through this system, the deaf individual can interact with an interpreter who will, in turn, translate to message to others. The concept is similar to that of the interpreter but, through this system the deaf individual does not need to be accompanied full time by someone who communicates through the usage of sign language. Basically, Viavel assures that an interpreter is always at hand to translate (Carneiro et al. 2018).

Although this is a well conceived strategy, most public spaces (for instance attending counters) still do not possess the technology. A problem that derives from this overlooking is the minimization of the need to dominate the national sign language system, a very negative aspect, since this population is becoming increasingly differentiated. In what pertains to Tecnofacil, one, obviously, has to recognize that nowadays mobile phones and social networks do facilitate the communication with individuals suffering from hearing impairments, not exclusively facilitating the communication among individuals that are geographically apart. To the population with hearing impairments the communication with the support of technology is a possibility to communicate with someone who is physically present but does not know the national sign language system (Carneiroet al. 2018).

We present the perspective of an individual with hearing impairment in an interview with Consolo (2014, in Carneiro et al. 2018): " Technology is today a very useful resource in the life of the deaf. The main advantage deaf people get from technology is the contact with the Portuguese language and, through it, the written communication." Still, one must understand that communication is losing its significance. In Psychomotricity we value communication, corporal expression and believe that communication cannot be restricted to writing. We, therefore, appeal to the investigation of communication in all of its facets. One should not accommodate only to the solutions that are available today.

Psychomotricity should be able to intervene with people with hearing impairment although, for that to be possible, it is necessary to acquire more knowledge relating to hearing impairments. For any given therapeutic intervention to be efficient, it has to be supported by theory. One can, therefore, assume that any therapeutic procedure, specially psychomotor interventions with this population, will benefit if there is a true interest in acquiring knowledge on the sensorial impairment.

4   Final Considerations

Presbiacusia has consequences both a psychological and emotional level, generating feelings of frustration, anxiety and uselessness, causing, at a social level, the distancing between the elderly and society, therefore augmenting the problems of social interacting (Etcheverria et al. 2014).

As for the providing of health care services to the elderly patients with hearing impairment, the majority of the professionals do not possess the basic knowledge on sign language, having to make usage of other strategies. Still, all communication methods have disadvantages, the biggest being the distortion of information.

The technologies being used nowadays do make it much easier but one should not conform to the available solutions. One should aim for even more practical solutions when communicating with individuals suffering from hearing impairments.

At last, one should consider that the psychomotor intervention regarding the population with hearing impairments will benefit from an effective interest in finding out more about this sensorial deficiency, which, in turn, will provide more technological alternatives to the ones already in existence.

References

Barreto, J.: Envelhecimento e qualidade de vida: o desafio actual. Sociologia: Revista da Faculdade de Letras da Universidade do Porto, 15 (2017)

Carneiro, M., Nogueira, C., Silva, T.: Recursos tecnológicos nas interações cotidianas de adultos surdos. CIET: EnPED (2018)

Carneiro, R.S., Falcone, E.F.: Avaliação de um programa de promoção de habilidades sociais para idosos. Análise Psicológica 34(3), 279–291 (2016). https://doi.org/10.14417/ap.960

d'Araújo, M., Alpuim, M., Rivero, C., Marujo, H.: Possibilidades para envelhecer positivamente: Um estudo de caso com base na psicologia positiva. Revista E-Psi 5(1), 40–75 (2015)

Etcheverria, A., et al.: Estudo sobre a audição em idosos e associação com sintomatologia depressiva. Revista Brasileira de Ciências do Envelhecimento Humano 11(2) (2014)

Fernani, D., et al.: Análise do desenvolvimento psicomotor em indivíduos com deficiência auditiva. Colloquium Vitae 6(3), 19–26 (2015)

Nascimento, G., Fortes, L., Kessler, T.: Estratégias de comunicação como dispositivo para o atendimento humanizado em saúde da pessoa surda. Saúde (Santa Maria) 41(2), 241–250 (2015)

Oliveira, Y., Celino, S., Costa, G.: Comunicação como ferramenta essencial para assistência à saúde dos surdos. Physis: Revista De Saúde Coletiva 25(1), 307–320 (2015). https://doi.org/10.1590/s0103-73312015000100017

Paschoallin, H.C., Perensim, K.: A importância da comunicação e do estímulo para a qualidade de vida do idoso. Revista de Enfermagem da UFJF 1(1) (2016)

Rangel, G., Stunpf, M.: A pedagogia da diferença para o surdo. Letramento, bilinguismo e educação de surdos, 113–124 (2015)

Ribas, A., Kozlowski, L., Almeida, G., Marques, J.M., Silvestre, R., Mottecy, C.: Qualidade de vida: comparando resultados em idosos com e sem presbiacusia. Revista Brasileira de Geriatria e Gerontologia 17(2), 353–362 (2014)

Mobility Deficit – Rehabilitate,
An Opportunity for Functionality

Gorete Reis[1,2](✉) , Patrícia Páscoa Pereira[3] , Lena Sabino[4],
and Maria José Bule[1]

[1] University of Évora, Évora, Portugal
greis@uevora.pt
[2] Research Group AgeingC, Cintesis - Center for Health Technology and
Services Research, FMUP, Investigator POCTEP 0445_4IE_4_P, Porto, Portugal
[3] Polyvalent Intensive Care Unit of Hospital Espírito Santo, Évora, Portugal
[4] Local Health Unit of Baixo Alentejo, Beja, Portugal

Abstract. There are many pathological conditions that cause mobility deficits
and that ultimately influence someone's autonomy. To overcome these difficulties implies the patient's involvement and professional action, namely from a
rehabilitation nurse, whose target is to capacitate the patient. The person can be
capacitated and reach quality of life through organized and systematic rehabilitation programs, which can result in health gains. **Aims:** to evaluate patients
with mobility deficits functional status; to implement a Rehabilitation Nursing
intervention plan; to monitor health gains through mobility deficits rehabilitation; **Method:** Cross-sectional study, action research approximation. Non-
probability sampling, 9 patients admitted at an Intensive Care Unit and at a
Stroke Unit who fulfilled the inclusion criteria. The intervention plan included
two moments of formal evaluation: the initial (T1) and the final (T2) that relied
on specific instruments. **Results:** improvement and solving of rehabilitation
nursing diagnoses, increased balance and better transferring ability. Data suggest
that the implementation of an intervention plan decreased the level of dependence. **Conclusion:** Early intervention and the implementation of a nursing
rehabilitation intervention plan results in health gains (direct or indirect),
decreases the risk of developing Pressure Ulcers (PU) and the risk of developing
a situation of immobility that affects patients' autonomy and quality of life.

Keywords: Rehabilitation Nursing · Mobility limitation · Daily activities

1 Introduction

The admission at highly differentiated hospital units often forces the patients to a
therapeutic rest that naturally evolves to mobility restriction and consequently to its
negative effects. To understand the short- and long-term effects of immobility of
admitted patients in a post critical situation requires the development of specialized
care, focused on self-care. Given this scenario, an early nursing rehabilitation approach
is crucial for optimizing patients' functional status and for reducing their inabilities.
The problem here studied focuses on dependence, specifically concerning affected

© Springer Nature Switzerland AG 2019
J. García-Alonso and C. Fonseca (Eds.): IWoG 2018, CCIS 1016, pp. 162–172, 2019.
https://doi.org/10.1007/978-3-030-16028-9_15

mobility that restrains the performance of daily activities (DA). The main effects of immobility are: decreased functional mobility, decreased lean muscle mass and difficulty in recovering the functional status prior to hospital admission [1]. The loss of mobility affects the capacity of the individual to remain physically independent, to perform daily activities, resulting in a reduction of his/her quality of life [2].

Current literature highlights that the rehabilitation process after a stroke should start as early as possible [3, 4] as it is considered a major condition for recovery [5]. 30% of stroke survivors are estimated to develop some level of dependence that prevents them to perform basic daily activities [6]. Treatment at Intensive Care Units (ICU) and the period after a critical medical episode are also associated with increased physical and psychological morbidity [7]. When we focus on the patient functional rehabilitation, after patients, hemodynamic and respiratory stabilization, early rehabilitation has been seen as a positive intervention that works as an important treatment and modifies the probability of developing negative effects related to functional and physical morbidity. [8]. A study developed at an ICU shows that early rehabilitation reduces hospital stay time and delirium, increases muscle strength and the patient's motivation. Long term effects were also observed, namely the increase of self-care ability, a faster return to independent functioning, improvement of physical function and reduced risk of readmission and death [9]. Another study, with ventilated patients who took part on an exercise program, showed that these patients improved their ability to perform DAs (hygiene, eating, transferring from bed to a chair and using wc) and increased walking distances in comparison with the group of control (not performing the exercises). There was an improvement of objective measures, such as the FIM and the Barthel Index, among the participant group at the time of hospital discharge [10]. For these reasons, assessing the level of dependence in selfcare is an important skill for a nursing professional, as it will allow to plan an individualized care and implement realistic interventions adjusted to the patient's needs, leading to feasible outcomes. Rehabilitation should, therefore, been seen as an enabler and promoter of the patient's function outcomes, as evidence suggests that structured rehabilitation processes can avoid patient's mobility deterioration [11–13].

Considering the current situation and based on data from the last census [14], the population presented in this article is characterized as an aged population presenting difficulties performing DAs (20.85%) when compared with the national average (17,8%). Walking is one of the main limitations [14]. This way and to respond to the needs of patients at a Stroke and Intensive Care Units of a Central Hospital in the interior of Portugal, we propose to organize an intervention plan (IP) focused on mobility issues. Taking into account Rehabilitation Nursing diagnoses we aim to design a specific and individualized intervention plan that aims autonomy capacity building. The intervention plan targeted people with mobility deficits and included bed mobility and transfers, which are considered pillars for developing long term patients' autonomy.

2 Methods

The development of the IP is included in the Nursing Master's degree, Rehabilitation Field. Its implementation was previously authorized by the Central Hospital. The participants signed a voluntary and informed consent and ethical principles, data anonymity and confidentiality were respected.

The IP takes place within a research – action context and is based on participation and action as the researcher interacts with the individuals and can serve as a facilitator for behavioural change [15]. The cross-sectional plan took place between 14th October and 14th December in 2017. The selected patients were the ones admitted at the Stroke Unit and ICU and the inclusion criteria were the following: admission period at the unit inferior to 48 h; to show commitment with mobility; to be collaborative; to accept to participate in the project by signing the required consent; possibility to be part of the intervention plan for at least 3 days. The target population was 50 patients (n), 41 were excluded as they did not fulfil the required criteria. The sample was composed by 9 patients (n), 6 patients admitted at the Stroke Unit and 3 patients at the ICU.

It was created a data collection protocol, composed by two distinct parts. The first, characterization variables (age, sex, medical diagnoses, family unit and carer presence), the assessment of the level of conscience (Glasgow Coma Scale) and of the patient's function capacity (Functional Independence Measure – FIM score). The second, presented information related with the focuses Bed Mobility and Transfers. For the latter, direct observation was used for assessing the necessary variables and obtaining a RN diagnosis. Each focus group included 3 variables, with defined and sustained criteria according to standard documentation about nursing care for rehabilitation nursing [16]. The change in one of the criteria (Table 1) suggests making the diagnosis and implement the planned interventions.

Table 1. Diagnoses evaluation grid

Focus	Variable	Diagnoses criteria
Bed mobility	Muscle Tone	Shows contractures Shows an increased tone Shows joint stiffness Presence of Spasticity Presence of Hypotonia Modified Ashworth Scale
	Muscle Movement	Has movement control Has reduced movement Mobilizes actively
	Positioning	Can position him/herself Knows the adaptation technique for positioning Braden Scale

(*continued*)

Table 1. (*continued*)

Focus	Variable	Diagnoses criteria
Transferring	Body Balance	Has seated static balance Has seated dynamic balance Has static orthostatic seated balance Has dynamic orthostatic seated balance Has vicious postures Supports his/her own weight in different positions Berg Scale
	Transfers	Transfers from lying to sitting position Transfers from sitting to standing Needs an auxiliary device for transferring Knows the adaptation technique for transferring
	Standing	Can lift the SMs Can lift the IMs Supports his/her own weight while standing Is alert for security cautions while lifting Needs an auxiliary device for standing

For Bed Mobility the following variables were evaluated: *muscle tone, muscle movement and positioning*. The focus 'Transfers' included the variables *body balance, standing and transfers*. To support the evaluation, valid and objective measures were used, namely the Modified Ashworth Scale, the Berg Scale and also the Braden Scale.

Regarding the procedure, the evaluation was led in 2 different moments. In the first stage, the Initial Evaluation (T1) took place when the patient was first approached and in the second stage it took place by the end of the third day of intervention (T2). In general, the following stages were identified: Stage A - **Evaluation** - feedback was given for each variable (when changes occurred or not). When they were evaluated as positive, interventions were implemented. The Stage A coincides with the T1 moment. Stage B - **Intervention** - The Intervention Plan was composed by a set of exercises that aimed bed mobility and transfers. It included joint mobility, standard antispastic positioning, practising balance sitting in bed and in a chair. The intervention plan was adapted to each patient needs, with types of mobility and exercises appropriated to the patient's situation, with his/her cooperation. Stage C - **Reevaluation** - after three consecutive days of interventions of RN, the nursing diagnosis was reevaluated and the results presented. The reevaluation stage occurs during the T2 moment.

The data were inserted in a database and descriptive statistics was used to analyse them.

3 Results

The sample used in the IP was composed by 9 participants between 43 and 86 years old, from which we highlight the 60–69 years age group (n = 4). The majority were males (n = 6). The most common group was participants living with the spouse (56%)

and none of the participants had an informal carer at the time of the initial evaluation (n = 9). The diagnoses most observed were stroke (n = 7), 78%.

Regarding the level of conscience (Glasgow Coma Scale), the patients at the Stroke Unit had an average score of 15, whereas the patients at ICU presented an inferior average value, score = 11. Concerning functionality, a relatively low FIM score average was observed (54,78): there was a change on the patients' level of dependence and they needed assistance for performing at least 50% DA's tasks. Moreover, significant differences in the FIM score were also observed in patients of both services. Patients at the Stroke Unit presented an average score of 69 in opposition with an average score of 26 for patients at ICU, who had a change in their level of dependence and needed more assistance in 25% of the tasks compared with the patients at the Stroke Unit. In general, the total sample showed positive results regarding the FIM score between the moments T1 and T2, as presented in Fig. 1.

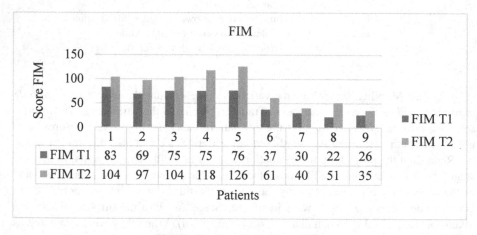

Fig. 1. Function Evolution – FIM

After the initial evaluation (T1), there were 6 associated nursing rehabilitation diagnoses, namely: *Presence of hypertonia* (n = 1), *Decreased muscle function* (n = 9), *Potential to improve knowledge about the adaptation technique for positioning* (n = 9), *Compromised body balance* (n = 9), *Compromised standing* (n = 9) and *Compromised adaptation technique for transferring* (n = 9). Looking at the results, there was only one patient diagnosed with hypertonia and the rest of the patients presented all the others diagnoses. Considering the interventions appropriated for each diagnoses and adapted to each patient, at T2 moment the diagnoses initially observed remained. However, there was a decrease in their prevalence. Therefore, in T2 the following could be observed: *Presence of hypertonia* (n = 1), *Decreased muscle function* (n = 4), *Potential to improve knowledge about the adaptation technique for positioning* (n = 1), *Compromised body balance* (n = 4), *Compromised standing* (n = 3) and *Compromised adaptation technique for transferring* (n = 4). Regarding objective measures, namely the risk of PU (Braden Scale) and balance (Berg Scale), the patients showed clear improvements in T2 in comparison with T1, as it is presented in Figs. 2 and 3.

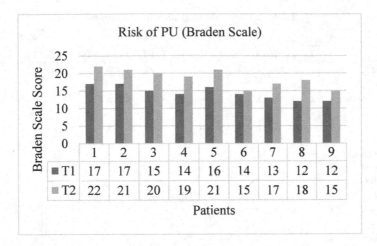

Fig. 2. Risk of PU (Braden Scale)

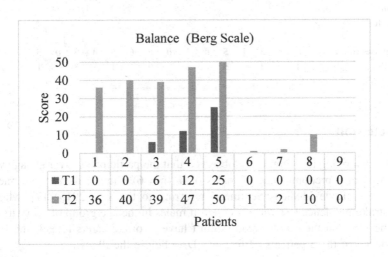

Fig. 3. Balance (Berg Scale)

After implementing the designed IP and after the participant patients' final evaluation (T2), there was approximately a reduction of 29 diagnosis of RN in comparison with T1, which means that 63% the diagnoses were solved. These data are illustrated in Table 2.

Table 2. Rehabilitation nursing diagnoses

Patient	1		2		3		4		5		6		7		8		9		Total	
Evaluation	T_1	T_2	T_1	T_2	T_1	T_2	T_1	T_2	T_1	T_2	T_1	T_2	T_1	T_2	T_1	T_2	T_1	T_2	T_1	T_2
Presence of hypertonia	–	–	–	–	–	–	–	–	–	–	x	x	–	–	–	–	–	–	1	1
Decreased muscle function	x	x	x	–	x	x	x	–	x	–	x	x	x	x	x	–	x	–	9	4
Potential to improve knowledge about the adaptation technique for positioning	x	–	x	–	x	–	x	–	x	–	x	x	x	–	x	–	x	x	9	1
Compromised body balance	x	–	x	x	x	–	x	–	x	–	x	x	x	x	x	–	x	x	9	4
Compromised standing	x	–	x	–	x	–	x	–	x	–	x	x	x	x	x	–	x	x	9	3
Compromised adaptation technique for transfers	x	–	x	–	x	–	x	–	x	–	x	x	x	x	x	–	x	x	9	4
RN Diagnoses (n)	**5**	1	**5**	1	**5**	1	**5**	0	**5**	0	**6**	6	**5**	4	**5**	0	**5**	4	**46**	17
Solved RN Diagnoses (n)	4		4		4		5		5		0		1		5		1		29 (63%)	

4   Discussion

While characterizing the sample, we observed that the participants' average age was 65 years old, with a predominance of males 67% (n = 6). Similar data to the ones collected by the 'Rede Médicos Sentinela' referring to the year 2015 [17], where the highest stroke incidence rate was observed in males in the age group of 75 years old or more. The fact that the sample group didn't have informal carers reveals the level of independence of these patients performing DAs before the illness.

Regarding the functionality, a change in the patients' FIM score after the intervention plan (T2) was observed. Results that are congruent with the study developed by Kinoshita et al. [18], where the FIM score in patients with acute stroke before and after the intervention plan were evaluated. The results showed that functionality (FIM score) improved significantly in the three groups of the study and the gains (FIM) were more evident in the group that initiated the program within the first 24 h. The authors concluded that an intervention plan was valuable and helped the patients with acute stroke to improve their ability for performing DAs.

As referred previously, after T2, the RN diagnoses were still observed but with decreased prevalence. We remind that most patients presented a stroke diagnosis. Depaul, Moreland and Dehueck [19], reinforce the idea that this type of population has great needs related to mobility. However, keeping in mind the duration of the intervention plan, a significant number of RN diagnoses were solved in T2.

Referring specifically to the variable of muscle tone, presence of hypertonia, we realized that the short duration of the IP could have had influence on its evolution, revealing that it is insufficient for this variable. Studies in this area present durations of 6 weeks or more [20]. However, the aggravation of the patient's level of hypertonia was not observed. Such fact reveals the need to keep implementing the IP focusing more on standard antispastic body positioning.

Benefits for the other diagnosis were also observed: *Decreased Muscle Function, Potential to improve knowledge about the adaptation technique for positioning, Compromised body balance, Compromised standing and Compromised adaptation technique for compromised for transferring.* 63% of the RN diagnoses were solved (n = 29). Studies show that such interventions result in benefits for patients' mobility, as they favour the functional recovery in the acute phase and improve the quality of life of the patient after being discharged. The passive, active mobilization or the combination of both is associated with increased muscle strength, less days of in-hospital stay, less duration of delirium, less days of invasive mechanical ventilation dependence, higher probability to walk without medical assistance after discharge and a better functional status when discharged [21, 22]. Moreover, provide care to positioning also reveals to result positively regarding passive mobility and comfort [23]. Considering the developed IP, we observe that taking care of the positioning led to the reduction of risk of developing UP.

An intervention plan focused on *body balance commitment* can become valuable. After four weeks of study, Moghe and Kanase [24], concluded that initial interventions for controlling the trunk are effective and improved the balance in individuals with stroke and that, together with structured exercises, they contribute for a faster recovery in acute and subacute stages of stroke [24]. Buyukavci et al. [25], obtained similar results. Conventional exercises, or these combined with exercises of trunk balance, can result in significant balance, functional condition and ambulation improvements [25]. The IP sample group showed identical results after its implementation. By evaluating with the Berg Scale, we observe in T1 a total of 6 patients with a score = 0 and in T2 a global improvement of the body balance, although with low scores.

As for the variable *standing*, it was observed that improving muscle function and balance was crucial for the gains obtained in the IP in T2 and, therefore, we argue for the importance of the IP regarding this variable. This is also present in Thomsen, Snow, Rodriguez and Hopkins [26], study. The aim of the study was to increase the patients' ambulation with acute respiratory failure, who were transferred from different ICU to a specific ICU, where the activity was focused on care. The mobility activities began in the first 24 h until the moment of discharge. The patients were submitted to an early action protocol, where interventions such as early standing and practising standing took place. In the first 24 h the authors observed an increase of the percentage of patients sitting in bed, sitting in a chair and of the ones who started walking [26]. Morris et al. [27], also corroborate these conclusions in their study. The authors divided two groups of patients in an ICU. One group was submitted to a mobility protocol and the other only to medical general care. The results demonstrated that patients under the mobility protocol started to stand earlier than the other group, within a difference of 5 days [27].

The difficulty with transfers motivated Alexander, Grunawalt, Carlos and Augustine [28], to design a set of exercises for bed mobility to test key movements, such as arms, legs and trunk movements that could probably contribute to the success of moving from one place to another. The study suggested that to improve bed mobility in older adults, the exercises should go beyond the improvement of the trunk function and therefore more exercises for bed mobility and training about the superior members positioning should been included, as these would be essential for straightening the trunk [28]. The IP results suggest that the integration of the exercises mentioned above was essential for the gains observed in the ability of the patient to go from the lying position to the seated position and from this to standing.

5 Conclusion

The effectiveness of the IP was evidenced by the Nursing Rehabilitation diagnoses being solved and reduced. Data suggest that the implementation of an IP focusing on people with mobility deficits decreased their level of dependence. We realised that when improving functional mobility, we are improving indirectly other variables, namely body balance, ability to transfer and the risk for developing UP. To improve muscle function and balance, implement exercises and provide information to the patient about procedures were crucial factors that enabled the patient to stand, easing the transfers and contributing to their independence.

Considering the results obtained, we believe that small evolutions should not be underestimate as, in the long run, they can result in great gains. It is not enough to evidence the partial gains, but also the gains that will contribute for self-care capacity building and for the highest possible level of independence.

We believe that the protocol for evaluating functionality, namely mobility, should be made available electronically. This allows the evaluations to be carried out by remote access, from the place where the evaluator is located. We then have the conditions to obtain nursing diagnoses, while keeping a history that traces the care process.

References

1. Booth, K., et al.: Progressive mobility protocol reduces venous thromboembolism rate in trauma intensive care patients: a quality improvement project. J. Trauma Nurs. Official J. Soc. Trauma Nurses 23(5), 284–289 (2016)
2. Kneafsey, R.: A systematic review of nursing contributions to mobility rehabilitation: examining the quality and content of the evidence. J. Clin. Nurs. 16, 325–340 (2007)
3. Hernández, B., Benjumea, P., Tuso, L.: Indicadores del desempeño clínico fisioterapéutico en el manejo hospitalario temprano del accidente cerebrovascular (ACV). Revista Ciencias De La Salud 11(1), 7–34 (2013)
4. Svendsen, M., Ehlers, L., Hundborg, H., Ingeman, A., Johnsen, S.: Processes of early stroke care and hospital costs. Int. J. Stroke Official J. Int. Stroke Soc. 9(6), 777–782 (2014)
5. Kutlubaev, M., Akhmadeeva, L.: The early post-stroke mobilization. Vopr. Kurortol. Fizioter. Lech. Fiz. Kult. 92(1), 46–50 (2015)
6. Oliveira, A., Araújo, T., Costa, A., Morais, H., Silva, V., Lopes, M.: Evaluation of patients with stroke monitored by home care programs. Revista da Escola de Enfermagem da USP 47(5), 1143–1149 (2013)

7. Schmidt, U., Knecht, l., MacIntyre, M.: Should early mobilization be routine in mechanically ventilated patients? Respir. Care **61**(6), 867–875 (2016)
8. Azevedo, P., Gomes, B.: Efeitos da mobilização precoce na reabilitação funcional em doentes críticos: uma revisão sistemática. Revista de Enfermagem Referência **IV**(5), 129–138 (2015)
9. Hopkins, R., Mitchell, L., Thomsen, G., Schafer, M., Link, M., Brown, S.M.: Implementing a mobility program to minimize post-intensive care syndrome. AACN Adv. Crit. Care **27**(2), 187–203 (2016)
10. Schweickert, W., et al.: Physical and occupational therapy in mechanically ventilated, critically ill patients: a randomised controlled trial. Lancet **373**(9678), 1874–1882 (2009)
11. Mudge, A., Giebel, A., Cutler, A.: Exercising body and mind: an integrated approach to functional independence in hospitalized older people. J. Am. Geriatr. Soc. **56**(4), 630–635 (2008)
12. Said, C., Morris, M., Woodward, M., Churilov, L., Bernhardt, J.: Enhancing physical activity in older adults receiving hospital based rehabilitation: a phase II feasibility study. BMC Geriatr. **12**, 26 (2012)
13. Folden, S., Tappen, R.: Factors influencing function and recovery following hip repair surgery. Orthop. Nurs. **26**(4), 234–241 (2007)
14. Instituto Nacional de Estatística: Censos 2011 Resultados Definitivos – Região Alentejo (2012). http://censos.ine.pt/ngt_server/attachfileu.jsp?look_parentBoui=156656957&att_display=n&att_download=y. Accessed 01 Oct 2018
15. Carvalho e Silva, J., Ribeiro de Morais, E., Figueiredo, M., Tyrrell, M.: Pesquisa-acção: concepções e aplicabilidade nos estudos em Enfermagem. Rev. Bras. Enferm. **64**(3), 592–595 (2011)
16. Ordem dos Enfermeiros: Padrão Documental dos Cuidados de Enfermagem da Especialidade de Enfermagem de Reabilitação. Colégio de Especialidade de Enfermagem de Reabilitação, Porto, pp. 1–60 (2015). http://www.ordemenfermeiros.pt/colegios/Documents/2015/MCEER_Assembleia/PadraoDocumental_EER.pdf. Accessed 01 Oct 2018
17. Rodrigues, A.P., Batista, I., Sousa-Uva, M., Pereira, S.: Médicos-sentinela: o que se fez em 2015. Instituto Nacional de saúde Doutor Ricardo Jorge, IP, Lisboa (2016)
18. Kinoshita, T., et al.: Effects of physiatrist and registered therapist operating acute rehabilitation (PROr) in patients with stroke. PLoS ONE **12**(10), e0187099 (2017)
19. Depaul, V.P., Moreland, J.D., Dehueck, A.L.: Physiotherapy needs assessment of people with stroke following discharge from hospital, stratified by acute functional independence measure score. Physiotherapie Can **65**(3), 204–214 (2013)
20. Krishnamoorthy, K., Varadharajulu, G., Kanase, S.: Effect of close kinematic chain exercises on upper limb spasticity in hemiparetic adult. Indian J. Physiother. Occup. Ther. **11**(2), 146–152 (2017)
21. Tipping, C., et al.: The effects of active mobilisation and rehabilitation in ICU on mortality and function: a systematic review. Intensive Care Med. **43**(2), 171–183 (2017)
22. Rosa, D., Olgiati, T.: Revisione narrativa della letteratura sulla mobilizzazione precoce in corso di ventilazione meccanica (A narrative review of early mobilization during mechanical ventilation). SCENARIO Off. Italian J. ANIARTI **34**(3), 32–38 (2017)
23. Pickenbrock, H., Ludwig, V.U., Zapf, A., Dressler, D.: Conventional versus neutral positioning in central neurological disease: a multicenter randomized controlled trial. Deutsches Arzteblatt Int. **112**(3), 35–42 (2015)
24. Moghe, D.M., Kanase, S.: Effect of early intervention for trunk control in stroke patients. Indian J. Physiother. Occup. Ther. **11**(3), 177–182 (2017)

25. Buyukavci, R., Şahin, F., Sağ, S., Doğu, B., Kuran, B.: The impact of additional trunk balance exercises on balance, functional condition and ambulation in early stroke patients: randomized controlled trial. Turkish J. Phys. Med. Rehabil. **62**(3), 248–256 (2016)
26. Thomsen, G., Snow, G., Rodriguez, L., Hopkins, R.: Patients with respiratory failure increase ambulation after transfer to an intensive care unit where early activity is a priority. Crit. Care Med. **36**(4), 1119–1124 (2008)
27. Morris, P., et al.: Early intensive care unit mobility therapy in the treatment of acute respiratory failure. Crit. Care Med. **36**(8), 1–8 (2008)
28. Alexander, N.B., Grunawalt, J.C., Carlos, S., Augustine, J.: Bed mobility task performance in older adults. J. Rehabil. Res. Dev. **37**(5), 633–638 (2000)

"Making the Invisible Visible": Intelligent Recovery Monitoring of Aortic Arch Repair Surgery Proposal

Mercedes de Dios[1,4] ⓘ, David Mendes[3,4(✉)] ⓘ,
Sagrario G. Cantarino[2,4] ⓘ, and Margarida Sim Sim[3,4] ⓘ

[1] Health Service of Castilla-La Mancha (SESCAM),
Talavera de la Reina, Toledo, Spain
[2] ENDOCU Group, University School of Nursing and Physiotherapy Toledo
(Nursing, Pain and Care), Avda. Carlos III s/n., 45071 Toledo, Spain
[3] School of Nursing S. João de Deus, University of Evora,
Largo do Senhor da Pobreza, 7000-811 Évora, Portugal
dmendes@uevora.pt
[4] Castilla-La Mancha University,
Toledo. Avda. Carlos III, s/n, 45071 Toledo, Spain

Abstract. Thoracic pain is a very frequent reason for consultation in the primary care nursing consultation. However, when the healthcare professional is facing a patient with intense and tearing pain in the chest that induces him to think that he is facing a possible aortic dissection, then it is in an emergency where the patient requires immediate attention and a referral without loss of time to a cardiac surgery unit. This study aims to publicize the misfortunes that may occur in the patient during the recovery of aortic arch repair surgery. The results were obtained through the analysis of the clinical history of patients with aortic pathology, all of them operated in the cardiac surgery unit of the Virgen de la Salud Hospital of Toledo (CHT) Spain. We are proposing a continuous monitoring solution that can ascertain the life quality of patients that went arch repair surgery. Life quality is difficult to measure quantitatively. We suggest threshold levels for a complex dataset that, when considered simultaneously through data fusion techniques applied with reinforcement learning algorithms can have a numeric output for quality of life as a whole. In this groundbreaking paper, the fundaments of the ontological structure for data acquisition, model definition, data acquisition and reasoning based in deep learning techniques are introduced.

Keywords: Aortic arch · Postsurgical complications · Perfusion ·
Primary care · Nursing · Continuous monitoring · Ontology · Disease model ·
Reinforcement learning · Data fusion

1 Introduction

Thoracic pain is a very frequent reason for consultation in primary care (PC). Several studies carried out in this field reveal that, although chest pain is associated with serious pathologies, the most frequent etiology is usually a benign pathology, however, 2% of

© Springer Nature Switzerland AG 2019
J. García-Alonso and C. Fonseca (Eds.): IWoG 2018, CCIS 1016, pp. 173–184, 2019.
https://doi.org/10.1007/978-3-030-16028-9_16

these consultations is for serious pathology [1]. These include the acquired pathologies of the aorta: acute dissection, intramural hematoma, penetrating ulcer, aneurysms of the aorta and traumatic rupture. The etiology of these pathologies has changed throughout history, in ancient times they were traumatisms, in the 15th century it was the epidemic of syphilis and in the 18th century arteriosclerosis, being the most common etiology at present [2].

Today the control of modifiable cardiovascular risk factors: smoking, hypertension, diabetes, dyslipidemia, obesity, stress and sedentary lifestyle that influence the onset of arteriosclerosis, is a great burden of work and effort for primary care professionals as in hospital care. However, despite the efforts of professionals and prevention campaigns, today, patients still have not assumed as their own risk to their health to keep these factors out of healthy limits of risk [1, 2].

A patient with intense and tearing chest pain that does not change with postural changes or with respiratory movements, and also has asymmetry or absence of peripheral pulses with high blood pressure, can lead the healthcare professional to face an aortic dissection and, therefore, to an emergency, where the seconds count. To date, the coordination between primary care and hospital care with protocols of joint action and evacuation of the patient in the shortest possible time, have managed to reduce the possible complications associated with the emergency [1].

There are several classifications regarding the dissection and rupture of the aorta, it can be commented as DeBakey, in the year 1965 [3] classified the dissections in relation to the site of rupture of the intima and the extent of the dissection:

- Type I: the dissection begins in the ascending aorta extending to the arch and the descending aorta;
- Type II: the dissection affects only the ascending aorta, frequently occurs in the Marfan syndrome.
- Type III: subdivided into IIIa, the dissection begins distal to the left subclavian and extends to the diaphragm; and IIIb, in which the dissection extends to the abdominal aorta.

The Stanford classification proposed by Daily, also widely used, groups the dissection into two types: Type A affects the ascending aorta and Type B affects any segment of the distal aorta from the left subclavian outlet, without affecting the ascending aorta. However, the classification that is considered most useful at present is the one proposed by Crawford who classifies the dissection into: proximal, that which affects the intrapericardial aorta and may affect the arch; and the distal one that begins distal to the left subclavian artery and can retrogradely affect the aortic arch [4]. According to Torregrosa [5], the indication of surgical treatment of aortic arch aneurysm (AAA) dissection depends on the estimated risk of complications for the patient in relation to the surgical risk (Table 1).

In cerebral aortic surgery, cerebral protection is vital, because the Supra Aortic trunks (TSA) and the brain are exposed to a period of ischemia when the anterograde cerebral circulation is interrupted [7]. Then, the selective anterograde arterial perfusion described by Kazui, is the technique that best preserves cerebral metabolism by maintaining intracellular pH, enzymatic function and energy reserves. It also allows to extend the safety time of the stop, up to 80–100 min, the only potential drawback being

Table 1. Estimated risk of complications for the patient in relation to the surgical risk.

Classification	Affection
DeBakey Classification	
Type I	Ascending, crooked and descending aorta
Type II	Ascending aorta
Type III	Descending aorta
IIIa	Up to the diaphragm
IIIb	Below the diaphragm
Stanford classification	
Type A	Ascending aorta
Type B	Aorta from the left subclavian outlet
Crawford classification	
Proximal	Intrapericardial aorta to the arch
Distal	It starts distal to the subclavian artery left

Cardiac Surgery is a specialty that was developed in the second half of the 20th century. Aortic arch repair, nowadays, is performed in visceral circulatory arrest with moderate hypothermia; said surgical treatment is performed worldwide with excellent results. In order to reduce morbidity, mortality and achieve greater success in aortic arch repair surgery, changes have been required that respond to the needs of each historical stage and, in addition, have been necessary. A deep knowledge of the physiopathology of the cerebral circulation, of the surgical technique of perfusion, of the technical and technological advances in the control and preservation of brain tissue, of the repercussion of the cessation during some minutes of the systemic circulation in other organs and structures involved, as well as notoriously the evolution throughout the years [6].

the risk of tampering with the TSA, minimized after the modern techniques of individual reimplantation [8, 9]. The main causes of neurological damage are secondary to two main causes: cerebral hypoperfusion, and the existence of micro/macroembolisms. It has been found that during the Extracorporeal Circulation (ECC) there are alterations of the cerebral blood flow and platelet microcoagulae that can cause neurological lesions during the postoperative period. At present there are no conclusive studies on the cause and this can be related to intraoperative factors during the CEC (acid-base management, systemic flow, cerebral perfusion pressure, hematocrit, glycemic control, time of CPB, etc.) and/or with preoperative factors (diabetes, previous cerebrovascular disease, etc.) [8]. Therefore, while the anesthetic awakening occurs, it is very important to assess the presence of focal neurological deficits, as well as delay in said awakening.

The appearance of neurological sequelae ranges between 3% and 92%, depending on whether only major neurological lesions are considered or are included as such, mild neuropsychological deficits. So much is the variability that in some studies diffuse brain damage affects 80% of individuals undergoing CPB. Considering minor neurological manifestations, the alteration of the level of consciousness, concentration, memory, and learning, alteration of the character and the speed of visual-motor response. In addition, it produces a significant number of alterations manifested as psychiatric symptoms of the post-CEC delirium type, anxiety, depression [10, 11].

Hypothermia is the technique most commonly used to protect the Central Nervous System (CNS) when the perfusion of the organ most sensitive to ischemia is reduced. When the temperature is lowered, a decrease in brain metabolism is observed when enzymatic reactions are reduced, as well as the predicted minimum flow, increasing the period of tolerated ischemia.

The complete suppression of brain activity is a good indicator of the minimal cellular metabolic activity.

With hypothermia, the non-eflow phenomenon occurs: The microcirculation closes at the multifocal level, causing incomplete reperfusion. The cause is not known, but may involve increased blood viscosity, vasoconstriction, precapillary shunt with response to hypo-anoxia.

The reduction of cerebral metabolism and the reduction of surgical time are the two fundamental measures for brain protection. In any case, preservation of brain metabolism is not synonymous with brain protection, so the technique must be selected individually for each case.

Hypothermia slows down all biochemical processes and reactions, especially enzymatic reactions. There is a relationship with direct dependence between the degree of activity of biochemical reactions and temperature. The slowing down of metabolic activities significantly reduces the consumption of metabolic and oxygen substrates. Oxygen consumption can be considered as a measure of metabolic activity.

Chemists use the symbol Q10, defined as the increase or decrease in the speed of reactions or metabolic processes in relation to temperature, for a change of 10 °C. Most reactions, including oxygen consumption, have a Q10 of 2 to 3.

Michenfedler and Theyer showed that normal oxygen consumption in normothermia, which is $150/ml/min/m^2$, decreases up to 50% with moderate hypothermia of 28 °C and up to 30% with hypothermia of 25 °C. Approximately conclude that the oxygen consumption decreases exponentially around 9% for each degree of temperature reduction [10, 11].

The tolerance to ischemia is variable according to the different organs. The kidney can tolerate 50 to 60 min of ischemia, and the liver 20–30 min; however, the spinal cord and the brain are much more sensitive. The kidney and the liver have an enormous reserve and regeneration capacity that does not exist in the marrow or in the central nervous system.

Hypothermia can delay, but not prevent indefinitely, the appearance of structural metabolic changes that lead to a functional neurological deterioration.

At present, there are multiple studies, which analyze in detail the results of cardiac interventions from the technical point of view, focusing exclusively on the effectiveness of surgical, anesthetic and perfusion techniques. These studies provide such amount of data that sometimes the professional feels overwhelmed and bombed without knowing very well how the patient evolves at home.

To this day, people usually do not accept the terms: illness, aging, disability or death. Likewise, the perception they have about postoperative recovery is unreal, because in most cases the patient is unable to think about the possible surgical sequels, the bad condition that may occur after surgery, the limitations in his life work, but think about the complete restoration of the person's capacity, obviating that during the rest of his life he will be subject to controls and medical follow-ups. In addition, it is convenient to emphasize that medicine is a science subject to limitations and uncertainties, facts that lead, in multiple occasions, to the impossibility of curing a pathology which will force the person to live with a disability.

2 Objectives

To know the misfortunes that can happen to the patient during his/her recovery derived from the repair surgery of the aortic arch. Propose a methodology of measuring the QoL (quality of Life) when such misfortunes occur.

3 Methodology

3.1 Method

The surgical technique under study is reconstructive surgery of the aortic arch with moderate hypothermia, the period-investigated being between 2012 and 2015. The results were obtained through the analysis of the clinical history of patients with aortic pathology, operated in the cardiac surgery unit of the Hospital Virgen de la Salud (HVS) of Toledo, and whose postoperative was carried out in the Health Service of Castilla-la Mancha (SESCAM). For the search of results, all the surgeries that were carried out in this service were reviewed, all the visits that the patients made to the cardiac surgery service were reviewed until they were referred to the cardiology service, and all the visits they made to the cardiology service were analyzed in primary care during the recovery of said pathology. Therefore, it is a descriptive study of case series, longitudinal and retrospective.

3.2 Procedure

The review of the patient's history was carried out thanks to the joint work between hospital care and primary care. All the patients who made their recovery in the SESCAM were included in the study; therefore, the study excluded patients who, although undergoing surgery in the HVS cardiac surgery service, did not perform the postoperative period in Castilla la Mancha when they were residents of another autonomous community. Obviously, patients who did not achieve hospital discharge were excluded from the study.

3.3 Variables

The study focused on postoperative complications arising from repair surgery of the aortic arch, analyzing the immediate postoperative period, the first year of postoperative recovery and the period of time that elapses until the patient is referred to the HVS cardiology service.

3.4 Reference Population

The total number of patients studied was 25 (15 men and 10 women), whose mean age was 61.19 years (SD). During the first postoperative year, 3 patients died, a fact considered in the research as experimental progressive mortality. The death of both patients took place during the immediate postoperative period because of the complications derived from the surgery.

4 Monitoring the Patient

Evaluating the QoL is by itself a mischievous task. What are the parameters, features that influence the apparent QoL of any individual? Our proposal is trying to render such QoL measureable by definition and evaluation (monitoring) several characteristics that, when measured simultaneously, can confidently suggest a richer or poorer QoL. Many factors are subjective by themselves, mostly psychological issues and can only be measured by form filling of carefully crafted questionnaires. Some, however, when considered as information fusion [12, 13] can deliver some powerful insights into the absolute discomfort and, thus, QoL.

4.1 Measuring QoL (Quality of Life)

We intend to grab measureable sensor data to profile the ADL (activities of daily living), extract some patterns and compare them against a golden standard of comfortable living. That Golden Standard is built using QoL public datasets that render our comparison matrix. That matrix has to be compared to the monitored data using a multi feature threshold comparison technique that can't be described algorithmically. It can be, however, automatically built using the most recent Machine Learning (ML) techniques [14–16] for multi-perceptron using like Deep Learning [12, 17–20] using Recurrent Neural Networks (RNNs) enhanced by Reinforcement Learning [21, 22] using our monitored post chirurgical patients.

4.2 QoL Dataset

A usable dataset in what concerns to deep learning is a labeled set of features big enough to have subsets for training and validation, commonly referred as model development.

5 Deep and Reinforcement Learning Techniques

The proposed model development not only uses the bare data in the above referred dataset but has the knowledge complemented with the Elderly Virtual Model Ontology (EVMO) developed in the International Institute for Research and Innovation of the Elderly (4IE – Instituto Internacional de Investigação e Inovação do Envelhecimento). The ontology complements the dataset defining the "acceptable values" for the elderly living model. Those acceptable values, when considered in fusion, render a picture of a measureable QoL.

5.1 Data Fusion Thresholds

Threshold definition is automatically developed by the multi labeled classification machine that is produced by the DL RNN [20, 22, 23] and reinforced a posteriori by the continuous usage [21, 22].

6 Results

The analyzed documentation reveals that the preoperative diagnosis in 19 patients was type A acute aortic dissection, while in another 6 patients the diagnosis was thoracic aortic aneurysm without mention of rupture. In all surgeries, a dissection of the right axillary artery was carried out, a median sternotomy was performed and the ECC was performed with a centrifuge and membrane oxygenator. Of the 25 patients studied, complete CEC was established through cannulation of: right axillary artery, right atrium (atrial cavity) and coronary sinus, in 23 of them. In one patient, the axillary artery could not be cannulated due to inadequate caliber and tortuous path, with complete CPB being initiated through the cannulation of the distal ascending aorta, right atrium and coronary sinus. In another patient, due to hemodynamic instability, emergent surgery was started with partial ECC through cannulation of the right axillary artery and the femoral vein, once the patient was stabilized, complete ECC was performed through cannulation of the right atrium and of the coronary sinus.

In all cases, to reach an optimal circulatory stop with deep systemic hypothermia, a gradual decrease in temperature of 1 °C per minute was performed. Of the 25 patients under study, 12 reached the esophageal temperature of 25°, 4 of them reached 26°, and in the remaining 9, hypothermia only reached 28°. The surgical procedure analyzed was the repair of the aortic arch in visceral circulatory arrest and hypothermia; 16 patients underwent resection and replacement of thoracic vessels and replacement of the aortic valve. In the other 9 patients, thoracic vessels were resected with replacement. Cerebral perfusion (CP) during visceral circulatory arrest was performed following the protocol established in the HVS cardiac surgery service; 21 of them underwent visceral circulatory arrest with anterograde PC through both carotids and in the other 4 patients the CP was performed through the trunkbrachicephalic, left carotid and left subclavian.

The analysis of the results in relation to postoperative complications in the Cardiac Care Unit (CCU) showed that 4 patients presented acute renal failure with elevated creatinine. 8 patients presented respiratory failure requiring prolonged mechanical ventilation and tracheotomy. 5 patients presented temporary neurological dysfunction, 3 patients profuse hemorrhage that required transfusion of haemoderivatives and haemostatic, 13 patients presented fever of inflammatory origin with negative blood cultures and phase reactants in descending curve, 2 patients suffered cerebrovascular accident and one patient in the course of her immediate postoperative period had to be urgently intervened due to esophageal perforation secondary to a transesophageal echocardiographic study. None of the patients presented lesion in the skin that could be related to the adverse effect of controlled hypothermia (Table 2).

Table 2. Origins of skin lesions.

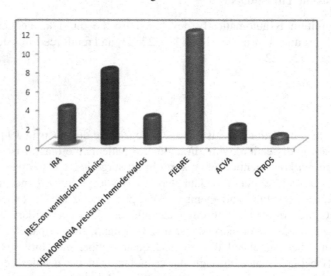

After reviewing all the documentation, it was observed in all patients that the closure of stereotomy and surgical wounds was performed in the primary care setting and therefore they did not present infection. All periodically go to their health center to perform the control of cardiovascular risk factors and to maintain the syntrom in therapeutic range, in addition it is observed that, one year after surgery, in four patients of the 25 studied, their postoperative course was without incidents.

Eight patients needed pharmacological treatment for paresthesia, musculoskeletal pain and vertigo, requiring referral to rehabilitation to treat pain with physiotherapy, even being a patient diagnosed with immobility syndrome, which motivated its institutionalization to be able to recover mobility.

In relation to infections occurred during the first year after surgery, three patients needed treatment for herpes Zoster.

The family doctor detected cognitive impairment in four patients, without there being any previous record of this alteration, it was in the course of his postoperative recovery where the deterioration arose.

All patients successfully underwent the annual postoperative control performed by the cardiac surgery service of the HVS. However, six of them, at present, remain in charge of the Vascular Surgery service of the HVS as a consequence of the pathologies associated with the descending thoracic aorta and the abdominal aorta. Four of this present intimal flap, which translates into vascularization problems in the arteries: mesenteric, celiac trunk and iliac arteries; and the other two people need placement of a thoracic stent due to associated pathologies.

Finally, the analysis reveals that eight patients needed to go to the psychiatry unit for evaluation of anxiety-depressive syndrome, five people are currently under treatment for depression and one of these eight people is institutionalized by autolysis attempt.

7 Discussion

Once the results were studied, it is observed that the fever of inflammatory origin stands out among the postoperative complications in the CCU. This complication described by Valenzuela [24], "Postoperative fever in the second and third days in patients with cardiac surgery, is accompanied by an increase in neutrophils, twice higher than the initial values", corresponds to the inflammatory response that It produces the contact of the blood with: the circuit of the ECC, oxygenator or the implanted prosthesis. The results support this theory because during the immediate postoperative period in all cases the blood cultures were negative and the reactants were in the phase of descending curve. The author says, "extracorporeal circulation can also cause susceptibility to infections." The CEC continues to be the trigger of the activation of neutrophils and consequently the cause of the alteration of the immune system after cardiac surgery. This explains in relation to the infection that no patient suffered a delay in the healing of the surgical wounds, although during the postoperative period three patients were diagnosed with Herpes Zoster made related to the alteration of immunity. The results of the study corroborate that the surgical asepsis standards established in the area of cardiac surgery, the protocols of action in relation to the patient during the stay in the unit, the vaccination campaign carried out in the health centers against influenza and pneumococcus in high-risk patients as well as the care carried out in primary care are adequate and of the highest quality.

Regarding mortality, as mentioned on page 2 of the document "the technical and technological advances in the control and preservation of brain tissue and other organs", make it possible for only one patient to die in the first two months of post-surgical recovery, due to a pump failure, fact that shows that: the surgical technique, the anesthetic techniques, as well as the perfusion techniques have reached very high quality and safety thresholds.

When studying the neurological sequelae it is important to remember that hypothermia has protective effects in the CNS; this statement, described on page 3 of the study, is supported by the results achieved, since only three patients suffered cognitive deterioration during their first year of postoperative recovery, and it is important to note that during the immediate postoperative period in the CCU only five patients suffered Temporary neurological dysfunction. This reality shows that antegrade arterial perfusion during surgery, together with the cerebral perfusion protocol used in the visceral circulatory arrest, protect the brain from possible neurological lesions associated with ischemia during repair of the aortic arch.

The study draws attention to the number of consultations made to his health center eight patients for the trinomial vertigo, paresthesia and musculoskeletal pain. These pathologies, although not serious, are generators of dissatisfaction on the part of the patient; the pain limits his movements and incapacitates him to carry out his activities of daily life, needing pharmacological treatment for the pain and even rehabilitation to mitigate the discomfort. However, it is possible to think that these pathologies are related: with the risk of perioperative injury when handling the patient during transfers from the bed to the surgical table and vice versa, with the position in the surgical table that can produce muscular distension in the scapular waist and neck; It may also be related to the surgical approach of the axillary artery, because the incision in the delto-pectoral sulcus can damage the branches of the brachial plexus and produce said trinomial. These results highlight the need to perform with great care all movements, manipulations and techniques practiced on the patient while remaining sedated and relaxed [25]. These simple actions would avoid many of the consultations that the patient makes to his health center, save money on treatments and ultimately provide a better quality of life to the patient.

The results obtained show that, during the postoperative recovery, the patient comes periodically to the health center to monitor their cardiovascular risk factors, shows adherence to the prescribed treatment and is able to carry out the recommendations prescribed by the health personnel. During the postoperative period, he becomes aware of the risk involved in not having the risk factors within limits and is ultimately responsible for his health. However, it should not be forgotten that the cardiovascular patient usually has a Type A and Type D personality pattern as described by Patrick [26], which corroborates that some patients in the study went to the psychiatric service because they presented anxiety-depressive syndrome. In addition, the results are faithfully adjusted to the following statement of the author "the negative affective state, which is a more general trait typified by negative emotional experiences, includes both anxiety and depression." and in relation to personality, the author says "Type D individuals experience more chronic levels of general discomfort, which are not easily detectable since they are not expressed." A statement that explains why a patient presents an attempt at autolysis even though he does not suffer severe complications, compared to another patient who still suffers multiple complications and is currently undergoing revision by vascular surgery. He does not need a referral to psychiatry, even though he is extremely fragile and vulnerable.

8   Conclusion

The research team considers that "Living with quality after repair of the aortic arch is a challenge subject to many misfortunes", so many that only four of the 25 patients studied managed to recover, which presupposes to the research team that living with quality was an achievable challenge. In addition, a patient of the 25, at present, is institutionalized by attempt of autolysis, what makes presuppose to the investigating team that this patient did not obtain the quality of life that he yearns.

Acknowledgements. To our patients, source of inspiration and wisdom. The work done with them provides us with the necessary knowledge to reduce their suffering and improve the quality of nursing care.

This work was supported by 4IE project (0045-4IE-4-P) funded by the Interreg V-A España-Portugal (POCTEP) 2014-2020 program by the European Regional Development Fund.

References

1. de Adana, R.: Manual de diagnóstico y terapéutica médica en atención primaria (2002)
2. Gosálbez Jordá, F., Llosa Cortina, J.C.: Principios de cirugía cardíaca. Universidad de Oviedo, Servicio de Publicaciones, Oviedo (2002)
3. Debakey, M.E., Henly, W.S., Cooley, D.A., Morris, G.C., Crawford, E.S., Beall, A.C.: Surgical management of dissecting aneurysms of the aorta. J. Thorac. Cardiovasc. Surg. **49**, 130–149 (1965)
4. Ricardo, F.J.N., et al.: Enfermedades de la Aorta y Vasos Periféricos Disección y hematoma aórtico Diagnóstico y tratamiento de la enfermedad vascular periférica Intervencionismo y endoprótesis Aneurismas de la aorta toracica descendente y toracoabdominales. Presented at the (2012)
5. Puerta, S., Martínez, F., Argudo, J.: Cirugía de los aneurismas del arco aórtico. Cir. Cardiovasc. **14**, 321–330 (2007). https://doi.org/10.1016/S1134-0096(07)70238-3
6. Mestres, C., Domenech, A.: Cirugía cardiovascular, pasado, presente y futuro. Rev. Fed. Arg. Cardiol. **44**, 57–63 (2015)
7. Suárez Gonzalo, L., García De Lorenzo y Mateos, A., Suárez Álvarez, J.R.: Lesiones neurológicas durante la circulación extracorpórea: fisiopatología, monitorización y protección neurológica. Med. Intens. **26**, 292–303 (2002)
8. Díez Castro, R., Reta Ajo, L., Rubia Martín, M., González Santos, J.M.: Perfusión cerebral y sistémica simultáneas en cirugía de arco aórtico con hipotermia moderada. In: XVII Congreso Asociacion Española de Perfusionistas, Sevilla (2012)
9. Griepp, R.B.: Cerebral protection during aortic arch surgery. J. Thorac. Cardiovasc. Surg. **121**, 425–427 (2001). https://doi.org/10.1067/MTC.2001.113594
10. Gomar Sancho, C., Mata, M.T., Pomar, J.L., Asociación Española de Perfusionistas: Fisiopatología y técnicas de circulación extracorpórea. Ergón (2012)
11. Rubio-Regidor, M., Pérez-Vela, J., Escriba-Barcena, A.: Complicaciones neurológicas en el postoperatorio de cirugia cardiaca. Med. Intens. **31**, 241–250 (2007)
12. Banos, O., et al.: Multi-sensor fusion based on asymmetric decision weighting for robust activity recognition. Neural Process. Lett. **42** (2015). https://doi.org/10.1007/s11063-014-9395-0
13. Gravina, R., Alinia, P., Ghasemzadeh, H., Fortino, G.: Multi-sensor fusion in body sensor networks: state-of-the-art and research challenges (2016). https://doi.org/10.1016/j.inffus.2016.09.005
14. Domingos, P.: The Master Algorithm: How the Quest for the Ultimate Learning Machine Will Remake Our World. Basic Books, New York (2015)
15. Goodman, K.: Ethics, Medicine, and Information Technology: Intelligent Machines and the Transformation of Health Care. Cambridge University Press, Cambridge (2015)

16. Catal, C., Tufekci, S., Pirmit, E., Kocabag, G.: On the use of ensemble of classifiers for accelerometer-based activity recognition. Appl. Soft Comput. J. **37** (2015). https://doi.org/10.1016/j.asoc.2015.01.025
17. Shoaib, M., et al.: Fusion of smartphone motion sensors for physical activity recognition. Sensors **14**, 10146–10176 (2014). https://doi.org/10.3390/s140610146
18. Rusk, N.: Deep learning. Nat. Methods **13**, 35 (2011). https://doi.org/10.1038/nmeth.3707
19. Hassan, M.M., Uddin, M.Z., Mohamed, A., Almogren, A.: A robust human activity recognition system using smartphone sensors and deep learning. Futur. Gener. Comput. Syst. **81** (2018). https://doi.org/10.1016/j.future.2017.11.029
20. Arifoglu, D., Bouchachia, A.: Activity recognition and abnormal behaviour detection with recurrent neural networks. Procedia Comput. Sci. **110**, 86–93 (2017)
21. Sutton, R.S., Barto, A.G.: Reinforcement learning: an introduction. IEEE Trans. Neural Netw. **9**, 1054 (1998). https://doi.org/10.1109/tnn.1998.712192
22. Schmidhuber, J.: Deep Learning in neural networks: an overview (2015)
23. Park, S.U., Park, J.H., Al-masni, M.A., Al-antari, M.A., Uddin, M.Z., Kim, T.-S.: A depth camera-based human activity recognition via deep learning recurrent neural network for health and social care services. Procedia Comput. Sci. **100**, 78–84 (2016). https://doi.org/10.1016/j.procs.2016.09.126
24. Valenzuela-Flores, A., Valenzuela-Flores, A.: Alteraciones fisiopatólogicas secundarias a circulación extracorpórea en cirugía cardíaca. Cir. Cir. **73**, 143–149 (2005)
25. de Dios Aguado, M.M.: Plan de cuidados de enfermería quirúrgica. Enferm. Cient. **250–251**, 57–61 (2003)
26. Smith, P.J., Blumenthal, J.A.: Aspectos psiquiátricos y conductuales de la enfermedad cardiovascular: epidemiología, mecanismos y tratamiento. Rev. Española Cardiol. **64**, 924–933 (2011). https://doi.org/10.1016/J.RECESP.2011.06.003

Study of the Innovative Characteristics of a New Technology for Bladder and Intestinal Elimination: An Empirical Study for the Evaluation of Ease of Use and Perceived Utility

Joana Parreira[1] , Daniela Fernandes[2] , Lisete Mónico[2] ,
Anabela Salgueiro-Oliveira[3] , Liliana Sousa[4] ,
Paulo Santos Costa[4] , Inês Marques[4] , Daniel Ventura[3],
Mónica Silva[3], Arménio Cruz[4] , César Fonseca[5] ,
Rafael Bernardes[4] , Carla Carvalho[2] , Luciene Braga[6] ,
and Pedro Parreira[4(✉)]

[1] Polytechnic School of Leiria, Leiria, Portugal
[2] Faculty of Psychology and Education Sciences of Coimbra University,
Coimbra, Portugal
[3] Nursing School of Coimbra, 3046-851 Coimbra, Portugal
[4] The Health Sciences Research Unit: Nursing, 3000-232 Coimbra, Portugal
parreira@esenfc.pt
[5] Nursing School of Évora, Évora, Portugal
[6] Medicine and Nursing Department of Federal University of Viçosa,
Viçosa, Brazil

Abstract. Background: Bedpans are medical devices usually used in the healthcare delivery to bedridden patients which health condition implies that bladder and/or intestinal elimination is done in bed. Physical and psychological discomfort experienced by patients in these situations it's a challenge to professionals to look for innovative proposals, looking for the reduction of negative impacts in many levels.

Objective: To evaluate the acceptance, by general population of (i) classical bedpans currently in the market and (ii) an inflatable proposal based on the Technology Acceptance Model. **Method:** The sample included 108 participants, aged between 19 and 81 years, caretakers/users of bedpans. The Technology Acceptance Model was used to evaluate the perception of utility and ease of use. All participants completed an online self-response questionnaire, later submitted to Exploratory Factor Analysis and Confirmatory and reliability study. **Results:** The results allow indicating a high degree of acceptance for the value proposition of the innovative bedpan, compared to the classic model. **Conclusion:** This study constitutes an important contribution to the human sciences, since it allows evaluating the ease of use and utility by users of bedpans, evidencing the importance of the innovative characteristics proposed to the new inflated bedpan.

© Springer Nature Switzerland AG 2019
J. García-Alonso and C. Fonseca (Eds.): IWoG 2018, CCIS 1016, pp. 185–200, 2019.
https://doi.org/10.1007/978-3-030-16028-9_17

Keywords: Classic bedpan · Insufflate bedpan ·
Technology Acceptance Model · Healthcare technology · Medical device

1   Introduction

The development of health promotion strategies is crucial as they build on the process by which people are empowered to improve their health and increase control over health, as advocated by the World Health Organization (WHO) in 1984 [1]. As regards to health professionals, this strategy should also be promoted through the creation of favorable environments [2], whether at home or in hospital. Hence, the mobilization of expertise linked to innovation is a key strategy to improve the quality of life of patients who need to regularly use the bedpans, promoting the health of bedridden patients, thus contributing to the development of a more favorable environment.

1.1   The Medical Device – Bedpans

According to the PORDATA (Portugal Contemporary Database), in Portugal in the year 2015/2016 there were 331.9 beds per 100.000 inhabitants, which makes a total of 34.522 beds in Portuguese hospitals [3]. Of these, a percentage of 25% of bedridden patients was calculated, making 8.630 beds with patients requiring a bedpan, estimating four patient/bed to cope with cleaning and disinfection times, making a total of 34.522 bedpans.

Bedpans are medical devices that are used to provide care for people who are bedridden and in homecare situations [5], who suffer from various clinical conditions that, by compromising their physical and/or mental state, limit their mobility or by clinical indication of bed rest due to safety concerns, long-term diseases, conduction of exams, or even for safety reasons.

In terms of comfort and accident prevention, bedpans with appropriate ergonomic characteristics are required. Already in the 1970s, Gibson [4] pointed out that bedpans should be ergonomically acceptable in order to ensure adequate levels of comfort and well-being in patients and should be a simple, effective, safe and harmless to be used by health professionals. We found that conventional bedpans are constructed from metal or hard plastic, with the purpose of being reused, after being properly washed and disinfected [5].

However, there have been numerous difficulties experienced by patients using them. The use of bedpans made of hard and cold plastic, and the need to raise the body before placing them, indicates inconvenience and discomfort.

A study by Mag, Werner and Saxer [6] aimed to describe patients' experiences when using the intensive care bedpans. Most felt very dependent on other people. Patients frequently reported pain and reported that the bedpans were cold and had hard surfaces and also reported having to assume uncomfortable positions. They also pointed out that health professionals feel the task difficult and uncomfortable, often because of a standardized size, not adapting to all patients. Difficulties in removing the bedpan without littering the bed are also referred to as one of the problems [6].

1.2   An Innovative Proposal of Inflatable Bedpan

Over time, some models with inflatable characteristics were developed to improve patient comfort. For example, some researchers [7] have developed a prototype of an inflatable body support for the use of bedpans [US4207633 (A)]. This inflatable body support is intended to facilitate the use of bedpans or access to the pelvic or anal area of the bedridden or wheelchair user. The prototype comprises a U-shaped inflatable hip support pad that occupies a space for receiving a bedpan or sanitary absorbent material when the hip support pad is inflated. It also incorporates a lumbar support cushion that is separately inflated. A waterproof flexible sheet extends under the hip support cushion and prevents any spilled matter from littering the bed.

In 1993, Royal [8] patented a disposable inflatable bedpan [patent US5224223 (A)], consisting of thermoplastic material. When inflated, it can withstand high pressure, supporting the weight of the bedridden patient. This device is larger than the conventional metallic wiper, providing more stability to the patient, in addition to presenting a collar that surrounds the seating area. The device has a wedge-shaped extension to support the lumbar region of a patient who cannot sit on it, and should wear it in the prone position. The remainder of the invention consisted of an absorbent pad inserted into the container, containing an odor suppressant, preferable activated by the presence of body fluids.

In 2008, an inflatable bedpan was developed [patent CN201108556 (Y)], the structure of which comprises a U-shaped inflation pad. It contains a channel for collecting and holding the squatting tray. In comparison with the primary technique, the inflatable casket frame has convenient usability characteristics, preventing patient cooling.

More recently, in 2016, a bedpan was developed [patent CN204972015 (U)], especially for post-operative patients, to give support to the lumbar vertebrae, including the pelvic floor and the basin limit. The utility model reveals that it does not need to be lifted to the patient's buttock, thus maintaining the stability of the lumbar vertebrae, removing discomfort during intestinal elimination. Thus, constipation can be prevented, improving the level of comfort and quality of life of the patient.

1.3   Innovative Proposal – Inflatable Bedpan: Innovative Features and Competitive Advantages

The product under development will have a reduced height, to facilitate its placement underneath the patient. Thereafter, the device will be inflated (by connecting the device to the compressed air ramps present in the tops of bed headboards of any hospital room). After the satisfaction of the fundamental human need for elimination, the bedpan is removed, and then deflated and cleaned (through sterilization by autoclaving), which will occupy a smaller space, allowing a greater number of bedpans available in the same physical space.

The target audience for this new proposal are patients who are bedridden with greater mobility and movement difficulties. The simplicity of the value proposition is based on the technical characteristics developed and the apparent ease of use, showing some advantages for patients with greater difficulty in mobilization or with greater functional limitations, as well as for the healthcare professionals (e.g., easier placement, less physical effort).

In general, the inflatable bedpan has the following advantages: (i) greater flexibility in presenting a moldable material, adapting to the patient's body, reducing the risk of friction and shear pressure ulcers (as for example with classic sweepers); (ii) the need for less physical effort in the positioning of the non-collaborative patient by health professionals, reducing the risk of low back pain in health professionals, contributing to the reduction of absenteeism rates; (iii) it is an environmentally friendly product; (iv) it takes advantage of waste from other polymers (recyclable); (v) is a reusable product; (vi) it's not aggressive to the patient's skin, since its surface has no edges or sharp edges; (vii) integrates "hot" materials and therefore is not a cold surface contrasting with the classic bedpan, therefore being more comfortable for the patient; (viii) supports high weights due to its ability to withstand high pressures with high elasticity; (ix) can be sterilized by wet heat; (x) integrates a deodorant incorporated through nanotechnology, reducing/neutralizing unpleasant odors for the patient and neighbors, which can positively impact the patient, reducing general embarrassment; (xi) it's more economical if acquired on a large scale; (xii) allows connection to a compressed air ramp, present in all hospital units; (xiii) facilitates the correct mobility and positioning of patients when they present physical limitations or presentation to mobilization; (xix) reduces hospital costs. In general, this value proposition can have a positive impact on the political, economic, social, technological, environmental, physical and mental health of patients, and health professionals.

1.4   The Technology Acceptance Model – TAM

In the last decades, multiple approaches have been used based on different models to evaluate the technology acceptance [9]. We especially note the Technology Acceptance Model (TAM), the Theory of Innovation Adoption (TIA), the Innovation Diffusion Theory (TDI), the Innovation Diffusion Theory (TDI) [10].

Recently, derivations of the TAM model have emerged, such as TAM2 [11, 12], Technology Readiness Acceptance Model (TRAM) and Unified Theory of Acceptance and Use of Technology (UTAUT) [9, 13].

The TAM (Technology Acceptance Model) model was proposed by Davis [14] in 1989 [14]. It aims to evaluate the acceptance of the technology by the future users, focusing on two fundamental dimensions: (i) perceived utility (PU), which seeks to understand to what extent the person believes that the use of technology will contribute to improving the performance [14], and (ii) perceived ease of use (PEU), regarding the degree to which the person believes that the use of the new system will be effortless [14]. Both dimensions have a positive influence on Behavioral Intent (BI) to use this new technology [15, 16].

The TAM model is one of the most used models to evaluate, explain or predict the acceptance of new technologies by possible users of this technology to implement [17]. The TAM model has also been used to improve understanding and acceptance of new services. It is thus considered one of the most powerful models regarding the ability to predict the acceptance by different groups about the context technology and/or service to be tested, being used in different contexts. Thus, to evaluate the acceptance of the technology, different dimensions inscribed in the TAM model can be evaluated, besides the commonly evaluated dimensions – Utility and Ease of Use. The TUAUT model

(Unified Theory of Acceptance and Use of Technology) (see Fig. 1) consists of an evolution of the TAM model, in which the acceptance by the end user of the technology appears inscribed within an integrated perspective, where new dimensions emerge: (i) expectation of its performance; (ii) expectation of effort; (iii) social influence and (iv) facilitating conditions. This new model presents 20 to 30% increase in explanatory power relative to TAM, which presents on average 40 to 50% of explanatory power over the behavior of the end user or the behavioral intention to use the technology [9, 13].

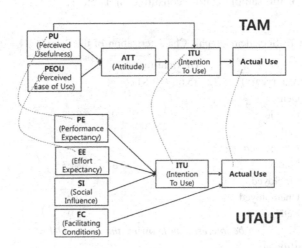

Fig. 1. TAM Model (Technology Acceptance Model) and UTAUT Model (Unified Theory of Acceptance and Use of Technology) [13].

2 Method

2.1 Search Strategy and Study Identification

This article, being part of a research project called "Inflatable Bedpan", intends to evaluate the potential of innovation in terms of the usefulness and ease of use related to a medical device – inflatable bedpan, by health professionals and users of bedpans, aiming to evaluate their acceptance by the market. To do so, a brief questionnaire was developed, based on the Technology Acceptance Model (TAM) [14], presented as a Likert scale.

The questionnaire intends to evaluate the following dimensions: (i) perceived utility (PU); (ii) perceived ease of use (PEU); (iii) subjective norm (SN); (iv) technological readiness (TR); (v) attitude (A); (vi) perceived behavioral control (PHC); (vii) intention of use/behavioral intension (IU/BI); (viii) experiment (E); (ix) image (I); (x) design (D); and (xi) innovative capacity (IC).

2.2   Data Synthesis

The sample of the present study is non-probabilistic of convenience. It comprises 108 participants, of both sexes (84.3% female and 15.7% male), aged between 19 and 81 years (M = 35.12, SD = 15.65). Regarding the professional status, 34.3% are students, 63% are employed, and 0.9% unemployed and 1.9% are retired. About 72.2% care for or have cared for someone in bed; 61.1% were hospitalized and 42.6% of the respondents needed to use a bedpan. Of the total sample, 95.4% of the respondents would be interested in knowing the new model of the bedpan. The sociodemographic characterization of the sample can be consulted in Table 1.

Table 1. Sociodemographic Characterization of the Sample [N = 108]

	M	DP (min-max.)	n	%
Age (years)	35.12	15.65 (19-81)		
Genre				
Female			91	84.3
Male			17	15.7
Professional status				
Student			37	34.3
Employed			68	63
Unemployed			1	0.9
Retires			2	1.9
Would you be interested in knowing the new model of dragging?				
Yes			103	95.4
No			5	4.6
Do you care or have you taken care of someone in bed?				
Yes			78	72.2
No			30	27.8
Have you ever been hospitalized?				
Sim			66	61.1
Não			42	38.9
Length of hospitalization (days)		14.16	51.49 (0–365)	
Have you ever had a bedpan?				
Yes			46	42.6
No			62	57.4

2.3   Instrument and Proceedings

The sample was collected through an online questionnaire, sent through the network of researchers who integrate nursing, physical therapy, psychology students and citizens who contact bedridden patients. The questionnaire, formulated by the research team, was available during one month and was open to the public, covering questions related to the classic bedpans present in the market and questions related to the characteristics to be incorporated in the new model. It was created through a panel of four experts, made up of doctorates and masters in the areas of Health, Management and Psychology. In addition to assessing respondents' satisfaction regarding the different types of bedpans and their characteristics, the questionnaire aimed to evaluate questions regarding the usability and satisfaction of the respondents of the classic bedpan and about the new proposal of value in development. It includes data on sociodemographic and personal experiences related to previous contacts with the use of a bedpan, whether related to a use by one's own by third parties. The collection of data and the procedures used have respected the ethical and deontological requirements inherent to such an investigation, guaranteeing the anonymity and confidentiality of individual responses. Before completing the questionnaire, an explanation was given to the participants about the goals, the context in which it is inserted, its confidential nature, as well as the anonymity of the data obtained.

2.4 Data Analysis

The research is of a non-experimental nature [18]. The data was analyzed with the Statistical Package for the Social Sciences (SPSS) version 22.0 and the Analysis of Moment Structures (Amos) version 22.0. The existence of outliers was evaluated by the quadratic distance of Mahalanobis [19], and no relevant extreme values were found.

Prior to conducting the factorial analysis (exploratory and confirmatory), a panel of experts was created to classify the questionnaire items, taking into account the two fundamental dimensions of the TAM model: ease of use and perceived utility. Then, the distribution of items by seven response options on a Likert scale (from 1 = unsatisfied to 7 = fully satisfied) was analyzed. The relative frequencies confirmed that the items were distributed across all response options of the scale, none of which significantly absorbed more than 50% responses.

The exploratory factorial analysis (EFA) was performed through a Principal Component Analysis (PCA) with SPSS version 22.0 with the entire sample. The assumptions of a correct PCA were tested through the sample size (N > 100 subjects), the normality and linearity of the variables, as well as the outliers, R- lettering and sample suitability [19]. We have chosen to use the Varimax rotation method, since we want to obtain as many different factors as possible.

In order to perform the EFA we followed the recommendations of Bryman and Cramer [20] and Gorsuch [21], authors who consider that at least the sample is required to consist of 100 participants, the number of observations per item should be higher than 10 and the relation between the number of participants and the number of items should not be less than 3:1, which was verified in our sample. Confirmatory factorial analyzes (CFA) were done with AMOS version 22.0 [22]. The maximum likelihood estimation method was used. The composite reliability and the mean variance extracted for each factor were analyzed as described in Fornell and Larcker [23]. The existence of outliers was evaluated by the quadratic distance of Mahalanobis [19], eliminating four outliers, corresponding to the highest quadratic distance of Mahalanobis (p < 0.001). The normality of the variables was analyzed by the coefficients of asymmetry (Sk) and kurtosis (Ku). None of the variables presented values of Sk and Ku that could indicate violations of the normal distribution, being that we obtained coefficients of $|Sk| < 2.0$ and of $|Ku_{univariate}| < 5.2$.

The quality of the overall adjustment of the factorial models was done by the NFI (Norma – Normed of Fit Index, good adjustment > 0.80) [24]; SRMR (Standardized Root Mean Square Residual; appropriate adjustment > 0.90) [25], CFI (Comparative Fit Index, good adjustment > 0.90) [26], RMSEA (Root Mean Square Error of Approximation, good adjustment < 0.05, acceptable adjustment < 0.08) [24, 27, 28] and X^2/gl (acceptable adjustment < 5; good adjustment < 2) [24, 28].

The refinement of the model adjustment was done by the modification indexes [29]. We followed the suggestion of Arbuckle [22], which indicates the analysis of the IMs by their statistical significance, considering the value of $\alpha = 0.05$. Another criterion used was centered in Marôco [28], which suggests that the parameter modification with IM higher than 11 ($p < 0.001$) is safer.

Reliability was assessed by calculating the Cronbach's Alpha coefficient [30], both for the global scale and for the constituent dimensions of each scale. We followed the indication of Hair, Anderson, Tatham, and Lack [31], which refers coefficients of internal consistency higher than 0.70 to indicate adequate convergence and internal consistency. Among other authors, Hill and Hill [32] point to the value of 0.80 as an indicator of good internal consistency. The composite reliability and the mean variance extracted for the extracted factors were analyzed as described in Fornell and Larcker [23].

3   Results

3.1   Descriptive Statistics

Descriptive statistics were initially carried out regarding the characteristics of classic bedpans (Table 2), which allowed us to evaluate the degree of average satisfaction in each of the characteristics present in these bedpans. It can be observed that, on a seven-point Likert scale, the respondents presented mean values significantly with the characteristics of the classic bedpan, especially with regard to patient comfort, odor and privacy, with mean values of M = 2.67, 2.67 and 2.63, respectively. It should be noted that stainless steel bedpans are considered more uncomfortable.

Table 2. Descriptive statistics about classic bedpan's characteristics (N = 108)

Characteristics	Min.	Max.	M	DP
p1_a – Comfort provided to the patient	1	7	**2.67**	1.45
p1_b – Odor	1	7	**2.67**	1.39
p1_c – Bedpan's height	1	7	2.78	1.42
p1_d – Provided privacy	1	7	**2.63**	1.63
p1_e – Safety for the patient	1	7	3.46	1.61
p1_f – Used material (metal bedpan)	1	7	2.69	1.62
p1_g – Material used (plastic bedpan)	1	7	3.18	1.48
p1_h – Ease of placement	1	7	2.89	1.52
p1_i – Ease of removing	1	7	2.80	1.48

Next, the overall satisfaction level for a classic bedpan's characteristics was calculated. Between a mean minimum value of one point and a maximum of 6.67, we found a score of M = 2.86 (SD = 1.13), marking a general satisfaction. This result allows us to conclude that the level of satisfaction with conventional bedpans is very low, indicating users' dissatisfaction and pointing out problems to deal with bedridden patients.

The same procedures were repeated with respect to the characteristics to be incorporated in the new bedpan to be developed (see Table 3). When evaluating the satisfaction with the characteristics of the bedpans to be included in this value proposal, there is an evident discrepancy, denoting mean values well above the midpoint of the scale, indicating more satisfactory characteristics, namely with regard to comfort, to relieve the load of who places them and withdraws them and their easy placement in the patient. The mean value of satisfaction with the characteristics of the new bedpan to be developed was M = 6.07 (SD = 0.98), a value very close to the maximum value, evidencing a high degree of acceptance/satisfaction with the new characteristics to be incorporated.

Table 3. Descriptive statistics relative to the characteristics to incorporate to the bedpan in development (N = 108)

Characteristics	Min.	Max.	M	DP
P2_a - Provide minimum height for easy placement	2	7	5.77	1.27
P2_b - Allow to be inflated (reaching the desired height)	2	7	5.85	1.36
P2_c - Being moldable to the body	2	7	6.32	1.11
P2_d - Be easy to place on the patient	2	7	**6.33**	1.03
P2_e - Be reusable	1	7	5.29	1.76
P2_f - Present odor reduction (built-in deodorant)	3	7	6.01	1.24
P2_g - Be more comfortable	3	7	**6.36**	1.07
P2_h - Allow sterilization	1	7	6.23	1.20
P2_i - Being recyclable	1	7	5.94	1.52
P2_j - Relieve the burden to those who put them	2	7	**6.32**	1.17
P2_k - Relieve the burden to those who remove them	2	7	**6.32**	1.15
P2_l - Reduce hospital costs	3	7	6.07	1.26
Global Score	2.83	7.00	6.07	0.98

When comparing the satisfaction with the characteristics of the classic bedpans with the satisfaction of the new characteristics to incorporate, we denote an acceptance by the new characteristics to the detriment of the classic bedpans.

3.2   Exploratory Factorial Analysis

In order to evaluate the dimensionality of the items indicative of the characteristics to be incorporated in the new bedpan, an Exploratory Factorial Analysis (EFA) was chosen. All requirements for a reliable interpretation of Principal Component Analysis (PCA) have been met. It was found that the intercorrelations matrix differed from the identity matrix in that the Bartlett test indicated a $\Sigma 2$ (66) = 1282.31, p < 0.001 and sampling was adequate, since the value obtained for the Kaiser-Meyer-Olkin (KMO) measurement was greater than 0.70 (KMO = 0.891).

Both the *eigenvalue* criterion superior to the unit and the scree plot indicated the retention of two factors, responsible for 74.07% of the total variance. The first factor explained 43.88% of the total variance and added items referring to the ease of use of the bedpan, so we called it EU – Ease of Use. The second factor explained 30.19% of the total variance and, since it refers to the utility that the respondent attributes to the characteristics that the device presents, was designated PU – Perceived Utility.

The factorial saturations and the commonalities (h^2) of each of the considered factors are presented in Table 4 and are arranged in descending order of magnitude within each factor. We found that the vast majority of items saturate their factor above the recommended value of s > 0.45 [19], being the lowest value of 0.604 and the highest value of 0.918.

The coefficient of internal consistency of Cronbach (see Table 4), presented an indicative value of excellent reliability, both for the FU – Facility of Use (α = .944) and for the UP – Perceived Utility (α = .874), both were already superior to 0.80 [30].

In the study concerning the number of factors to be retained, the Kaiser criterion (*eigenvalues* greater than one) was followed, and also the Cattell criterion, considering also criteria directly related to its degree of interpretability. An PCA was performed and the orthogonal varimax rotation was performed and a two- factor solution emerged according to the theoretical model TAM, which supported the creation of the instrument. The varimax rotation was selected to simplify the interpretation of the factors, minimizing the number of variables with high saturations in each factor.

From the refinement process, in order to give meaning, coherence and interpretability and considering only factorial saturations above 0.50, a matrix with two factors that explain 74.07% of the total variance resulted. The empirically generated dimensions are globally according to the TAM model. The retained items saturate properly in the dimensions to which they belong, presenting a positive value which indicates that the higher the value, the higher the respondents' acceptance of the dimension in question. Thus, the first factor called "Ease of Use" (EU) explains, 43.88% of the variance and the second factor "Perceived Utility" (PU) explains 30.19% of the variance (see Table 4).

Table 4. Influential bedpan questionnaire: percentage of explained variance, factorial saturations, commonalities (h^2) and internal consistencies of the dimensions "Ease of Use" (EU) and "Perceived Utility" (PU)

	Factor		
	FU 43.88%	UP 30.19%	h^2
p2_c - Being moldable to the body	.918		.858
p2_d - Be easy to place on the patient	.875		.832
p2_g - Be more comfortable	.832		.803
p2_k - Relieve the burden to those who remove them	.809		.821
p2_j - Relieve the burden to those who put them	.799		.818
p2_a - Provide minimum height for easy placement	.740		.615
p2_b - Allow to be inflated (reaching the desired height)	.724		.650
p2_i - Being recyclable	.876		.823
p2_e - Be reusable		.816	.688
p2_h - Allow sterilization		.811	.758
p2_l - Reduce hospital costs		.659	.647
p2_f - Present odor reduction (built-in deodorant)		.604	.575
Eigenvalues:	5.27	3.62	
% explained variance	43.88	30.19	
Cronbach Alpha	.944	.874	
M (DP)	6.18 (1.01)	5.90 (1.15)	

3.3 Confirmatory Factor Analysis

The Confirmatory Factor Analysis (CFA) performed on the two-dimensional structure obtained in the PCA showed some fragility in the SRMR, TLI, IFC and RMSEA adjustment indices (Table 5, model 1). Thus, based on the highest modification indices within and with each factor, the errors associated to the observed variables were correlated. The quality of the adjustment of the model improved, showing an excellent adjustment of the NFI, TLI, CFI indexes, an acceptable adjustment of the SRMR and χ^2/gl indices, while an inadequate adjustment considering the RMSEA index (cf. indexes of adjustment of the model 2 in Table 5).

The composite good reliability (FC) obtained in both factors (FC = .938 for F1 and FC = .890 for F2), both of them exceeding the value of 0.70 [31].

The extracted mean variance (EMV) for Factor 1 was EMV = 0.72 and for Factor 2 of 0.58, being above 0.50, a value equal to or above which, it is considered an acceptable value for the extracted variance [33], illustrating the existence of convergent validity in the constituent items of each factor [23]. The calculation of the coefficient of determination between the factors (R2 = .67) suggests that we are in the presence of discriminant validity for Factor 1, since the proportion of variance extracted in this factor exceeded the square of the correlations between both factors [23].

The graphical representation of the estimated one-dimensional model is shown in Fig. 2. The standardized regression coefficients ranged from 0.60 to 0.99.

Table 5. Adjustment indices obtained in the confirmatory factor analysis of the Inflatable Bedpan Questionnaire

Model	NFI	SRMR	TLI	CFI	χ^2/gl	RMSEA	RMSEA confidence interval 90%
1	.827	.091	.823	.858	4.57*** (gl = 53)	.186	.163–.210*
2	.916	.074	.926	.947	2.67*** (gl = 48)	.120	.093–.148*

* $p < .001$

AFC Modelo TAM;X2(47)=117,267; p=,000; X2/df=2,495;CFI=,947; GFI=,842 ;RMSEA=,120; P(rmsea<.05)=,000; IC90%],093; ,148[

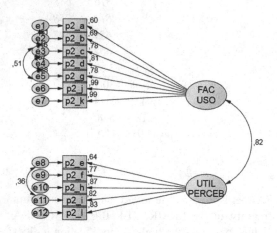

Fig. 2. Model 2, estimated for the Inflatable Bedpan Questionnaire: Standardized Regression Coefficients (λ) and proportions of variance explained (R2)

4 Discussion

The results of this study were in agreement with the advantages presented by the authors, especially regarding the comfort, ease of placement and lower physical load for those responsible for their placement (e.g., health professionals), by correctly positioning bedridden patients without the potential to assist in the placement of the bedpan.

In order to fulfill the above mentioned objective, an exploratory and confirmatory factorial analysis was carried out on the items of a questionnaire that aimed to evaluate the degree of satisfaction regarding several bedpan characteristics, classic and inflatable (innovative proposal in the present manuscript).

When evaluating the average degree of satisfaction in each of the characteristics present in the classic bedpans, we can conclude that the respondents present a global dissatisfaction, especially with regard to patient comfort, odor and privacy. The overall satisfaction level presented, related to the characteristics of classic drawers, is also low, reinforcing a lack of satisfaction on the part of the users. It's possible to verify this, since the average global value with classic bedpans was 2.86, in a scale ranging from 1–7 values. We can also note that the dissatisfaction with the classic stainless bedpans presents higher values of dissatisfaction than the classic plastic drawers.

When evaluating the satisfaction of the characteristics of the product that we intend to develop (the inflatable bedpan), we can verify more positive evaluations, therefore, more satisfactory, with respect to the classic bedpans, namely with regard to the comfort, to relieve the load of the one who places them and withdraws and easy placement on the patient. When the overall satisfaction with this product was evaluated, there was a high level of satisfaction on the part of the population, since the average value obtained was very close to the maximum value (6.07, on a scale of 1–7).

When comparing the satisfaction with the characteristics of the classic bedpans with the satisfaction of the new characteristics to incorporate, we denote an acceptance by the new characteristics to the detriment of the classic bedpans.

With the accomplishment of the factorial analyzes it was possible to retain the items of the scale in two factors: (i) ease of Use (EU) and (ii) Perceived Utility (PU). The first factor aggregates the items referring to ease of use and the second factor to the utility that the respondent gives to the characteristics of the device. Of all the characteristics included in the TAM model, only two fundamental dimensions were used in the present study [14].

The results suggest the importance and necessity of development of the inflatable bedpan, reinforcing the dissatisfaction presented by the consumers and users of the existing bedpans. The statistical analyzes evidenced the importance of the TAM model in the evaluation, explanation and prediction of the acceptance [17] by future users.

4.1 Limitations of the Study

As a limitation of the study it is mentioned, besides a non-probabilistic sample, its representativeness, since it was collected only by an online questionnaire. Future studies should seek to cover more participants from different geographic areas of the country. In addition, most of the sample has already taken care of someone in bed, which may be influencing the results. Therefore, future studies should control this variable.

5   Conclusion

To our knowledge, this is the first study in Portugal, which intends to develop a new proposal for inflatable bedpan, with clear competitive advantages (for customers and for consumers) in relation to existing bedpans. Likewise, this study is a pioneer in the evaluation of the acceptability of the general population, in relation to the bedpans currently in market and the new proposal.

The present research team is developing its prototype and aims to verify its acceptability by the general population, through the physical and face-to-face experimentation of the same.

These results have important practical implications. At the political level, they can influence the existing health policies, which value the increase of patient comfort, encouraging the national production of medical devices and reducing health costs. At an economic level, our product presents clear competitive advantages over existing products, by reducing sterilization costs, as it allows a greater number of units to be sterilized per square meter, compared to classic bedpans that cannot be deflated. At the social level, given the aging of the Portuguese population and the significant increase of bedridden patients, this product allows the improvement of the quality of life, promoting the social value of the needs of the citizen, being a useful and effective solution to respond to health problems. At the technological level, this proposal requires simple technological processes, which allows the reduction/neutralization of odors. Finally, at the environmental level, by presenting ecological, reusable and recyclable characteristics, it reduces hospital costs while minimizing the negative environmental impact.

The aim of this research was to evaluate the potential of an innovation in terms of the usefulness and ease of use related to an inflatable medical device, by caregivers and users of bedpans, with a view to their acceptance by the market.

The results obtained were in accordance with the expectations of the researchers, since the characteristics presented by the new proposal of bedpan denoted a degree of acceptance much superior to the one obtained with the classic bedpans.

In conclusion, this study constitutes an important and innovative contribution, highlighting the importance of the development of this prototype, with implications for its clients and consumers, at the political, economic, social, technological and environmental level.

References

1. World Health Organization. A discussion document on the concept and principles of health promotion, Copenhagen, 9–13 July 1984. http://www.who.int/healthpromotion/milestones_yellowdocument.pdf
2. Buss, P.: Uma introdução ao conceito de promoção da saúde. In: Czeresnia, D., Freitas, C.M. (orgs.) Promoção da Saúde: Conceitos, Reflexões, Tendências, pp. 15–38. Fiocruz, Rio de Janeiro (2003)
3. PORDATA (a) - Base de dados Portugal Contemporâneo: Camas nos estabelecimentos de saúde por 100 mil habitantes - Continente Portugal (2017). http://www.pordata.pt/
4. Gibson, G.L.: Bacteriological hazards of disposable bedpan systems. J. Clin. Pathol. **26**(2), 146–153 (1973). https://doi.org/10.1136/jcp.26.2.146
5. Young, J.: Inflatable, disposable bedpan apparatus and method. United States Pattern (1990)
6. Mag, H., Werner, B., Saxer, S.: Patient experience with bedpans in acute care: a cross-sectional study. J. Clin. Nurs. **22**(15–16), 2216–2224 (2013). https://doi.org/10.1111/jocn.12203
7. Smith, R.E., Wash, R., Imel, M.: Inflatable body support for use with bedpan. United States Patent [US4207633(A)] (1980)

8. Royal, G.S.: Disposable inflatable bedpan. United States Patent [US5224223 (A)] (1993)
9. Venkatesh, V., Morris, M.G., Davis, G.B., Davis, F.D.: User acceptance of information technology: toward a unified view. MIS Q. **27**, 425–478 (2003)
10. Hoque, M.R.: An empirical study of mHealth adoption in a developing country: the moderating effect of gender concern. BMC Med. Inform. Decis. Mak. **16**, 51 (2016). https://doi.org/10.1186/s12911-016-0289-0
11. Venkatesh, V.: Determinants of perceived ease of use: integrating control, intrinsic motivation, and emotion into the technology acceptance model. Inf. Syst. Res. **11**(4), 342–365 (2000). https://doi.org/10.1287/isre.11.4.342.11872
12. Venkatesh, V., Davis, F.D.: A theoretical extension of the technology acceptance model: four longitudinal field studies. Manag. Sci. **46**(2), 186–204 (2000). https://doi.org/10.1287/mnsc.46.2.186.11926
13. Kim, S., Lee, K., Hwang, H., Yoo, S.: Analysis of the factors influencing healthcare professionals' adoption of mobile electronic medical record (EMR) using the unified theory of acceptance and use of technology (UTAUT) in a tertiary hospital. BMC Med. Inform. Decis. Mak. 16(12) (2016). https://doi.org/10.1186/s12911-016-0249-8
14. Davis, F.D.: Perceived usefulness, perceived ease of use, and user acceptance of information technology. MIS Q. **13**(3), 319–340 (1989). https://doi.org/10.2307/249008
15. Nysveen, H., Pedersen, P.E., Thorbjørnsen, H.: Intentions to use mobile services: antecedents and cross-service comparisons. J. Acad. Mark. Sci. **33**(3), 330–346 (2005)
16. Bao, Y., Xiong, T., Hu, Z., Kibelloh, M.: Exploring gender differences on general and specific computer self-efficacy in mobile learning adoption. J. Educ. Comput. Res. **49**(1), 111–132 (2013)
17. Chang, C.: The technology acceptance model and its application in a telehealth program for the elderly with chronic illnesses. Hu Li Za Zhi J. Nurs. **62**(3), 11–16 (2015). https://doi.org/10.6224/JN.62.3.11
18. Alferes, V.R.: Methods of Randomization in Experimental Design. Sage, Thousand Oaks (2012)
19. Tabachnick, B., Fidell, L.: Using Multivariate Statistics. Pearson Education, Upper Saddle River (2013)
20. Bryman, A., Cramer, D.: Análise de Dados em Ciências Sociais: Introdução às Técnicas Utilizando o SPSS, 2nd edn. Celta, Oeiras (1993)
21. Gorsuch, R.: Factor Analysis, 2nd edn. Erlbaum, Hillsdale (1983)
22. Arbuckle, J.L.: Amos 22 User's Guide. SPSS, Chicago (2013)
23. Fornell, C., Larcker, D.: Evaluating structural equation models with unobservable variables and measurement error. J. Mark. Res. **18**(1), 39–50 (1981)
24. Schumacker, R.E., Lomax, R.G.: A Beginner's Guide to Structural Equation Modeling. Routledge Academic, New York (2012)
25. Brown, T.: Confirmatory Factor Analysis for Applied Research. The Gilford Press, New York (2006)
26. Bentler, P.: Quantitative methods in psychology: comparative fit indexes in structural models. Psychol. Bull. **107**, 238–246 (1990)
27. Kline, R.B.: Principles and Practice of Structural Equation Modeling, 3rd edn. The Guilford Press, New York (2011)
28. Marôco, J.: Análise Estatística com o SPSS Statistics, 5th edn. ReportNumber, Lisboa (2011)

29. Bollen, K.: Sample size and Bentler and Bonett's nonnormed fit index. Psychometrika **51**, 375–377 (1986)
30. Nunnally, J.: Psychometric Theory, 2nd edn. McGraw- Hill, New York (1978)
31. Hair, J., Anderson, R., Tatham, R., Black, W.: Multivariate Data Analysis, 7th edn. Pearson Prentice-Hall, Upper Saddle River (2008)
32. Hill, M., Hill, A.: Investigação por Questionário. Edições Sílabo, Lisboa (2012)
33. Bagozzi, R., Yi, Y.: On the evaluation of structural equation models. J. Acad. Mark. Sci. **16**, 74–94 (1988)

Emotional Intelligence and Life Satisfaction in Adulthood

Lisete dos Santos Mendes Mónico[1](✉)[iD],
Patrícia Isabel Valente dos Santos[4],
Carla Maria Santos de Carvalho[1][iD], Joana Íris Lopes Parreira[2][iD],
Paulo Jorge dos Santos Costa[3][iD], and Pedro Miguel Dinis Parreira[3][iD]

[1] Faculty of Psychology and Education Sciences,
University of Coimbra, 3001-802 Coimbra, Portugal
lisetemonico@gmail.com
[2] The Health Sciences Research Unit: Nursing, 3000-232 Coimbra, Portugal
[3] Nursing School of Coimbra, 3046-851 Coimbra, Portugal
[4] Psychology and Life Sciences - Universidade Lusófona, Lisboa, Portugal

Abstract. The aim of this study was to analyze the relationship between Emotional Intelligence (EI) and Life Satisfaction (LS) (18 to 60 years) as a repertoire of acquired psychological competences and intelligent adaptive behavior through the promotion of personal success, happiness and general well-being and explore their contributions to LS. Three research hypotheses were formulated for young adulthood (18–39 years) and advanced adulthood (40–60 years), aiming at comparing the magnitude of these two life phases: (H1) EI and LS are positively related; (H2) EI and self-esteem are positively related; and, (H3) EI is a predictor of LS. The sample study is composed of 200 participants aged 18–60 years. The results did not indicate differences between EI in young and elderly adults, although the latter were significantly less satisfied with their life and reported going through a less favorable life period. The three hypotheses found statistical support, with greater magnitude in advanced adulthood. For young adults, EI accounted for 15% of their overall well-being and for older adults this proportion increased to 43%.

Keywords: Emotional intelligence · Life satisfaction · Adulthood

1 Introduction

This study aims to analyze the relationship between Emotional Intelligence (EI) and Life Satisfaction (LS) in two groups of adults. In other words, it is sought to ascertain whether EI constitutes a positive predictor of LS in different life stages of adulthood - young adulthood and advanced adulthood.

1.1 Brief Historical Review on the Concept of Emotional Intelligence

The concept of EI has motivated a large amount of research in recent decades. As a target of diverse debates and discussions, EI generated some discord among

© Springer Nature Switzerland AG 2019
J. García-Alonso and C. Fonseca (Eds.): IWoG 2018, CCIS 1016, pp. 201–215, 2019.
https://doi.org/10.1007/978-3-030-16028-9_18

researchers, namely as to the definition of the concept and its validity and utility [1], but also a considerable amount of research in this area.

The roots of the EI construct go back to Thorndike who in 1920 proposed the term *social intelligence*, defined as the ability to understand and manage people and to act wisely in human relationships [2]. Afterwards, Gardner [3] introduced the concept of *multiple intelligences*, contributing to the conceptualization of the EI construct as a set of social skills that relate to the individual's ability to know and discriminate their feelings, developing the notions of *intrapersonal intelligence* and *interpersonal intelligence*. According to Gardner [3], multiple intelligences are as important as the intellectual quotient (IQ), since people are provided with a wide spectrum of skills that allow them to solve problems. Thus, the "first steps" were being taken to conceptualize EI as a construct [4].

Literature is prolific in definitions about EI. In 1990, Salovey and Mayer [2] defined EI as a subcategory of social intelligence that involves the ability to monitor one's feelings and emotions and those of others by distinguishing them and using that information to guide their thinking and actions. For Bar-On [5], EI refers to a type of emotional-social intelligence that interrelates emotional and social skills and competences that determine how effectively individuals understand and express themselves, as well as the degree of effectiveness with which they understand and relate to each other, and their ability to cope with daily demands at this level.

According to Bar-On [5], EI can be defined as a set of personal, emotional and social skills as well as a set of faculties that influence the ability to be successful in dealing with environmental demands and pressures. This author divides EI into five areas of skills and competences: (1) Intrapersonal skills: emotional self-awareness; self-realization; independence; self-respect and assertiveness; (2) Interpersonal skills: relationships, empathy and social responsibility; (3) Adaptability: ability to solve problems, flexibility: (4) Stress Management: Impulse management and tolerance; (5) General Humor: happiness and optimism.

The IE construct became popular with Daniel Goleman's book *Emotional intelligence: Why it can matter more than IQ* [6]. In this work, Goleman, like Gardner, attached great importance to IE, stimulating research and eliciting the general public's curiosity about this construct, namely its potential benefits [7].

EI can be seen as a competency model. In this context, according to Goleman [6], for an individual to be skilled in a given emotional competence, competency skills determine the "potential" that an individual has to "optimize" a given ability, and emotional skills are learned skills, and this individual can use them to control impulses, deal with frustrations, postpone rewards, regulate his own state of mind, and prevent discouragement from intermingling in his ability to think, to empathize, or to hope. Continuing his studies, in 1995, Goleman [6] simplified the concepts previously developed for a set of important skills such as: self-control; enthusiasm; empathy; perseverance and self-motivation. Petrides and Furnham [8, 9] distinguished the construct as a trait, measured through self-report, as well as a capacity, evaluated by performance tests where one tries to measure the cognitive capacity to process information loaded with emotion.

In 2004, Van Rooy and Viswesvaran [10] define the construct as a set of verbal and nonverbal abilities that enables the individuals to generate, recognize, express, understand and evaluate their own and others' emotions with the objective to direct their thinking and their actions, in order to handle them successfully, with the demands and the pressures of the surrounding environment. EI is, for many, seen as an individual's competence to recognize, express, rationalize and manage one's own emotions as well as those of others [11].

Despite the diversity of EI definitions, these have some points in common [12]. In this context, Bar-On [5] lists the following common points of most definitions of the construct: (1) ability to recognize, understand and express emotions and feelings; (2) an ability to understand others' emotions and relate to them; (3) ability to manage and control emotions; (4) ability to deal with change and to solve personal and interpersonal problems; and (5) ability to generate positive emotions and self-motivation.

Regardless of the definition or even of the EI model in which each research is supported, it should be noted that several studies have found interesting results between IE and other constructs, namely with life satisfaction.

1.2   Life Satisfaction and Subjective Well-Being

In the literature, LS often emerges as synonymous with Subjective Well-being. LS and Subjective Well-being (SWB), is a domain that addresses general well-being, being evaluated from the results referring to the dimensions of LS and Happiness, which are differentiated by the specificity of the involved psychological processes. According to Novo [13], LS can be considered a dimension of a more cognitive nature, which represents the psychological balance that each individual makes of his/her life in general; while Happiness, of a more emotional nature, represents each individual's assessment of their positive and negative emotional experiences. This construct has been structured in two areas of approach. A strand in the development of the adult and mental health and another aspect in the psychosocial context, with respect to quality and satisfaction according to the conditions and circumstances of life. According to the same author [13], in spite of the apparent similarity of objectives, there are different forms of conceptualization: on the one hand we have research on the SWB, whose focus is Happiness, Satisfaction and Emotional Experiences; and, on the other hand, we have research on psychological well-being, which is of interest to the areas of developmental psychology, clinical psychology and mental health.

LS is a phenomenon of great complexity and difficult to measure, since it is, by nature, a subjective process. It assesses the individual's state of life with respect to his life in general and to certain specific areas of his life, such as health, family life, love relationships, economic conditions, social relations, autonomy, among others [14, 15]. It is a cognitive evaluation favoring life according to criteria pre-established by the individual. LS, in general terms, can be dismissed as an overall assessment of the SWB of the individual according to his or her own criteria. It concerns the individual's perception of their position in life, within the context of the culture systems and values in which they are included and in relation to their objectives, expectations, standards and concerns (psychological, regarding levels of independence, social relationship, environmental characteristics, spiritual pattern) [16–18].

LS is, therefore, a multidimensional construct and a process of cognitive evaluation based on an appreciation that each person makes about their life in general, or in more specific domains, according to a set of criteria considered valid for themselves; nonetheless, there is a set of factors that can decisively influence this LS (e.g., personality, work, school, religious or spiritual life, learning and growth or leisure, group of friends, stipulated or achieved personal or professional goals, etc.).

It refers to a process of personal judgment, in which each individual evaluates the quality of his life based on a comparison between the circumstances of his current life and the ideal or standard circumstances. From the greater or lesser correspondence between the two, there is a greater or lesser satisfaction with life [17].

A study by Carvalho, Gerrero and Chambel [19], with a sample of young adults that aimed to analyze the role of EI as a predictor of the well-being of these students (i.e., burnout and LS), over a period of time, evidenced that the evaluations of the emotions of others and the use of emotion had a positive direct effect in LS.

Some studies have shown that LS, in addition to varying from individual to individual, due to the aforementioned criteria, varies considerably at different times in life, according to certain criteria.

1.3   Adulthood and Life Satisfaction

The great transformations that have affected the world in the last decades have required the introduction of profound changes and political, economic, social, cultural, etc. reforms in the various countries. We see great changes at various levels, including human development and adaptability (plasticity, Baltes [20]) to the ever-changing world. The goals and priorities of life are also compulsively reformulated: young people study later, find employment later, become a family later, leave their parents/family later, all their dreams and goals are not uncommonly postponed. All this has an impact on your satisfaction with life, your well-being and happiness.

According to Levinson [21], adulthood (young adulthood) is a sequence of stable and transitional phases or periods, not a single phase, which the author calls the seasons of man's life. The essential character of this sequence is the same for all. At this stage, the ability to create a sufficiently stable structure to exploit the available possibilities becomes extremely important. Given that responsibilities will fall on their choices, a balance will have to be struck, and one of the main tasks is related to the clarification of objectives and the achievement of greater self-definition as an individual adult. Important milestones such as marriage, childbirth, divorce, among others, can take great importance in this phase as crucial choices. According to Marchand [22], around the 30 years transition, the Young Adult often has to correct and reassess the options and positions that he/she has previously taken, and this moment can be of great stress for him/her, if there are moderate changes in the lifestyle, or of great tension if there are major breakdowns in relation to what was previously built.

For Marchand [22] the third life structure develops between the 33 and 45 years. At this point, individuals seek to invest in various dimensions (family, community, individual interests, friendships) while pursuing their aspirations and goals. At the end of this phase the adult is expected to be more aware of his abilities, more self-sufficient and more independent in the face of the control exercised by others. All of these changes can affect LS, depending on several factors internal and external to the individual.

The period from 40 to 45 years is seen as the Mid-life Transition, and for Levinson [21] the Middle Age lasts until about 65 years. It is at this stage that the individual, as a rule, becomes more compassionate and judicious, less tyrannized by internal conflicts and external demands. Finally, the author [21] defines the Late Adult Transition period, between the ages of 60 and 65, representing the beginning of the late adulthood (Late Adulthood). The author does not consider that the sequence of these life structuring periods derives solely from a maturational process or from the socializing influence of a single social system, but rather as the product of their combination and the influence of bio-psycho-social sources.

According to Craig [23], the tasks of the Middle-age concern: (1) to have civic and social responsibilities; (2) establish and maintain an economic standard of living; (3) helping teens to be responsible and happy future adults; (4) developing adult leisure activities; (5) establish relationship with his/her spouse as a person; (6) to accept and adjust to physical changes of middle age and last (7) to adjust to elderly parents. Although biologically it is possible to verify a thin decline, at this stage individuals are still sufficient to lead an energetic and socially active life in order to provide a high personal satisfaction. We can say that this is an opportunity phase to work towards individuation and self-realization, making a deeper understanding of oneself and realizing its place and its relationship with the world and with others.

Given the above, what is the relationship between EI and LS in young adulthood (18–39 years) and in advanced adulthood (40–60 years)?

2 Objective

The main objective of this study was to analyze the relationship between EI and LS in young adulthood (18–39 years) and in advanced adulthood (40–60 years).

3 Hypotheses

Based on the previously mentioned objectives, three research hypotheses were formulated: EI and LS are positively related (H1); EI and self-esteem are positively related (H2); and it is possible, from the EI predict LS in young adulthood (18–39 years) and in advanced adulthood (40–60 years) (H3).

4 Method

4.1 Sample

The sample is non-probabilistic, of convenience and in "snowball" format. It is composed of 200 subjects living in mainland Portugal, 55 (27.5%) men and 145 (72.5%) women. The age of the sample varies between 18 and 60 years, with the mean (M) being 25.26 and the standard deviation (SD) of 8.53 years. With regard to men, ages vary between 18 and 60 years, with M = 30.12 and SD = 9.98 years. Age among women varies between 19 and 53 years, with M = 23.42 and SD = 7.12 years. In young adulthood (18–39 years) the mean age was M = 22.90 years (SD = 4.59 years), whereas in advanced adulthood (40–60 years) the mean was M = 46.55 years (SD = 5.91 years).

Regarding academic qualifications, the majority of the participants have Secondary Education (n = 117, 58.1%), followed by the Baccalaureate (n = 72, 36%), Basic Education (n = 8, 4.0%) and Master's degree (n = 3; 1.5%).

4.2 Instruments

The following measurement instruments were used to perform the present study: (1) the Emotional Intelligence Scale (in Portuguese, Escala de Inteligência Emocional) [24], a seven-point Likert type scale (from 1 = The statement does not strictly apply to me to 7 = The statement applies completely to me) comprising 23 descriptors, distributed by six factors [24]: understanding of own emotions, self-control in the face of criticism, self-encouragement, emotional self-control, empathy and emotional contagion, and understanding the emotions of others); (2) Satisfaction with Life Scale (in Portuguese, Escala de satisfação com a vida) [17], composed of five items measured on a seven-point Likert scale (from 1 = I disagree at all to 7 = I agree at all); (3) a question regarding the self-perception of life situation, measured by a five-point Likert scale: "Currently, you are experiencing a life situation" (from 1 = very bad to 5 = very good); (4) Measure of self-esteem, in which the question "Do you like yourself?" was elaborated, answered on a five-point Likert scale (from 1 = Absolutely no to 5 = Always); and (5) sociodemographic questionnaire, with questions about sex, age, literacy and data concerning the professional situation.

4.3 Procedure

The distribution of the questionnaires occurred in a "snowball" format. During data collection, all precautions were taken to ensure the anonymity of the respondents and the confidentiality of the data. To analyze the data, we used version 22.0 of the SPSS (Statistical Package for the Social Sciences) and Amos (Analysis of Moment Structures) software. The descriptive and inferential analyzes were performed based on Alferes [25], Andrews, Klem, Davidson, O'Malley, and Rodgers [26], Fink [27], Howell [28], and Pestana and Gageiro [29]. All the assumptions of a correct use of the statistical analyzes were tested and obeyed.

4.4   Instruments Validation

Emotional Intelligence Scale. For the validation of the construct, the scale was submitted to a confirmatory factorial analysis. Taking into account the relationships between the latent constructs and the variables examined, the measurement model was specified according to Rego and associates [24]. Then, the degree of being observed in the trajectory diagram, we have six first-order latent constructs (that is, the six dimensions of the Emotional Intelligence Scale), and a second order one, referring to the construct of global EI. Given the quality of the adjustment, we found a good adjustment considering the indexes CMIN/164 = 1.89, p < .001, Normed of Fit Index – NFI = .828 (since it is considered a good adjustment when NFI > .80; [30]), Comparative Fit Index – CFI = .910 (since it is considered as a good indicator when it exceeds the .90 value; [31]). Given the RMSEA we found the value .067, being in compliance with the requirement RMSEA < .08 [32]). Considering the mentioned criteria for the quality of the adjustment, we conclude that the model is perfectly adjusted. The regression coefficients related to the scale items varied between a minimum of β = .33 and a maximum of β = .93, all of them being statistically significant. We conclude that the hexafatorial structure was confirmed. The scale dimensions presented acceptable reliability. The global scale presented an internal consistency coefficient of α = .87, indicative of a good measure reliability.

The alpha of Factor 1 - Understanding of Own Emotions was .70, that of Factor 2 - Self-control in the face of criticism was .77, that of Factor 3 - Self-encouragement was .83, that of Factor 4 - Emotional Self-Control was .61, that of 5 - Empathy and Emotional Contagion was .83, and that of Factor 6 - Understanding the Emotions of Others was .86.

Satisfaction with Life Scale. The unifactory structure of the Life Satisfaction Scale was submitted to a confirmatory factorial analysis. A coefficient was found CMIN/DF = 1.89, p = .640, indicative of a good adjustment. We also achieved a good adjustment considering the indexes NFI = .992, CFI = .999) and RMSEA = .001. The Cronbach's alpha was α = .85, indicative of good internal consistency.

5   Results

Table 1 presents the minimum (Min.) and maximum (Max.) values, the mean scores (M), the standard deviations (SD) and errors (PE) of the measures under study and constituent factors for the global sample and for the subsamples of young adulthood (18–39 years) and advanced adulthood (40–60 years).

Considering the central tendency measure of the six EI factors, the highest mean score found was Emotional Empathy and Contagion (M = 5.78), and the lowest was Emotional Self-Control (M = 4.36). The highest scoring factor was found at the level of Empathy and emotional contagion (F5), followed by the level of Self-Encouragement (F3) and successively by the level of Understanding of Own Emotions (F1), Understanding the Emotions of Others (F6), Self-Control in the face of criticism (F2) and, finally, Emotional self-control (F4).

Table 1. Minimum and maximum values, mean scores and standard deviations of the measures under study according to age group (young adulthood vs. advanced adulthood): comparative tests between means.

Sample [N = 200]

	Min.	Max.	Total (18–60 years)		Young adulthood (18–39 years)		Advanced adulthood (40–60 years)		F (1, 198) t (198)
			M	DP	M	DP	M	DP	
Emotional Intelligence (global scale)	2.55	6.83	5.00	0.63	5.03	.62	4.75	.67	
F1: Understanding of Own Emotions	2.75	7.00	5.00	0.83	5.02	.82	4.84	.95	F = 0.89
F2: Self-control in the face of criticism	1.00	7.00	4.71	1.10	4.76	1.11	4.25	.90	F = 3.87
F3: Self-encouragement	2.67	7.00	5.14	1.01	5.15	1.02	5.07	.98	F = 0.13
F4: Emotional Self-Control	1.25	6.75	4.36	0.90	4.37	.91	4.29	.78	F = 0.16
F5: Empathy and Emotional Contagion	1.80	7.00	5.78	0.86	5.82	.83	5.47	1.08	F = 2.92
F6: Understanding the Emotions of Others	2.00	7.00	4.99	0.99	5.04	.97	4.60	1.13	F = 3.54
Satisfaction with life (global scale)	1.60	6.80	4.72	1.03	4.80	.99	4.01	1.14	t = 3.31***
Currently, you are experiencing a life situation	2.00	5.00	3.38	0.65	3.44	.64	2.85	.59	t = 3.96***
Do you like yourself? (self-esteem)	2.00	5.00	3.79	0.72	3.82	.71	3.50	.76	t = 1.91

* p < .05, *** p < .001

The comparison between the two age groups led to a MANOVA Variance Multivariate Analysis (General Linear Model), with the independent variable (IV) being the age group (1 = young adulthood, 2 = advanced adulthood) and as dependent variables (DVs) each of the dimensions of the EI scale. The multivariate test did not indicate the presence of a significant effect of the age group (young adulthood vs. advanced adulthood) on the participants' perception of emotional intelligence, Λ Wilks = 0.931, $F_{(6.193)} = 1.17$, p = .326, $\eta p^2 = .035$. The results of univariate tests $F_{(1, 198)}$ are shown in Table 1. No difference was statistically significant.

In relation to the Life Satisfaction Scale, the value obtained (M = 4.72) is close to the answer alternative number 5 (in a total of 7 points), meaning that, in general, the participants are satisfied with their lives. The comparison test between means indicated a statistically significant difference between young adulthood (M = 4.80) and advanced adulthood (M = 4.01), since adults of an advanced age were less satisfied with their lives, Cohen's d = 0.74, R2 = 12% of Life Satisfaction variance, on the basis of young adulthood vs. advanced adulthood. Likewise, these participants reported that they were experiencing a less favorable life situation (M = 2.85) compared to young adults (M = 3.44), Cohen's d = 0.96, R2 = 19% explained variance. Regarding their self-esteem, no statistically significant differences were recorded.

Table 2. Correlation coefficients and classification of the magnitude (from nil to strong) between the Emotional Intelligence scale and constituent factors with the three measures of Life Satisfaction for young and advanced adulthood.

	r					
	Measures of Life Satisfaction					
	Young adulthood (18–39 years)			Advanced adulthood (40–60 years)		
Emotional Intelligence:	LS Scale (r)	Self-perception of the life situation (rho)	Self-esteem (rho)	LS Scale	Self-perception of the life situation	Self-esteem
F1 - Understanding of Own Emotions	.16 (weak)	.19 (weak)	.27 (weak)	.25 (weak)	.21 (weak)	**.65 (strong)**
F2 - Self-control in the face of criticism	.06 (null)	.01 (null)	.15 (weak)	.03 (null)	−.01 (null)	.37 (moderate)
F3 - Self-encouragement	.23 (weak)	.09 (null)	.34 (moderate)	.19 (weak)	.27 (weak)	**.56 (strong)**
F4 - Emotional Self-Control	.12 (weak)	.11 (weak)	.30 (moderate)	.28 (weak)	.09 (null)	.20 (weak)
F5 - Empathy and Emotional Contagion	.2 2 (weak)	.15 (weak)	.18 (weak)	.34 (moderate)	−.03 (null)	.43 (moderate)
F6 - Understanding the Emotions of Others	.2 7 (weak)	.28 (weak)	.25 (weak)	.20 (weak)	.11 (weak)	.47 (moderate)
IE_global	.26 (weak)	.17 (weak)	.37 (moderate)	.32 (weak)	.03 (null)	**.67 (strong)**

Table 2 presents the results of the association between EI, LS and self-esteem. We calculated the Pearson and Spearman correlation coefficients (for the ordinal variables Self-perception of Life Situation and Self-esteem) between the emotional intelligence scale and constituent factors with the three measures of satisfaction with life. The interpretation of the results will be carried out considering the classification of Cohen: | r | < .10 correlation of null magnitude; .10 < | r | < .30 weak magnitude correlation; .30 < | r | < .50 correlation of moderate magnitude; and r | > .50 correlation of strong magnitude.

We found that, in general terms, the relationships between emotional intelligence and satisfaction with life are positive, which gives statistical support to the H1 hypothesis (EI and LS are positively related). Considering the magnitude of the correlation coefficients, we found that the assigning associations oscillate between weak and moderate for both age groups.

Regarding the item that evaluates the Self-perception of life situation, the relationships found are of null or weak magnitude, indicating a tenuous positive association between EI and self-perception of the life situation (from very poor to very good). However, the association of global scale was only significant for younger adults (rho = .17).

The second hypothesis (H2 = EI and self-esteem are positively related), found empirical support. Considering the measure of self-esteem, we found that the correlations with the EI scale are the highest, which indicates that the more emotionally intelligent the more self-esteem the individual has. The comparison between younger and older adults has allowed us to ascertain that it is in the latter that the association between self-esteem and EI is the highest, assuming strong magnitudes (rho > .50).

We submit the three measures of satisfaction with life (Life Satisfaction Scale, Self-Perception of Life Situation, and Self-Esteem) to a Principal Components Analysis (PCA), since we wanted to investigate the emergence of only one factor, which we called the composite measure of satisfaction with life.

The requirements for a reliable interpretation of PCA were met: the intercorrelations matrix differs from the identity matrix [the Bartlett test indicates a χ^2 (3) = 103.17, p < .001] and sampling is adequate, since that the Kaiser-Meyer-Olkin measure is greater than .70 (KMO = .708). We verified the emergence of a single factor, according to the eigenvalue superior to the unit criterion (eigenvalue = 1.82), so we began to use the composite measure of satisfaction with life (calculation of the average score after standardization of all measures for the scale of 5 points).

Table 3. Multiple regression analysis of the Factor Satisfaction with life predicted from the six factors of the Emotional Intelligence scale for young and advanced adulthood.

Predictors	Factor Satisfaction with Life					
	Young adulthood (18–39 years)			Advanced adulthood (40–60 years)		
	b	EP	β	b	EP	β
F1 - Understanding of Own Emotions	.03	.06	.05	.04	.18	.08
F2 - Self-control in the face of criticism	−.01	.04	−.02	−.12	.14	−.21*
F3 - Self-encouragement	.07	.04	.13	.24	.15	.47***
F4 - Emotional Self-Control	.07	.04	.11	.12	.15	.19*
F5 - Empathy and Emotional Contagion	.04	.05	.06	.11	.13	.25*
F6 - Understanding the Emotions of Others	.11	.05	.20*	−.02	.14	−.05
R	.39			.66		
R^2	.15			.43		

* p < .05, *** p < .001

We performed a multiple regression analysis using the enter method, considering as predictors the six factors of the emotional intelligence scale and as a criterion variable the composite measure of satisfaction with life. We present the results in Table 3. We found that for young adults the 6 factors of EI explain 15% of their LS, while for adults in older age this proportion increased to 43%. Considering the regression coefficients indicated in Table 3 and, in particular, their significance levels, we found that in young adults, only F6 (Understanding the Emotions of Others) emerges as statistically significant, while in older adults, the positive predictors found were F3 (Self-encouragement), F4 (Emotional self-control) and F5 (Empathy and Emotional Contagion); however, F2 (Self-control in the face of criticism) showed a negative predictive ability.

The analysis of the standardized regression coefficients (β) in older adults indicates that the most significant predictor relates to F3 (Self-encouragement), followed by F5 (Empathy and Emotional Contagion), F2 (Self-control in the face of criticism) and, finally, F4 (Emotional Self-Control). In this context, we can establish that the empirical support for the third hypothesis was found (H3 = it is possible to predict the individuals' LS through their EI).

6 Discussion and Conclusions

The aim of this research was to evaluate the relationship and predictive power of Emotional Intelligence (through its six factors) in Life Satisfaction in two groups: young adulthood (18–39 years) and advanced adulthood (40–60 years). Descriptive statistics showed that the two groups were similar in terms of Emotional Intelligence. Older adults were less satisfied with their lives, indicating that they were experiencing a significantly less favorable life situation, contrasting with some investigations showing that in advanced adulthood higher levels of subjective well-being appear with more LS [33], life meaning [34] and less negative affects [35–39]. However, other research efforts evidence nonlinear patterns of subjective well-being and LS in adulthood resulting from the capacity for emotional regulation and/or ability to generate adaptive responses to positive events culminating in differences in subjective well-being and LS. Hence Ramsey and Gentzler [40] state that levels of LS change throughout life.

Dias [41] points out that LS is an important cognitive component that represents the psychological balance that each person makes about their life in general. Thus, the personal evaluation that the individual makes about his/her life mirrors the judgment of his/her experiences, culminating in greater or lesser satisfaction that "depends on a comparison between the individual's life circumstances and a standard established by the individual" [14]. Satisfaction reflects, therefore, individual subjective well-being, in other words, the motives and the way that lead people to live their life experiences in a positive way [14]. Thus, high levels of LS mirror high levels of positive affect and low levels of negative affect that translate subjective well-being [42].

In our research it is interesting to note that in young adulthood the Understanding of the Emotions of Others is a predictor of LS. This fact can be sustained in the appreciation and importance of sociability for the understanding of the emotions of others, an important dimension of EI that generates LS. Such predictor effect may reflect a greater satisfaction based on the intensification of relations established with friends, in which a higher level of complicity occurs, culminating in greater LS, due to a greater capacity for understanding, support and aid by the established network of relationships. It is a period in which dyad - to give and receive - is part of the process of socialization as a form of social interaction, culminating in satisfaction.

This ability to understand the emotions of others evidences a form of interpersonal intelligence that translates into social nature competences [3], a type of social intelligence important for the development of human relations. Understanding the Emotions of Others translates the ability to monitor the feelings and emotions of the individual and of others, guiding their thinking and actions [2]. Bar-On [5] considers this type of intelligence as an emotional-social intelligence, translating the degree of effectiveness of understanding and relating to others. In young adulthood, the individual fosters and nourishes a greater social participation, being expected a higher level in this competence to be socially better integrated and more successful. Van Rooy and Viswesvaran [10] draw attention to this competence in recognizing, expressing, understanding and evaluating their own and others' emotions as a strategy of directing thinking and action, in order to successfully deal with the pressures and demands of the environment that surrounds them. Palmer, Gignac, Ekermans and Stough [11] identify this competence as necessary to manage their own emotions and understand the emotions of others.

In turn, Silva, Carvalho and Lourenço [43] attribute to this competence a more sophisticated way of dealing with emotions (the regulation of emotions), implying the ability to monitor and regulate the emotions of oneself and others, with the goal of promoting emotional and intellectual growth [44].

On the other hand, we found in advanced adulthood different predictors of LS, based on the factors Self-Encouragement, Emotional Self-Control, Empathy and Emotional Contagion, and Self-Control in the Face of Criticism. It is a time in life where friendship relationships are more stabilized, which is why these individuals value factors that increase the ability to trigger positive feelings that generate LS. Salovey and Mayer [2] consider it as a form of positive emotional regulation [44]. Accordingly, Goleman [6, 45, 46] refers to the ability to recognize our feelings and of others, to motivate ourselves and to manage our emotions and our relationships well [47] as an EI competence. Thus, empathy is valued as a way to generate a positive effect on the other while stimulating participatory social interaction, valuing positive experiences. In turn, Emotional Self-Control capability translates maturity and stability into how each individual expresses himself/herself, while social desirability ceases to be the standard for assertive behavior, and in which the less Self-control in the face of Criticism generates greater LS.

It is interesting to note that the great majority of the factors that support the construct of EI are predictors of LS in advanced adulthood, although this is not the case for the younger adulthood group. In young individuals it is understandable that there are a diversity of factors based on other concepts and constructs that can be generators of LS. In advanced adulthood, the portfolio of acquired skills and life experiences contribute to the enrichment of the cognitive-affective map that determines emotional intelligence [48, 49]. Knowing how to act, to be weighed, to understand their emotions and that of others, to have emotional self-control by demonstrating maturity in the regulation of emotions, to be able to control criticism and to use emotions to generate self-encouragement, to be empathetic and cause emotional contagion, are factors that generate nuclei of sense that later support a predictor effect in LS, AS ALSO IN Psychological capital [50, 51]. In this line of thought, we emphasize the importance of offering programs for the development of EI in the academy [52], organizations [51, 53], peer-education and in-service training with the objective of preventing psychiatric morbidity [53], by improving the mental health of the population, with positive effects in the advanced adulthood that generates greater LS.

References

1. Mayer, J., Roberts, R., Barsade, S.: Human abilities: emotional intelligence. Annu. Rev. Psychol. **59**, 507–536 (2008)
2. Salovey, P., Mayer, J.: Emotional intelligence. Imagin. Cogn. Pers. **9**, 185–211 (1990)
3. Gardner, H.: Frames of Mind: The Theory of Multiple Intelligences. Basic Books, New York (1983)
4. Brackett, M., Rivers, S., Salovey, P.: Emotional intelligence: implications for personal, social, academic, and workplace success. Soc. Pers. Psychol. Compass **5**, 88–103 (2011)
5. Bar-On, R.: The Bar-On model of emotional-social intelligence (ESI). Psicothema **18**, 13–25 (2006)
6. Goleman, D.: Emotional Intelligence. Bantam, New York (1995)
7. Kafetsios, K., Maridaki-Kassotaki, A., Zammuner, V., Zampetakis, L., Vouzas, F.: Emotional intelligence abilities and traits in different career paths. J. Career Assess. **17**, 367–383 (2009)
8. Petrides, K., Furnham, A.: Trait emotional intelligence: psychometric investigation with reference to established trait taxonomies. Eur. J. Pers. **15**, 425–448 (2001)
9. Petrides, K., Furnham, A.: Trait emotional intelligence: Behavioural validation in two studies of emotion recognition and reactivity to mood induction. Eur. J. Pers. **17**, 39–57 (2003)
10. Van Rooy, D., Viswesvaran, C.: Emotional intelligence: A meta-analytic investigation of predictive validity and nomological net. J. Vocat. Behav. **65**, 71–95 (2004)
11. Palmer, B., Gignac, G., Ekermans, G., Stough, C.: A comprehensive framework for emotional intelligence. In: Emerling, R., Shanwal, V., Mandal, M. (eds.) Emotional Intelligence: Theoretical and Cultural Perspectives, pp. 17–38. Nova Science Publishers, New York (2008)
12. Ciarrochi, J., Chan, A., Caputi, P.: A critical evaluation of the emotional intelligence concept. Pers. Individ. Differ. **28**, 539–561 (2000)
13. Novo, R.: Para além da eudaimonia: O Bem-estar psicológico em mulheres na idade adulta avançada. Fundação Calouste Gulbenkian: Fundação para a Ciência e a Tecnologia, Lisboa (2003)
14. Joia, L.C., Ruiz, T., Donalisio, M.R.: Condições Associadas ao Grau de Satisfação com a Vida entre a População de Idosos. Rev. Saúde Pública **41**, 131–138 (2007)
15. Mookherjee, H.N.: Effects of religiosity and selected variables on the perception of well-being. J. Soc. Psychol. **134**, 403–405 (1994)
16. Moberg, D.O.: Subjective measures of spiritual well-being. Rev. Relig. Res. **25**, 351–359 (1984)
17. Pavot, W., Diener, E.: Review of the satisfaction with life scale. Psychol. Assess. **2**, 164–172 (1993)
18. Pavot, W., Diener, E.: The satisfaction with life scale and emerging construct of life satisfaction. J. Posit. Psychol. **3**, 137–152 (2008)
19. Carvalho, V., Guerrero, E., Chambel, M.: Emotional intelligence and health students' well-being: a two-wave study with students of medicine, physiotherapy and nursing. Nurse Educ. Today **63**, 35–42 (2018)
20. Baltes, P.: Theoretical propositions of life-span developmental psychology: on the dynamics between growth and decline. Dev. Psychol. **23**, 611–626 (1987)
21. Levinson, D.: The seasons of a man's life. Alfred A. Knoff, New York (1997)
22. Marchand, H.: Temas de desenvolvimento psicológico do adulto. Editora Quarteto, Coimbra (2005)

23. Craig, G.J.: Human development. Prentice Hall, Upper Saddle River (1996)
24. Rego, A., Sousa, F., Cunha, M.P., Correia, A., Saur-Amaral, I.: Leader self-reported emotional intelligence and perceived employee creativity: Na exploratory study. Creat. Innov. Manag. **16**, 250–264 (2007)
25. Alferes, V.: Methods of randomization in experimental design. SAGE, Los Angeles (2012)
26. Andrews, F., Kem, L., Davidson, T., O'Malley, P., Rodgers, W.: A guide for selecting statistical techniques for analyzing social science data. Institute for Social Research, Ann Arbor (2000)
27. Fink, A.: How to Ask Survey Questions. SAGE, London (1995)
28. Howell, D.C.: Statistics Methods for Psychology. Duxbury Press, Belmont (1997)
29. Pestana, M.H., Gageiro, J.N.: Análise de dados para ciências sociais: A complementaridade do SPSS, 2nd edn. Edições Sílabo, Lisboa (2000)
30. Schumacker, R.E., Lomax, R.G.: A beginner's guide to structural equation modeling. In: Hatcher, L. (ed.) A Step-By-Step Approach to Using the SAS System for Factor Analysis and Structural Equation Modelling. SAS Institute, Cary NC. Lawrence Erlbaum Associates, Mahwah (1996)
31. Bentler, P., Weeks, G.: Linear structural equations with latent variables. Psychometria **45**, 289–308 (1980)
32. Schumacker, R.E., Lomax, R.G.: A Beginner's Guide to Structural Equation Modeling. Routledge Academic, New York (2012)
33. Hamarat, E., Thompson, D., Zabrucky, K., Steele, D., Matheny, K., Aysan, F.: Perceived stress and coping resource availability as predictors of life satisfaction in young, middle-aged, and older adults. Exp. Aging Res. **27**, 181–196 (2001)
34. Steger, M.F., Oishi, S., Kashdan, T.B.: Meaning in life across the life span: levels and correlates of meaning in life from emerging adulthood to older adulthood. J. Posit. Psychol. **4**, 43–52 (2009)
35. Carstensen, L., Pasupathi, M., Mayr, U., Nesselroade, J.: Emotional experience in everyday life across the adult life span. J. Pers. Soc. Psychol. **79**, 644–655 (2000)
36. Gross, J., Carstensen, L., Pasupathi, M., Tsai, J., Skorpen, C., Hsu, A.: Emotion and aging: experience, expression, and control. Psychol. Aging **12**, 590–599 (1997)
37. Mroczek, D., Almeida, D.: The effect of daily stress, personality, and age on daily negative affect. J. Pers. **72**, 355–378 (2004)
38. Carstensen, L., et al.: Emotional experience improves with age: evidence based on over 10 years of experience sampling. Psychol. Aging **26**, 21–33 (2011)
39. Charles, S., Reynolds, C., Gatz, M.: Age-related differences and change in positive and negative affect over 23 years. J. Pers. Soc. Psychol. **80**, 136–151 (2001)
40. Ramsey, M., Gentzler, A.: Age differences in subjective well-being across adulthood: the roles of savoring and future time perspective. Int. J. Aging Hum. Dev. **78**, 3–22 (2014)
41. Dias, M.A.R.: Qualidade de Vida Relacionada com a Saúde e Satisfação com a Vida: Um Estudo em indivíduos amputados do membro inferior (2006)
42. Diener, E., Suh, E., Lucas, R., Smith, H.: Subjective well-being: three decades of progress. Psychol. Bull. **125**, 276–302 (1999)
43. Silva, N., Carvalho, C., Lourenço, P.: A emoção na organização: A complementaridade da inteligência emocional e do trabalho emocional. In: Carvalho, C., Lourenço, P., Peralta, C. (eds.) Emoção nas Organizações, pp. 11–28. PsicoSoma, Viseu (2012)
44. Mayer, J., Salovey, P.: What is emotional intelligence? In: Salovey, P., Sluyter, D.J. (eds.) Emotional Development and Emotional Intelligence: Educational Implications, pp. 3–34. Basic Books, New York (1997)

45. Goleman, D.: Emotional Intelligence: Issues in Paradigm Building. In: Cherniss, C., Goleman, D. (eds.) The Emotionally Intelligent Workplace, pp. 13–28. Jossey-Bass, San Francisco (2001)
46. Goleman, D.: An EI-based theory of performance. In: Cherniss, C., Goleman, D. (eds.) The Emotionally Intelligent Workplace, pp. 27–44. Jossey-Bass, San Francisco (2001)
47. Goleman, D.: Working with Emotional Intelligence. Bantam, New York (1998)
48. Mónico, L.S., Santos, P.I., Lima, L.N.: The implications of emotional intelligence in self-esteem. Rev. Saúde Pública 48, 264 (2014)
49. Franca, L.A., Mónico, L.S.: The role of emotional intelligence in job satisfaction of individuals. Int. J. Dev. Educ. Psychol. 1(7), 203–212 (2014)
50. Mónico, L.S., Mellão, N., Nobre-Lima, L., Parreira, P., Carvalho, C.: Emotional intelligence and psychological capital: What is the role of workplace spirituality? Rev. Port. Enferm. Saúde Mental 3, 45–50 (2016)
51. Mellão, N., Mónico, L.S.: The relation between emotional intelligence and psychological capital of employees. Int. J. Dev. Educ. Psychol. 2(1), 545–550 (2013)
52. Mónico, L.S., Lucas, H.M., Jordão, E.G.: Emotional and behavioural problems of adolescents in a school context. J. Psychol. Soc. Behav. Res. 2(1), 12–19 (2014)
53. Lucas, H.M., Mónico, L.S.: Emotional intelligence and the protection of organizational stress. Int. J. Dev. Educ. Psychol. 2(1), 551–560 (2013)

Psychomotor Intervention Using Biofeedback Technology for the Elderly with Chronic Obstructive Pulmonary Disease

Maria Santos[1], Rafaela Moreira[1], Ricardo Saldanha[1(✉)],
Salomé Palmeiro[1], and César Fonseca[2] (iD)

[1] Évora University, Évora, Portugal
saldanha05@gmail.com
[2] Évora University, Investigator POCTEP 0445_4IE_4_P, Évora, Portugal

Abstract. When we talk about aging we must take into account not only chronological age, but also a complex and dynamic process of biological, psychological and social changes. Chronic Obstructive Pulmonary Disease (COPD) is highlighted in this study, as it is one of the most common and one of the leading causes of worldwide mortality in the elderly. Thus, the importance of psychomotricity in this case, since it acts on the awareness and regulation of the physiological and psychological systems, facilitating the learning process (according to the principles of learning theory and cognitive behavioral). In addition, it is also proposed the use of support technology based on the therapeutic strategies of the biofeedback system. Therefore, through the application of the goals proposed by the psychomotricity and use of the technology associated with biofeedback, the individual with COPD becomes capable of controlling the symptoms associated with the disease, and consequently acquiring more autonomy in the daily life (essential to promote their quality of life).

Keywords: Elderly · Chronic Obstructive Pulmonary Disease ·
Psychomotricity · Respiratory disturbances · Biofeedback

1 Introduction

A set of bibliographical researches was developed with the objective of exposing the problem of respiratory alterations in the elderly, more specifically Chronic Obstructive Pulmonary Disease (COPD), since this is one of the most common in advanced ages. Therefore, it is proposed a psychomotor intervention articulated with the use of biofeedback technology in order to act on the problems that may be associated with this pathology.

Aging is associated with multiple modifications, namely respiratory problems that influence the elderly in the different contexts in which they are inserted (Matos 2016). COPD, characterized by airflow obstruction, is one of the respiratory changes that most affects this age group. With the proven need to improve the quality of life of the elderly with this pathology, psychomotor intervention and biofeedback can prevent and intervene in motor, psychological and social factors (Phipps 2004). In addition, they offer a

© Springer Nature Switzerland AG 2019
J. García-Alonso and C. Fonseca (Eds.): IWoG 2018, CCIS 1016, pp. 216–221, 2019.
https://doi.org/10.1007/978-3-030-16028-9_19

set of instruments that allow the elderly to have a greater awareness and control of the psychological and physiological processes associated with COPD, thus giving them more independence (Schwartz and Andrasik 2017). After several researches, it is verified that psychomotor therapy in agreement with the use of biofeedback technology can effectively help significantly by optimizing the care of these clients (Spruit et al. 2015).

Methodology. The methodology used in the construction of this study was based on the bibliographic research of the publication system (EBSCO, SciELO, Medline), in which the following keywords were introduced: Elderly, Aging, Respiratory Disorders, Chronic Obstructive Pulmonary Disease, Intervention, Psychomotricity, Physical Activity, Relaxation and Biofeedback.

After this search, an analysis was made of articles on COPD and the respective forms of intervention. This analysis provided a collection of information on the pathology and on different intervention proposals. These recommendations presented, for the most part, functional models (physical activity). This way, other concepts related to psychomotor therapies were introduced and the applicability of therapies by biofeedback was explored. The main proposal was to collect a set of ideas applied to preventive, interventional (motor, psychological and social) situations and to promote the quality of life of the elderly through body mediation techniques.

Discussion. When talking about aging, we must take into account not only chronological age, but also a complex and dynamic process of biological, psychological and social changes (Matos 2016). It is confirmed that pulmonary respiratory changes are one of the most recurrent changes in this age group. At the level of biological aging there are alterations in both the structure (chest wall morphology, decrease in height and increase of body weight, predominantly in the abdominal area), and in the function of organic constituents responsible for the respiratory process (Ruivo et al. 2009). In addition, a nutrient deficient diet often leads to weakness of respiratory muscles and muscles more susceptible to fatigue and thus to changes in lung mechanics (Ruivo et al. 2009).

According to Ruivo et al. (2009), the loss of elasticity typical of the elderly and the decrease in the number of alveoli, compromise the quality of pulmonary ventilation and cause a decrease in voluntary maximum ventilation. It is possible to affirm that the aforementioned corporal transformations may be the cause of these pulmonary difficulties (global aging of the thorax and the lung), (Ruivo et al. 2009).

In Portugal, according to the National Statistics Institute (INE) (2015), there was a large increase in the percentage of the elderly population from 9.7% to 20.3%. According to these data, there is a significant increase in the elderly population, which is proportional to the increase of diseases related to respiratory changes in this age group (McCarthy et al. 2015). In this sense, the implementation of interventions to counteract this evolution will emerge, and the psychomotricity associated with the resources offered by biofeedback may be a viable body mediation therapy to deal with this problem.

Chronic obstructive pulmonary disease (COPD), asthma, interstitial lung disease and cystic fibrosis are the respiratory changes related to the elderly population, which are highlighted in the literature. However, COPD is evidenced in this study, as it is one of the most common diseases and one of the leading causes of worldwide mortality in the elderly (McCarthy et al. 2015). Thus a psychomotor and social-emotional intervention is proposed, in order to promote the quality of life of the elderly.

An estimated 210 million people are living with COPD, and by 2030, this pathology is the third most frequent cause of death globally (McCarthy et al. 2015). According to the DGS in 2005, COPD is "the pathological condition characterized by a limitation of airflow that is not fully reversible. Ventilatory limitation is generally progressive and is associated with an abnormal inflammatory response of the lungs to the inhalation of noxious particles or gases". This pathology results from chronic bronchitis or emphysema, in which airflow obstruction may be accompanied by hyperreactivity bronchial (Phipps 2004).

Psychomotricity and Biofeedback

According to the International Organization for Psychomotricity and Relaxation, Psychomotricity is seen as an expressive body-measurement therapy in which the therapist is able to understand and balance inadequate or maladaptive motor conducts. With this, the specificity of Psychomotricity aims to provide a re-encounter of harmony and the "I", as well as the satisfaction of making it work, through the capacity to be and to act for the body in relation, through movement (Fonseca and Martins 2001).

Regarding the biofeedback method, this is conceptually defined as a set of therapeutic processes that uses electronic technology to obtain information about the patient's physiological behaviors (autonomic and neuromuscular activity). These data are collected through sensors placed in strategic places of the body, not causing any shock, allowing only to gather information non-invasive and not influenced by physical pain (Costa 2016).

These results can be measured analogically or digitally, either sonically or visually, and allow both the patient and the therapist to gather a set of useful information about the individual's psychomotor and psycho-emotional behavior. In this way it is simpler to assist the elderly in the awareness of their own physiological and emotional processes, thus promoting an increase in self-image and self-confidence (Neto 2018).

At the level of the consciousness of the physiological processes, this can be fundamental in the voluntary control of the respiratory alterations. While controlling for emotional (anxiety or stress) deregulations, it is important that there is a mastery of psychological processes. This being the great participation of psychomotricity and biofeedback, for prevention, reduction or even stopping the symptoms.

On the other hand, the contribution of motor activity to its stimulation is also a fundamental element in the prevention process. Several studies have reported that elderly people with COPD demonstrate low levels of daily physical activity compared to those without COPD (Spruit et al. 2015). In addition, the time they spend on the move, especially in walking, is significantly lower, as well as their intensity, and that much of this population does not reach recommended physical activity standards (Spruit et al. 2015). In this way, psychomotricity can act to strengthen the muscles that are associated with the respiratory process, through specific functional activities (Kawagoshi et al. 2015).

According to Spruit et al. (2015), in order to promote the functioning of the pulmonary system, it is essential to insert regular physical activity into the daily context of the elderly, as sedentary lifestyle is currently one of the factors responsible for the reduction of their functional capacity.

In this case, the application of group mediation interventions is advised, since the practice of physical activity in clients with COPD depends on physiological, behavioral, social, environmental and cultural factors that influence their daily life (Spruit et al. 2015). This way, psychomotricity can be an adequate response to the problem, through psychomotor activities (such as gait, balance and throwing and grabbing) that promote peer relationships (play activities and expressive group therapies) (Spruit et al. 2015).

In order to promote the quality of life of this type of population it is necessary to act on this disease also in a preventive way. According to Spruit, in a study carried out in 2013, this can be achieved through a holistic approach of the individual, which includes physical, educational and behavioral training therapies, aimed at improving the physical and psychological condition of people with COPD, promoting long-term adherence to behaviors that improve health (Spruit et al. 2015).

Studies show that there are beneficial effects of relaxation (one of the techniques used in psychomotricity), in the ventilatory dynamics, which in turn can improve the condition of COPD, acting on airflow obstruction, characteristic of this pathology. The advantages associated with relaxation in this population are "30 to 60% decrease in respiratory rate," "significant increase in inspiration and expiration" and "increase in inspiratory/expiratory quotient" (Rissardi and Godoy 2004) (Fig. 1).

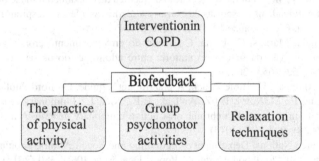

Fig. 1. Bases and intervention strategies for people with COPD

In summary, we can emphasize the importance of psychomotricity in the preventive, interventional level in several factors (motor, psychological and social) as well as the use of biofeedback as a complementary therapeutic resource, being this fundamental for the cognitive-behavioral therapies supported to the theories of learning and self-regulation.

For this type of population is advised: the practice of physical activity, with the purpose of counteracting the sedentary lifestyle, which causes the decrease of its functional capacity; group psychomotor activities since the practice of physical activity in these clients, depends on physiological, behavioral, social, environmental and cultural factors; relaxation techniques in order to be able to strengthen the muscles associated with the respiratory process; knowledge about your physical and psychological condition so as to provide full bodily awareness and definition of your own self-image. This process is fundamental for self-regulation and self-confidence, which are important factors for greater peer interaction and social participation.

References

Costa, A.M.P.: Analysis of pulmonary airflow on a smartphone application (2016)

DGS (Direcção Geral de Saúde): Programa Nacional de Prevenção e Controlo da Doença Pulmonar Obstrutiva Crónica. Lisboa: DGS (2005). https://www.dgs.pt/documentos-epublicacoes/programa-nacional-de-prevencao-e-controlo-da-doenca-pulmonar-obstrutiva-cronica-pdf.aspx. acedido em 2018. Journal 2(5), 99–110 (2016)

Fonseca, V., Martins, R.F.R.: Progressos em psicomotricidade (2001)

Kawagoshi, A., et al.: Effects of low-intensity exercise and home-based pulmonary rehabilitation with pedometer feedback on physical activity in elderly patients with chronic obstructive pulmonary disease. Respir. Med. 109(3), 364–371 (2015)

Matos, M.L.P.D.: Efeito de dois programas de reabilitação psicomotora (atividade contínua versus atividade intervalada) na capacidade neuromotora de idosos institucionalizados. Master's thesis, Universidade de Évora (2016)

McCarthy, B., Casey, D., Devane, D., Murphy, K., Murphy, E., Lacasse, Y.: Pulmonary rehabilitation for chronic obstructive pulmonary disease. The Cochrane Library (2015)

Neto, A.R.N.: Biofeedback em terapia cognitivo-comportamental. Arq. Méd. Hosp. Fac. Ciênc. Méd. Santa Casa São Paulo 55(3), 127–132 (2018)

Phipps, W.J.: Enfermagem Médico-Cirúrgica, Conceitos e Prática Clínica, 6ª Edição. Lusodidacta (Livro) (2004)

Rissardi, G.G., Godoy, M.F.: Estudo da aplicação da técnica de relaxamento muscular progressivo de Jacobson modificada nas respostas das variáveis cardiovasculares e respiratórias de clientes hansenianos. Arq. Ciênc. Saúde 14(3), 175–180 (2004)

Ruivo, S., Viana, P., Martins, C., Baeta, C.: Efeito do envelhecimento cronológico na função pulmonar. Comparação da função respiratória entre adultos e idosos saudáveis. Rev. Port. Pneumol. 15(4), 629–653 (2009)

Schwartz, M.S., Andrasik, F.: Biofeedback: A practitioner's guide. Guilford Publications (2017)

Spruit, M.A., Pitta, F., McAuley, E., ZuWallack, R.L., Nici, L.: Pulmonary rehabilitation and physical activity in patients with chronic obstructive pulmonary disease. Am. J. Respir. Crit. Care Med. 192(8), 924–933 (2015)

Bongaarts, J.: United Nations, Department of Economic and Social Affairs, Population Division, Sex Differentials in Childhood Mortality. Popul. Dev. Rev. 40(2), 380 (2014)

Burke, D., Gorman, E., Stokes, D., Lennon, O.: An evaluation of neuromuscular electrical stimulation in critical care using the ICF framework: a systematic review and meta-analysis. Clin. Respir. J. (2014)

Direcção-Geral da Saúde (DGS) Translation of: World Health Organization (resolution WHA54.21). International classification of functioning, disability and health (2004)

European Commission (EC): Population, Key figures on Europe – 2014 edn. Publications Office of the European Union, Luxembourg (2014). ISSN 2315-201X

Florin, J., Ehrenberg, A., Ehnfors, M., Björvell, C.: A comparison between the VIPS model and the ICF for expressing nursing content in the health care record. Int. J. Med. Inform. 82(2), 108–117 (2013)

José Lopes, M., et al.: Evaluation of elderly persons' functionality and care needs. Rev. Lat. Am. Enferm. (RLAE) 21, 52–60 (2013)

Maric, M., de Haan, E., Hogendoorn, S.M., Wolters, L.H., Huizenga, H.M.: Evaluating statistical and clinical significance of intervention effects in single-case experimental designs: an SPSS method to analyse univariate data. Behav. Therapy 46(2), 230–241 (2015)

Marôco, J.: Análise Estatística com Utilização do SPSS [Statistical Analysis using SPSS], 6th edn. Edições Silabo, p. 990 (2014). ISBN: 9789899676343

Meskell, P., Murphy, K., Shaw, D.G., Casey, D.: Insights into the use and complexities of the Policy Delphi technique. Nurse Res. **21**(3), 32–39 (2014)

Orem, D.E.: Nursing: Concepts of Practice, 6th edn. Mosby, St. Louis (2001)

Pereira, C., Fonseca, C., Escoval, A., Lopes, M.: Contributo para a classificação da funcionalidade na população com mais de 65 anos, segundo a classificação internacional de funcionalidade. Rev. Port. Saúde Pública **19**(1), 52–62 (2011)

Shen, P., Chen, C.: The WHO's international classification of functioning, disability, and health (ICF): essential knowledge for nurses. Hu Li Za Zhi J. Nurs. **59**(6), 92–97 (2012)

Sidani, S.: Effects of patient-centered care on patient outcomes: an evaluation. Res. Theory Nurs. Pract. **22**(1), 24–37 (2008)

So, H., Kim, H., Ju, K.: Prediction model of quality of life in elderly based on ICF model. J. Korean Acad. Nurs. **41**(4), 481–490 (2011)

The United Nations 2012 Population Projections. (UN) Population & Development Review **39**(3), 551–555 (2013)

World Bank (WB): The World Bank Annual Report 2014: Year in Review, p. 67 (2014)

Zhu, H.: Correctly selection methods of building up a model function of known categories in SPSS 16.0. J. Cap. Inst. Phys. Educ. **26**(1), 91–96 (2014)

Solutions for Active Aging, Social Integration and Self-care

Self-care Needs for Symptom Management and Medication in Elderly Person and Skills of Informal Caregiver to Care Him

Maria dos Anjos Dixe[1] , Ana Maria Vaz[2] ,
and Eugénia Nunes Grilo[3($\boxtimes$)]

[1] Center for Innovative Care and Health Technology (ciTechCare),
Escola Superior de Saúde de Leiria,
Instituto Politécnico de Leiria, Leiria, Portugal
maria.dixe@ipleiria.pt
[2] Health Sciences Research Unit: Nursing-UICISA:
E, Escola Superior de Saúde Dr. Lopes Dias,
Instituto Politécnico de Castelo Branco, Castelo Branco, Portugal
ana.maria@ipcb.pt
[3] Interdisciplinary Research Unit on Building Functional Ageing Communities
Communities - AGE.COMM and Collaborator, NURSE'IN -Nursing Research
Unit of the South and Islands, Escola Superior de Saúde Dr. Lopes Dias,
Instituto Politécnico de Castelo Branco, Castelo Branco, Portugal
eugenia@ipcb.pt

Abstract. Inadequate evaluation and support for dependent elderly people and their caregivers and health service practices often not adequate to the needs of elderly dependents and their caregivers justify a greater investment in this dyad.

This study aims to evaluate the clinical and self-care needs in the management of symptoms and medication of the elderly dependent people; relate their needs to self-care in medication and symptom management with sex and age; to assess the socio-demographic characteristics family and capacities to care for their relatives in the self-management of symptoms and medication management and to value the information received on how to manage the symptoms and medication and the professional who transmitted them. A correlational study of 135 dependent elderly and their informal caregivers through a face-to-face interview consisting of characterization variables and cause of dependence, self-care needs assessment in symptom management and medication.

Most of dependent elderly were women, mean age 83.4 ± 6.7 years and the main cause of dependence were respiratory diseases. Informal caregivers were mostly female, daughters, mean age of 59.1 ± 15.5 years. It was found that on average women were less dependent than men on self-care. Most informal caregivers considered that they were given the necessary information regarding symptom and medication management. Nurses were the professionals who provided them more information.

We concluded that this study brought relevant information regarding the dependent elderly and their caregivers in the identification of their difficulties and adequate information about the best way to manage these difficulties.

© Springer Nature Switzerland AG 2019
J. García-Alonso and C. Fonseca (Eds.): IWoG 2018, CCIS 1016, pp. 225–235, 2019.
https://doi.org/10.1007/978-3-030-16028-9_20

Keywords: Self-care needs · Informal caregiver · Elderly ·
Symptom management · Medication management

1 Background

Informal caregivers (IC) or simply caregivers, as they are usually designated, are part of the group of individuals who provide care and assistance to relatives and friends in an unpaid way [1]. One of the main characteristics of this care is the continuous assistance in activities of daily living (ADLs) or instrumental activities of daily living (IADLs) to a person with a chronic illness or disability [2] who are often elderly. Frequently women are who assume responsibility for caring for their dependents [3] and is considered dependent any person who regardless of age requires care for long periods of time [4]. Caregivers can be called upon to provide a wide variety of care such as assistance in the activities of daily living, including bathing, toilet help, dressing, change to another place, cooking, eating, home management, and medication management [1]. In addition, IC can also perform other functions such as stimulate cognitively their elderly relative, promote activities of motor stimulation and promotion of a safe and comfortable environment, and under the guidance of health professionals and in conjunction with them can also provide more differentiated care [5].

The issue of IC is closely linked to the growing number of elderly people since the mid-twentieth century, with increasing trends. In Portugal, the National Institute of Statistics (INE) projections suggest that this trend should be maintained in the next 40 years, and that in the year 2080 there will be 317 elderly people per 100 young people [6]. And while it is recognized that increasing life expectancy is one of the greatest human achievements of the last decades, living longer brings with it the higher probability of suffering diseases involving increased dependence [7]. The functional decline of the elderly and the consequent dependence are often related to the fragility syndrome involving the interaction of biological, psychological and social factors [8] and associated with an increased risk of adverse effects, such as falls and hospitalization.

There is already a significant amount of evidence on the potential and effective vulnerability of IC, yet formal supports for caregivers of the elderly are often inadequate [9] and their needs are neglected, underscore the effort that both the elderly and the caregivers make to improve and maintain autonomy, the perception of increasing dependence and decline of the loved one's capacities generates frustration and discouragement [10].

In Portugal most of the non-professional care that is provided on an ongoing basis to dependent people on long-term health condition is performed by IC [5]. In most European Union countries, public policy has not yet available formal responses to long-term care accessible to all. And this reality forces family and friends, especially women, to alleviate this gap [11]. Caring in an informal setting is a high-demand, often continuous, high-specificity care [4, 5, 8] and requires formal support and integration and cooperation from health services and social services [12]. Although the studies also report satisfaction derived from the act of taking care of their own's and caregivers say that they do it for affective reasons and love [13], a recent report from the European Commission [4] underlines the lack of formal support for caregivers of dependents and reinforces the need for greater investment in IC. Most countries offer training, psychological counseling and guidance, resources that vary widely, both in terms of availability and quality [4]. As in most European countries, in Portugal the orientation of health and social policies is aimed at favoring the permanence of dependent people at home, through the creation of proximity services, discouraging the institutionalization [5–12]. The overload and stress that result from caring for a close dependent is common. Authors highlight the concern and uncertainty both in relation to the present and in relation to the future as a constant. But knowledge about the illness of his relative increases the perception of effectiveness in the management of care [14].

From the systematic review conducted on the effectiveness of support given to caregivers of people with dementia Vandepitte et al. [15] emphasize psychoeducational interventions such as those that can produce positive results in IC and even delay permanent institutionalization [15]. However, other authors [16] point to the complexity of some activities often performed by IC, such as management of therapy, which both due to the complexity of the therapeutic regimens themselves, as well as to health system practices and lack of information and/or training available to the caregiver are mentioned by these as difficult to manage. In a more recent study on this experiences authors conclude that they are complex and experienced as fragmented and poorly focused on the elderly and in the family as a whole [17] which attests to the need for a better understanding of these experiences and requires the evaluation of the capacities of IC, their strengths and limitations difficulties and perceptions, both in the context of primary health care and in the context of secondary health care [12–15]. From this state of art the following objectives were defined: to evaluate clinical sociodemographic characteristics and self-care needs in the area of symptom management and medication of the dependent elderly person; relate self-care needs in medication management and management of symptoms of the elderly dependent on sex and age; to evaluate the sociodemographic characteristics, family and capacities of the caregiver to care for the dependent elderly person in the areas of self-care in the area of symptom management and medication of the elderly dependent person; to evaluate the information received by the informal caregiver on how to manage the symptoms and medication of the person they care for and the professional who transmitted the information.

2 Methods

This study is reported in line with the STROBE statement.

2.1 Study Design

This correlational study was performed using a face-to-face interview.

2.2 Participants and Setting

The sample consisted of 135 elderly people and their respective informal caregivers, who were interviewed at the time of discharge of the users of the medical services of a

Hospital Center in the Central Zone of Portugal for the home and during a home visit by the nurses of the Primary Health Care of a ULS in the Central Zone of Portugal. The selection of the users was performed by the nurses who accompanied the users and their caregivers based on the following inclusion criteria: Being dependent on at least one of the self-care needs (evaluated through the Barthel index), being able to answer the questions health professionals), ability to consent to participate in the study, or to have authorization from the legal representative and to have an informal caregiver. This was selected based on the following selection criteria: to be the main caregiver and to be present at the time of the interview with the patient. Data were collected during the months of March to May 2018. Patient and caregiver´s interviews where performed by nurses and nursing students who did not work at the unit to prevent bias by influencing patients' answers. A standardized protocol was followed. Participants were given information about the study, reinforced they were free to withdraw from the study at any time for any reason, with no obligation to give the reason for withdrawal. The names and any other identifying details of participants were not collected in any of the surveys, assuring confidentiality of the data collected.

2.3   Variables/Instruments

The interview was made up of two groups: Group I am consisting of sociodemographic and clinical characterization data (age, sex) and cause of dependence according to the international classification of diseases - ICD-10 and time of dependence; Group II, consisting of the evaluation of self-care needs in the area of symptom management and medication. These two domains of self-care were evaluated by 8 items (6 for symptom management and 2 for the medication management area) organized on a Likert-type response scale with 5 options: Dependent/non-participant; Needs help from one person; Needs help from a person and equipment; Needs equipment; Completely independent. These two dimensions are part of a multidimensional scale (allowing the use of several subscales autonomously) to assess self-care needs. These two subscales have good internal consistency: taking medication (2 items; $\alpha = 0.831$) and management of symptoms (6 items; $\alpha = 0.968$). The higher values of quotation of subscales correspond to greater independence in self-care activities. The caregiver interview was composed of two groups: sociodemographic and family characterization data, number of hours per week spent on care, information received on how to manage the symptoms and medication of the person they care for, and the professional who transmitted the information to them.

2.4   Ethical Approval

Research protocol, participant information and informed consent forms were submitted to CNPD (n° 3289/2017) and to the Ethic Committee of Centro Hospitalar de Leiria, who approved the study (04 - 2017/05/02). An appropriate location for data collection was always ensured and the Ethical Principles for Medical Research Involving Human Subjects were met, according to Helsinki Declaration [18].

2.5 Data Processing

Descriptive and inferential statistics were used. Considering the size of the sample and subsamples, non-parametric statistical techniques were used, according to the type of variables under study, namely the Mann Whitney test and the Spearman's correlation.

3 Results

Sociodemographic and Clinic Characteristics of Dependent People

Most of the elderly dependents are women 51,9% (70) with a mean age of 83.4 ± 6.7 years and there is no statistical difference in the mean age according to sex (U = 1934,50, p > 0, 05) when compared with males (81,45 ± 7,8). The women are dependent on the average there are 35,5 ± 45,7 and the men there are 24,2 ± 27,6 months not having the differences statistical significance (U = 1577,00; p > 0,05). The main cause of dependence is respiratory diseases (47,3%) (Table 1).

Table 1. Distribution of elderly dependent responses as to what has caused the dependence

	N°	%
Some infectious and parasitic diseases	1	,8
Neoplasms (tumors)	2	1,5
Diseases blood organs hemat and transt immune	1	,8
Nutritional and Metabolic Endocrine Diseases	1	,8
Mental and behavioral disorders	4	3,1
Diseases of the nervous system	3	2,3
Diseases of the circulatory system	21	16,0
Diseases of the respiratory tract	62	47,3
Diseases of the digestive system	3	2,3
Systemic musculoskeletal and connective tissue disorders	2	1,5
Diseases of the genitourinary system	16	12,2
Others	15	11,5

Self-care Needs in Medication Management and Symptom Management

Regarding symptom management and medication management we can verify that on average women are more autonomous than men, not having these statistical significance (p > 0,05). It should be noted that is the control of nausea, vomiting and anxiety where women are more dependent and in men the control of intestinal changes.

Men are more dependent on adequate preparation of medications as well as women (Table 2).

We also verified that the increase in age was not correlated, with statistical significance, with a greater dependence on medication management self-care (rs = -, 089; p > 0.05) or symptom management (rs = -, 069; p > 0.05). It should be pointed out that the dependent elderly person with greater dependence on symptom management also has greater dependence on medication management (rs = -, 711, p < 0.001).

Table 2. Mann Whitney U test results to self-care needs in medication management and symptom management according to the sex of the dependent person

	Male			Female			U	P
	Average	Medians	SD	Average	Medians	SD		
Prepare the medicines properly	1,54	1,00	,663	1,76	2,00	1,028	1895,000	,065
Take the medicines according to the hour and dose indicated	1,68	2,00	,886	2,16	2,00	1,379	2099,000	,381
Total Take Medication	1,60	1,5	0,7	1,9	2	1,1	1941,000	,113
Pain control	2,05	2,00	1,35	2,51	2,00	1,65	1987,000	,176
Control of respiratory distress	2,05	2,00	1,28	2,30	2,00	1,50	2138,500	,517
Control of nausea and vomiting	2,00	2,00	1,22	2,43	1,593	2,00	2042,000	,269
Control of intestinal changes	1,92	2,00	1,17	2,33	2,00	1,53	2036,000	,255
Anxiety control	1,98	2,00	1,23	2,34	1,58	2,00	2122,000	,468
Body temperature control	1,98	2,00	1,23	2,37	2,00	1,57	2065,000	,319
Management of symptoms	1,90	2	1,1	2,3	2	1,4	2011,000	,223

Taking into account the median value not only of each of the indicators (2.5) but also the weighted average of each of the subscales, we can also state that, on average, dependent people need help from one person (value 2).

The IC that help these elderlies have a mean age of 59.1 ± 15.5 years, are mostly female (111; 82.2%), are children (52.6%); spouses (35.3%) and other relatives (10.1%). Most live with the dependent person (65.9%) and use an average of 89 ± 50 h per week to care for their relative. Regarding the necessary information transmitted to caregivers to support self-care in the management of symptoms and the medication of the caregiver, we found that the majority (80,7%) of the IC considered that they were given the necessary as well as medication management (80,0%) (Table 3).

Table 3. Distribution of informal caregiver responses to information needed for caregivers to support self-care

Informations about	The necessary		Not enough		None		Not applicable	
	N°	%	N°	%	N°	%	N°	%
Managing Symptoms	109	80,7	23	17	3	2,3		
Self-care takes medication	108	80,0	16	11,9	1	0,7	10	7,4

Regarding the caregiver's source of information to support self-care of the elderly dependent, among the valid answers, we can verify that the nurse was the professional who provided the caregiver more information on medication management, but not on symptom management (Table 4).

Table 4. Distribution of informal caregiver responses to information given to caregivers to support self-care

Informations about	Doctor		Nurse		Doctor and nurse		Nurse and caregiver		Caregiver	
	N°	%	Nⁿ	%	N°	%	N°	%	N°	%
Managing Symptoms (n = 140)	100	74,0	7	5,2	17	12,6	0	0,0	11	8,2
Self-care takes medication (n = 132)	16	12,9	36	29,0	26	21,0	43	34,7	3	2,4

4 Discussion

The nature of informal care such as formal care is distinct whether the person being cared for is a child, an adult or an elderly adult, and the elderly are the most caring people in the world [12, 19] which reinforces the importance of knowing their needs for self-care in the management of symptoms and medication as well as the capacities of their caregivers. The elderly in this study needed help from a person for having dependence on at least one of the activities of daily living evaluated through the Barthel Index. In the elderly the dependence and the need for care arises when functional capacity declines and people are no longer able, without help, to guarantee the basic tasks necessary for their daily life [12].

Consistent with the available demographic information and the relative percentages of young and old in developed countries, the elderly in this study were mostly women with a mean age of 83.4 years, slightly higher than the mean age of men that was at 81, 45 following the trend of the average life expectancy at birth in the western world and that in Portugal in the triennium 2014–2016 was 80.62 years [20].

Regarding the time of dependence, the women in the study had a mean of 35.5 ± 45.7 months and in men this time was 24.2 ± 27.6 confirming that the informal care provision lasts in time [4]. Although this study did not show a significant relationship between age and greater dependence on the elderly, the World Health Organization (WHO) and other studies [12–17, 22] highlight the relationship between the greater prolongation of life expectancy and the increase in the number of elderly people with multiple chronic conditions and dependencies. The main cause of dependence of the elderly in this study were diseases of the respiratory (47.3%) and circulatory system, data consistent with that described in the official reports according to which Portuguese live longer but live with more, comorbidities among them diabetes, cardiovascular diseases, respiratory diseases, obesity and oncological diseases [21].

In relation to perceived need for self-care in symptom management, both men and women in the sample reported less independence in controlling intestinal changes and anxiety, thus perceiving a greater need for help. Other self-care in which the men in the sample manifested more dependence was on control of body temperature and women in managing respiratory difficulty. Regarding medication management both men and women perceived greater difficulty in proper preparation of medications, self-care management difficult both among elderly and also caregivers [17]. In the study by Ploeg et al. [17] elderly and caregivers reported that a large part of their communication with health professionals is about the management of therapy and one of the difficulties mentioned is managing the change in medications, especially when there are changes in prescription that occur after hospitalization, difficulty that can be better managed with adequate information and the use of pill dispensers [17].

In this study, there was no significant relationship between dependence on self-management of medication management and age increase. This can be explained from knowledge about health and disease. Health literacy understood as the individual's ability to access, understand, evaluate and use health-related information to make informed decisions [23] is increasingly considered a key aspect in chronic disease management and interventions that enable people to acquire skills and resources to manage their disease have shown results in a variety of these conditions [14–23].

The informal caregivers had a mean age of 59.1 ± 15.5 years; they were mostly female (111; 82.2%), daughters (52.6%); spouses (35.3%) and other relatives (10.1%). The majority lived with the dependent person (65.9%). These characteristics of IC are consistent with the available evidence. The studies [7–17, 19] describe the typical IC of dependent elderly people: it is generally female (usually daughter or daughter-in-law) of middle-aged upper or lower education and who spends more than 20 h per week in informal care activities that accumulates with full or part-time professionals. In this study, the IC reported that they used an average of 89 ± 50 h per week to care for their family member, largely exceeding the one described so far. Caregivers often assume the role of caring as a need without prior knowledge of the skills needed [1] for the self-care of their elderly relative. The majority of IC sample indicated they had received information necessary to support the self-care of their relative, both for self-care taking medication and for self-management symptom management, yet a significant percentage reported that the information received had been insufficient to manage the symptoms (17%) and to manage the self-care of medication (11,9%). Regarding the information source of the IC to support the self-care of his dependent elderly relative, it was verified that the nurses were the health professionals who provided more information to the caregiver in the management of the medication, but the information received on the symptomatic management was provided mostly by the physician.

Although there is not much evidence on the capabilities of IC, there is a documented importance of information and knowledge of caregivers in the perceived effectiveness of disease management [14] and the relevance of investing in caregiver training. Sullivan and Miller [1] recognized and highlighted the significant impact that informal care delivery has on caregivers particularly in social relations, physical and mental health and finances, reinforcing their need to be cared for and valued in their needs. They also emphasized the need to be well informed about their family member's disease process and not to fear increasing their knowledge, caring for themselves and maintaining a healthy life, maintaining social relations, accepting help, and recognizing their emotions as the healthy expression of their families. their feelings and allow themselves to rest from the care and still encourage the independence of their family member and seek help in community resources [1].

The literature review allowed to identify the complexity of informal care for dependent elderly people, but also the need to provide elderly and caregivers with greater formal support, which is recognized as insufficient in most European countries [4] including Portugal [5]. This gap in health care identified in this study is acknowledged by the WHO, stresses the importance of care assessment in a systematic way and recommends that a social worker or a nurse, are responsible for the assessment, because more important than the professional status of who evaluates, is their attitudes and capacity of relationship with the caregivers in a nonjudgmental way [12]. Support, psychological intervention and training should be offered to IC of dependent elderly people particularly when the need for care is complex and extensive, which is only possible with evaluation [12], thus allowing home-based care to be used flexibly and proactively, with the aim of avoiding further functional decline and unnecessary hospitalizations [24].

5 Conclusion

Given the current trend of care for elderly dependents in the context of home care and the recognition of the multiplicity of their needs and the duration of these care, with this study it was possible to identify the self-care needs of elderly dependent and the needs of their caregivers in self-care, symptoms and medication management and the ability of caregivers to manage this self-care. Although most caregivers realized that they had received adequate information to cope with such care, a significant number of informal caregivers expressed that they had insufficient knowledge to manage the self-care of their dependent elderly relative. The data obtained in the study interpreted with the literature review and the evidences found about the information needs and support to caregivers in an informal way reinforce the importance of a greater investment in informal caregivers in order to identify their difficulties in the daily routine to care for their elderly relatives and to provide them with information and support according to the needs identified in an integrated health care perspective, making possible to contribute to the elderly reduction of hospitalizations.

Acknowledgements. This work was supported by Fundação para a Ciência e Tecnologia FCT - Portugal, under the scope of the Help2CARE project: Help2care – Help to care for users and caregivers (POCI-01-0145-FEDER-23762).

Compliance with Ethical Standards Conflict of Interest. All authors declare that they have no potential conflicts of interest.

References

1. Sullivan, B.A., Miller, D.: Who is taking care of the caregiver? J. Patient Exp. **2**(1), 7–12 (2015). https://doi.org/10.1177/237437431500200103
2. Roth, L.D., Fredman, L., Haley, E.W.: Informal caregiving and its impact on health: a reappraisal from population-based studies. Gerontologist **55**(2), 309–319 (2015). https://doi.org/10.1093/geront/gnu177
3. Health Organization Regional Office for Europe: Services for older people in Europe. Strategy and action plan for healthy ageing in Europe, 2012–2020. In: Regional Committee for Europe Sixty-Second Session Malta, 10–13 September 2012 (2008). www.euro.who.int/__data/assets/pdf.../RC62wd10Rev1-Eng.pdf
4. Bouget, D., Spasova, S., Vanhercke, B.: Work-life balance measures for persons of working age with dependent relatives in Europe. A study of national policies, European Social Policy Network (ESPN), European Commission, Brussels (2016). https://doi.org/10.2767/80471
5. Teixeira, A.L., et al.: Medidas de intervenção junto dos cuidadores informais- Documento Enquadrador, Perspetiva Nacional e Internacional. Documento elaborado no processo de criação do estatuto de cuidador informal, com a colaboração do Gabinete de Estratégia e Planeamento do MTSSS (2017). www.cuidadoresportugal.pt
6. INE: Projeções de População Residente – 2015–2080. Destaques à comunicação Social, 29 de março de 2017 (2017). www.ine.pt
7. Moral-Fernández, L., Frías-Osuna, A., Moreno-Cámara, S., Palomino-Moral, P.A., Del-Pino, C.R.: The start of caring for an elderly dependent family member: a qualitative metasynthesis. BMC Geriatr. **18**, 228 (2018). https://doi.org/10.1186/s12877-018-0922-0
8. Carneiro, J.A., et al.: Frailty in the elderly: prevalence and associated factors. Rev. Bras. Enferm. **70**(4), 747–752 (2017). https://doi.org/10.1590/0034-7167-2016-0633. Thematic Edition "Good Practices: Fundamentals of care in Gerontological Nursing"
9. Fabbricotti, I.N., Janse, B., Looman, W.M., Kuijper, R., van Winjngaardem, H., Reiffers, A.: Integrated care for frail elderly compared to usual care: a study protocol of a quasi-experiment on the effects on the frail elderly, their caregivers, health professionals and health care costs. BMC Geriatr. **13**(1), 31 (2013). https://doi.org/10.1186/1471-2318-13-31
10. Kendall, M., et al.: Different experiences and goals in different advanced diseases: comparing serial interviews with patients with cancer, organ failure, or frailty and their family and professional carers. J. Pain Symptom Manage. **50**(2), 216–224 (2015). https://doi.org/10.1016/j.jpainsymman.2015.02.017
11. Moral-Fernández, L., Frías-Osuna, A., Moreno-Cámara, S., Palomino-Moral, P.A., Del-Pino-Casado, R.: The start of caring for an elderly dependent family member. A qualitative metasynthesis. BMC Geriatr. **18**(1), 228 (2018). https://doi.org/10.1186/s12877-018-0922-0
12. WHO: Integrated Care for Older People: Guidelines on Community-Level Interventions to Manage Declines in Intrinsic Capacity. World Health Organization, Geneva (2017). https://www.ncbi.nlm.nih.gov/books/NBK488250/
13. Marques, M.J.F., Teixeira, H.J.C., de Souza, D.C.D.B.N.: Cuidadoras informais de Portugal: vivências do cuidar de idosos. Trabalho Educação e Saúde **10**(1), 147–159 (2012). https://doi.org/10.1590/S1981-77462012000100009
14. Prorok, J.C., Horgan, S., Seitz, D.P.: Health care experiences of people with dementia and their caregivers: a meta-ethnographic analysis of qualitative studies. CMAJ Canad. Med. Assoc. J. **185**(14), E669–E680 (2013). https://doi.org/10.1503/cmaj.121795

15. Vandepitte, S., Van Den Noortgate, N., Putman, K., Verhaeghe, S., Faes, K., Annemans, L.: Effectiveness of supporting informal caregivers of people with dementia: a systematic review of randomized and non-randomized controlled trials. J. Alzheimers Dis. **52**(3), 929–965 (2016). https://doi.org/10.3233/jad-151011

16. Gillespie, R., Mullan, J., Harrison, L.: Managing medications: the role of informal caregivers of older adults and people living with dementia. A review of the literature. J. Clin. Nurs. **23** (23-24), 3296–3308 (2014). https://doi.org/10.1111/jocn.12519

17. Ploeg, J., et al.: Managing multiple chronic conditions in the community: a Canadian qualitative study of the experiences of older adults, family caregivers and- healthcare providers. BMC Geriatr. **17**, 40 (2017). https://doi.org/10.1186/s12877-017-0431-6

18. Associação Médica Mundial: Declaração de Helsínquia da Associação Médica Mundial - Princípios Éticos para a Investigação Médica em Seres Humanos (2013). http://ispup.up.pt/docs/declaracao-de-helsinquia.pdf

19. National Research Council (US) Committee on the Role of Human Factors in Home Health Care: The Role of Human Factors in Home Health Care: Workshop Summary. National Academies Press (US), Washington (DC), 7, Informal Caregivers in the United States: Prevalence, Caregiver Characteristics, and Ability to Provide Care (2010). https://www.ncbi.nlm.nih.gov/books/NBK210048/

20. INE: Tábuas de Mortalidade para Portugal 2014–2016. Destaques à Comunicação Social de 29 de maio de 2017 (2017). http://www.peprobe.com/pe-content/uploads/2017/05/29TabuasMortalidade2014_2016-PT.pdf

21. Ministério da Saúde: Retrato da Saúde, Portugal (2018). https://www.sns.gov.pt/wp-content/uploads/2018/04/RETRATO-DA-SAUDE_2018_compressed.pdf

22. Pollina, D., et al.: Integrated care at home reduces unnecessary hospitalizations of community dwelling frail older adults: a prospective controlled trial. BMC Geriatr. **17**, 53 (2017). https://doi.org/10.1186/s12877-017-0449-9

23. van der Heidel, I., et al.: Health literacy in chronic disease management: a matter of interaction. J. Clin. Epidemiol. **102**, 134–138 (2018). https://doi.org/10.1016/j.jclinepi.2018.05.010

24. Næss, G., Kirkevold, M., Wenche Hammer, W., Straand, J., Torgeir Wyller, B.T.: Nursing care needs and services utilised by home-dwelling elderly with complex health problems: observational study. BMC Health Serv. Res. **17**(645), 1–10 (2017). https://doi.org/10.1186/s12913-017-2600-x

Virtual Assistant to Improve Self-care of Older People with Type 2 Diabetes: First Prototype

Susana Buinhas[1], Ana Paula Cláudio[1], Maria Beatriz Carmo[1],
João Balsa[1], Afonso Cavaco[2], Anabela Mendes[3], Isa Félix[3],
Nuno Pimenta[5], and Mara Pereira Guerreiro[3,4(✉)] [iD]

[1] Instituto de Biossistemas e Ciências Integrativas, Faculdade de Ciências,
Universidade de Lisboa, Lisbon, Portugal
susana_santos94@hotmail.com,
{apc,jbalsa}@di.fc.ul.pt, mbcarmo@fc.ul.pt
[2] Faculdade de Farmácia, Universidade de Lisboa, Lisbon, Portugal
acavaco@ff.ulisboa.pt
[3] Unidade de Investigação e Desenvolvimento em Enfermagem,
Escola Superior de Enfermagem de Lisboa, Lisbon, Portugal
{anabelapmendes,isafelix,mara.guerreiro}@esel.pt
[4] Centro de Investigação Interdisciplinar Egas Moniz (CiiEM), Instituto
Universitário Egas Moniz, Almada, Portugal
[5] Escola Superior de Desporto de Rio Maior, Instituto Politécnico de Santarém,
Santarém, Portugal
npimenta@esdrm.ipsantarem.pt

Abstract. Diabetes has significant clinical, economic and humanistic implications, both at a national and global level. Type 2 diabetes (T2D) is highly prevalent in older people. This paper describes a first prototype of an application intended to facilitate self-care of older people with T2D, supplementing appointments with healthcare professionals. The application is based on a virtual assistant with an anthropomorphic representation. The virtual assistant is capable of speaking and expressing emotions through facial and body animations; it has been designed to act as a relational agent, developing long-term relationships with users. It targets adherence to medication, physical activity and diet, tailoring the intervention to users' needs and characteristics. The Behavior Change Wheel was chosen as the theoretical approach to behaviour change and supports dialogue content. Built for Android devices, the architecture of the application first prototype includes a core component, a dialogue creator, a speech generator and a database. The first tests on the application contents and usability were conducted in a sample of ten academic nurses with expertise in primary care. Overall, these tests yielded a positive opinion, as well as suggestions for improvement. On-going work includes testing the first prototype with older people with T2D plus health professionals in primary care units of the Portuguese National Health Service, and incorporating a rule-based context-sensitive dialogue manager, which is expected to convey a more flexible dialogue flow.

Keywords: Virtual humans · Relational agents · Health care ·
Behavior change · Type 2 diabetes · Older people

© Springer Nature Switzerland AG 2019
J. García-Alonso and C. Fonseca (Eds.): IWoG 2018, CCIS 1016, pp. 236–248, 2019.
https://doi.org/10.1007/978-3-030-16028-9_21

1 Introduction

The global prevalence of diabetes in the adult population, age-standardized, has nearly doubled since 1980, reaching up to 8.5% in 2016 [1]. Around the world, 90% of the diabetic adults suffer from type 2 diabetes mellitus (T2D); the disease or its complications represent the 9th major cause of death [2]. In Portugal, 2015 data shows a total diabetes prevalence, adjusted to the estimated population, of 13.3% [3]. Ageing of the Portuguese population has resulted in a 13.5% increase in diabetes prevalence between 2009 and 2015 [3]. More than a quarter of the Portuguese population between 60 and 79 years old has diabetes [3].

Hyperglycaemia control in T2D involves an adequate diet, physical activity and medication [4, 5]. Difficulties in adhering to diabetes management, which requires behavioural changes maintained indefinitely, is associated with lack of glycaemic control in more than half of the patients [4]. Sustained hyperglycaemia, in turn, results in complications in the kidneys, eyes, vascular system and peripheral nerves, which can be fatal [3]. These complications are associated with considerable direct and indirect costs for the national health system [3]. Improving adherence to T2D management is therefore crucial, as it will result in improved health outcomes, cost reductions and increased life quality.

Adherence to medication and to lifestyle changes is possible with self-management training [6]. Information Technologies (IT) are one resource to help T2D patients in self-managing their condition; their advantages include not relying on the availability of overwhelmed healthcare professionals and convenience of access. Previous studies have produced evidence on IT-based interventions to self-manage T2D. For example, a meta-analysis showed that computer-based interventions produced a small beneficial effect on blood glucose control; such effect can have important public health implications in light of T2D prevalence [7]. Another meta-analysis showed that IT strategies combined with other elements of chronic care are associated with improved glycaemic control [8].

Supporting self-care in T2D requires interactions for long periods of time, spanning from weeks to years; creating an empathic relation between the user/patient and technology is therefore regarded as crucial. Relational agents emerge as an approach to build long-term relationships with users [9].

The VASelfCare project aims to develop and test a prototype of a relational agent application to assist older people with T2D in self-care. In this paper we present the first prototype of an application intended to improve behavior patterns regarding diet, physical activity and medication. The paper is organized as follows: in the next section we examine related work; then the VASelfCare first prototype is described. In the section "First Tests" we present and discuss the results of the user tests performed with academic nurses and, finally, we conclude and point out future work.

2 Related Work

Studies resorting to relational agents have been conducted in several areas.

For example, Bickmore et al. evaluated how patients with a high-level of depressive symptoms responded to a computer animated conversational agent in a hospital environment [10]. Another publication described the use of relational agents in health counselling and behaviour change interventions in clinical psychiatry [11]. Ring et al. reported a pilot study based on an affectively-aware virtual therapist for depression counselling [12]. Still in mental health interventions, Provoost et al. [13] reviewed the use of embodied conversational agents in clinical psychology, mostly focusing on autism and on social skills training. Relational agents have also been used in other areas, such as breastfeeding promotion [14].

These studies, although mostly in a preliminary stage, unanimously reported positive results. Benefit in patients with lower health literacy was also demonstrated [10].

Moreover, work with relational agents in areas closely related to the present project has been published. Bickmore and colleagues have conducted extensive work with relational agents to promote physical activity (PA) [15, 16, 18–20]. They showed that this approach is well accepted, including by older adults, and demonstrated increases in physical activity. In these intervention studies, physical activity was assessed by means of pedometers, using steps count per day as the main outcome measure. For instance, in a two months intervention the daily number of steps increased from 3500 steps/day to over 7000 steps/day [15, 16]. Despite the small sample (n = 8) the increase was statistically significant; the control group showed no changes in daily steps [15, 16]. The intervention allowed these subjects to achieve the suggested minimum recommended level of steps/day; it is reasonable to expect a relevant impact on health outcomes [21]. The beneficial effect of relational agents interventions in physical activity was confirmed in a randomized control trial (RCT) in older adults, but only in the short term; the effects seemed to wane by 12 months [18]. Studies from the same research group in other populations than older people have shown less impressive results. An RCT in overweight adults reached only maintenance of physical activity in the intervention group, while the control group showed decreases [17]. These results were recently confirmed in another RCT on healthy adults [20]. In summary, interventions based on relational agents have shown effectiveness in promoting physical activity in older adults, in particular in the short term. Data on the health benefits and cost-effectiveness of these interventions are lacking.

The literature also offers examples of multi-behavioral interventions, in recognition of the fact that improving health or the self-care of chronic conditions requires more than single behavior change. One example is a study carried out in patients with schizophrenia, to promote adherence to antipsychotic medication and PA. A pilot evaluation over the course of 31 days, in a sample of 20 patients, showed the intervention was well accepted; self-reported medication and physical activity adherence were also very high [22].

The use of relational agents in people with T2D has been little explored. One exception is an Australian study, which described the development of an intelligent lifestyle coach for self-management of diabetes patients [23]. However, this study lacks data on usability or the effect on endpoints of interest. More recently, an on-going study in the USA employed a relational agent as a health coach for adolescents with type 1 diabetes and their parents [24].

3   VASelfCare First Prototype

As previously mentioned, the application is intended to be used by people aged 65 years or more suffering from T2D. It targets adherence to medication, physical activity and diet by means of a relational agent, called Vitória, with an anthropomorphic representation. Vitória plays the role of virtual assistant and is capable of speaking and expressing emotions through facial and body animations, depending on the users' response. Vitória's speech is also displayed in the interface as subtitles.

The 3D scenario where Vitória changes according to the context of the dialogue (e.g. a kitchen scenario is presented when talking about the diet), the time of the day and season of the year.

The user communicates with Vitória using buttons or recording values, such as the daily number of steps. The application plots inputted data and Vitória gives feedback based on these plots (e.g. with the number of steps over time).

The application can be used in two modes: (i) daily interaction with Vitória, fed by past records and information inputted during the dialogue and (ii) *ad-hoc* access to other functionalities.

The application runs in tablets with Android system without Internet connection. This decision was grounded on the need to enable access to the application in instances where Internet is not available, such as users' homes. While recent data shows that 70% of households in Portugal have Internet connection, mostly with broadband, Internet penetration rate may be lower in older adults' homes [25].

Each tablet keeps the records of one user on a local database. The application is able to store all data related to the interactions between the user and Vitória in a *json* file; when Internet connection is detected it backs-up this file into the project server.

User registration in the application is made by nurses providing care in diabetes consultations. Registration includes clinical information, such as prescribed antidiabetic agents, height and weight. This information is mandatory, and the application provides a specific interface for this purpose.

3.1   Dialogues Content

Only the medication adherence intervention has been set up; the development of the physical activity and diet interventions is on-going. All interventions consist of two phases: (1) assessment and (2) follow-up. As described by others [26], the assessment phase has the purpose of tailoring the intervention in the subsequent phase. For the medication adherence, this first phase is split into three days; each daily interaction is structured in repeated sequential steps adapted from the literature (opening, social talk, assessment, feedback, pre-closing and closing) [27].

The follow-up phase starts after the completion of the assessment phase. The Behavior Change Wheel (BCW) was chosen as the theoretical approach to behavior change and supports the dialogue creation [28, 29]. The dialogues in this second phase are also structured in repeated sequential steps (opening, social talk, review tasks, assess, counselling, assign tasks, pre-closing and closing) [27].

3.2   The Architecture of the Solution

The architecture of the technological solution is depicted in Fig. 1. The VASelfCare Core component includes the scripts that control the interface and the flow of the execution. The Dialogue Creator is the component used to define the speech of Vitória and the choices presented to the user. Finally, the Speech Generator includes the process to create the audio and viseme files to support Vitória's speech. Built for Android devices, the application resorts to different software tools, as explained in the next sections.

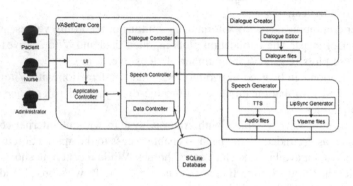

Fig. 1.   VASelfCare application architecture.

4   VASelfCare Core

The VASelfCare Core comprises the scripts responsible for the user interface and the logic of the app; it is implemented in Unity3D with C# scripts that control the entire flow of the interaction.

The flow of execution is managed by the Application Controller, which is responsible for the logical sequence of the application and for communicating with the other components of the VASelfCare Core, and with the local database. The other modules are the Dialogue Controller, the Speech Controller, and the Data Controller.

The Dialogue Controller is in charge of controlling the order of the dialogues, deciding which dialogue files should be used in a specific moment of the interaction. The Speech Controller is the module that allows Vitória to speak, searching and activating the audio and viseme files that correspond to the on-going dialogue. Data Controller has the responsibility of exchanging data with the local database. This embedded local database keeps track of clinical information inputted by the nurses and of all interactions with users. This information is relevant for the application to decide the flow of the dialogue, providing an adequate follow-up to the user.

4.1   Dialogue Creator

The dialogue editor Yarn is easily integrated into Unity3D projects and therefore was the chosen tool for building the dialogues. This open source software has been employed in well-known games, such as *Night in the Woods*[1] and *Knights and Bikes*[2], conferring credibility and status.

Yarn allows the insertion of few lines of code that influence the flow of dialogue. It is based on a graph system. Each node in the graph represents part of the dialogue and contains several response options, which are presented to users as buttons (Fig. 2).

4.2   Speech Generator

Criteria to choose the Text-To-Speech (TTS) software, which converts text to audio speech, were the following: (i) providing male and female voices in European Portuguese, (ii) minimal cost, (iii) unlimited service and (iv) no expiration date. In light of these criteria, Speech2Go from Harpo[3] (Ivona's voice), was the best option. Since currently the virtual assistant is represented by a female figure, only the female voice of Ivona has been used. The speech rate has been slowed down, taking in consideration the target population.

The LipSync Generator, developed in a previous project [30], is used to convert text to viseme files. These files are stored in the same folder as the audio files, since they are read simultaneously by the virtual character.

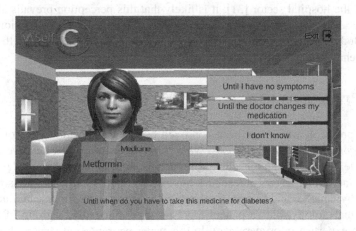

Fig. 2. Dialogue view.

---

[1] http://www.nightinthewoods.com/.

[2] http://foamswordgames.com/.

[3] https://harposoftware.com/en/2-main/s-1/index/brand-speech2goivona/language-portuguese.

4.3   Database

SQLite[4] was the database engine chosen. It is a popular choice as embedded database software, used for local/client storage by companies such as Apple, Mozilla Firefox and Skype. It is open source and encompasses a secure storage mechanism, which allows recording all the information in a single file without installation, except for the plugins that need to be integrated into the project.

4.4   VASelfCare Interaction

The application begins depicting Vitória in a living room scenario, which intends to provide a sense of comfort to the user. If the user logs in as a nurse, the button "Enter" redirects to the registration view. If the user logs in as patient, the button "Enter" redirects to a dialogue view, where the interaction with the virtual assistant begins.

Currently the app displays two charts in the history view. One shows the number of daily steps performed by the user; the other shows the number of days the user interacted with Vitória. Both charts can be viewed in different time periods: since the first time the app was accessed, the last 30 days or the last 7 days.

4.5   Virtual Assistant

The virtual assistant chosen for this first prototype is a female 3D model, obtained from Daz3D[5]. This choice was based on the traditional association of women with the role of "caring" in the hospital sector [31]; it is likely that this perception prevails also in the ambulatory sector. Other studies have also employed female figures as relational agents [15, 16]. Body animations and facial expressions are activated via scripts that control Vitória's behavior and verify the context of the on-going interaction.

5   First Tests

The study protocol, which has been approved by the Ethics Committee of *Administração Regional de Saúde de Lisboa e Vale do Tejo*, encompasses iterative tests with older people with T2D and health professionals during the software development phase. Two additional layers of feedback have been set up. Firstly, an Advisory Board, comprised by national and international experts in informatics, in research design and in clinical diabetology, plus a patient representative. Secondly, a group of academic nurses with expertise in primary care. In this paper we report on tests with the latter.

5.1   Participants and Procedure

Nurses were purposively sampled within the consortium lead Institution. Eleven academic nurses were invited. They all accepted to participate, but it was only possible to

---

[4] https://www.sqlite.org/index.html.

[5] https://www.daz3d.com/.

schedule sessions with ten nurses. No rewards were used. Respondents' age ranged between 39 and 62 years with a mean professional experience of 30.8 years (SD 7.3).

The data collection instrument was a self-administered questionnaire, comprised by three parts: socio-demographic questions, 15 closed-questions about the prototype and seven open-ended questions about the prototype and its use in older people with T2D. Experts responded to closed-questions on a 5-point Likert scale, with anchor points from (1) strongly disagree to strongly agree (5).

Data were collected in individual face-to-face sessions, which lasted for about 40 min. After a short introduction, respondents were asked to use the prototype independently, guided by a list of suggested tasks, which included talking to Vitória through a full interaction. The deployed tablets had the following characteristics: SO – Android 7.0; CPU - Snapdragon 435; RAM: 3 GB; ROM: 32 GB. In the end of the session a member of the research team went through the questions and probed for clarification if needed.

Data were entered into an Excel file and cross-checked for accuracy. Descriptive statistics was performed with the aid of SPSS v.24. Textual data were subjected to content analysis, by deriving main themes related to the open-ended questions and data, plus categories under these themes. Phrases or text segments were then labelled under each category.

5.2   Results and Discussion

A boxplot representing respondents' opinions on Vitória (Fig. 3) shows that, overall, responses were positive. The least encouraging opinions pertained to Vitória's look, as answers ranged from negative (n = 1) to neutral (n = 1) and positive (n = 8). Upon probing one academic nurse commented that "Vitória blinks too often" (ID5). On the contrary, the statements that Vitória's speech could be heard and understood well received only positive answers.

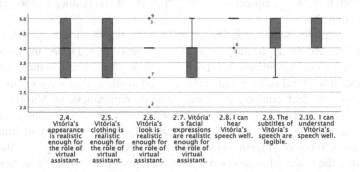

Fig. 3. Experts' views on aspects related to the virtual assistant

Respondents' opinions on other aspects of the interface were generally positive (Fig. 4). The least encouraging opinions pertained to the charts on the number of daily steps and on the application use, which received negative (n = 1) and neutral answers (n = 3), in addition to positive answers (n = 6). Upon probing one respondent (ID2) said that the information on what is a very good, good and insufficient number of daily steps should be available; another suggestion would be to have a line in the chart depicting the ideal or agreed goal (ID2).

Question 2.14 examined whether overall the application was easy to use. Respondents expressed agreement with this statement (median 4; minimum 4; maximum 5).

Globally, there were positive views on whether people with T2D would use the application often (median 4; minimum 3; maximum 5). Upon probing, the four neutral answers could be explained by a sense that the application use would largely depend on individual characteristics of patients.

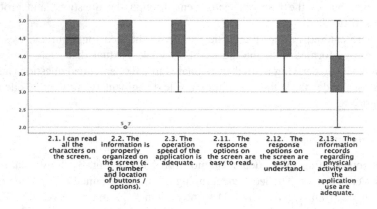

Fig. 4. Experts' views on other interface aspects

Over 100 comments were coded under six broad themes: "contents", "technology", "communication style", "frequency of use", "perceived motivating factors" and "perceived difficulties".

Several categories were identified in relation to the theme "technology". Three respondents labelled the application as intuitive. Aspects related to the interface and the synthetic voice were categorized into positive and negative. For instance, tables used for feedback on the level of knowledge about antidiabetic agents were regarded as too dense. One respondent complained about lack of naturalness in Vitória's speech: "Although understandable, it sounds a bit robotic" (ID6), whilst another took a divergent stance "(the voice) is pleasant" (ID8). Resorting to a virtual human as a relational agent received unanimous endorsement. Reasons underlying this positive view included the potential to develop a relationship with the virtual assistant and the possibility of a greater interactivity with users.

Under "communication style" the main findings pertain to appreciation about the use of simple language, the non-judgmental approach and the employment of positive reinforcement.

"Perceived motivating factors" pertain to aspects that may help older people using the application on a daily basis. For example, learning about topics of interest, effective problem-solving and monitoring the physical activity and self-monitored blood glucose via the application were put forward as motivating factors.

We found divergent views in respect to Vitória's synthetic voice. Less positive views are unsurprising, as expectations about synthetic voices may be somehow similar to the attributes exhibited by human voices. For example, Cabral et al. found that participants rated human voice as more expressive, understandable and likeable than the synthetic voice developed by the team [32]. Nonetheless, for the short one-way interaction tested in this study, different voices did not have a significant impact on character judgements, such as appeal and credibility [32]. Whether features such as smaller expressiveness of synthetic voices affect users in long-term two-way interactions, which is the situation envisaged for our application, merits further research.

Respondents considered that the ability of ascertaining progress over time via the application would motivate patients to use it daily. The patients' representative in our advisory board was of the same view. One of his suggestions was to have a plot of self-monitored blood glucose values, together with an indication of target values and records of physical activity and diet. In his view this would facilitate discerning relationships between lifestyle and outcomes.

The effect of self-monitoring of blood glucose in improving glycaemic control in people with T2D not treated with insulin is less clear than in their insulin-treated counterparts [33, 34]. International guidelines vary in their recommendations for self-monitoring of blood glucose in patients not using insulin or glucose-lowering medications that can cause hypoglycemia [35]. Nonetheless guidelines agree that, when recommended, self-monitoring of blood glucose should be part of an educational program, encompassing therapeutic interventions in response to blood glucose values [35]. Our prototype is envisaged to be used in non-insulin treated T2D patients and therefore offering functionalities related to self-monitoring of blood glucose was not a priority. The suggestions received both by the academic nurses and the patients' representative probably reflect the common use in Portugal of blood glucose test strips in patients treated with oral antidiabetics only [36]. Incorporating such functionalities in the application prototype deserves further discussion.

6 Conclusions and Future Work

We have developed a first prototype of a relational agent application to facilitate adherence to T2D management in older people. Built for Android devices, its architecture includes a core component, a dialogue creator, a speech generator and a database.

Testing this prototype with academic nurses provided valuable insights on the application contents and usability. Answers to closed-questions indicated, overall, a positive opinion about the application. Textual data yielded rich insights about opportunities for improvement. On-going work includes testing the first prototype with older people with T2D plus health professionals in primary care units of the Portuguese National Health Service. Upon completion of data collection, we will discuss the full range of suggestions and opportunities for improvement in terms of relevance and feasibility, followed by prioritization.

Additionally, we are exploring the incorporation of a rule-based component for the follow-up stage of the intervention. This is expected to convey a more flexible dialogue flow, in which each sentence/question produced by the virtual assistant results both from the user's previous answer and from additional contextual information.

Acknowledgements. The authors are indebted to Adriana Henriques and Isabel Costa e Silva for their work in the VASelfCare project, as team members.

The authors express their gratitude to the advisory board members and the academic nurses who participated in the tests.

This work was supported by FCT and Compete 2020 (grant number LISBOA-01-0145-FEDER-024250).

References

1. World Health Organization. Global report on diabetes (2016)
2. Zheng, Y., Ley, S.H., Hu, F.B.: Global aetiology and epidemiology of type 2 diabetes mellitus and its complications. Nat. Rev. Endocrinol. **14**(2), 88 (2018)
3. Observatório, Da Diabetes. Diabetes Factos e Números o ano de 2015-Relatório Anual do Observatório Nacional da Diabetes. Sociedade Portuguesa de Diabetologia (2016)
4. García-Pérez, L.E., Alvarez, M., Dilla, T., Gil-Guillén, V., Orozco-Beltrán, D.: Adherence to therapies in patients with type 2 diabetes. Diab. Ther. **4**(2), 175–194 (2013)
5. Lavie, C.J., et al.: Exercise is medicine—The importance of physical activity, exercise training, cardiorespiratory fitness, and obesity in the prevention and treatment of type 2 diabetes. Eur. Endocrinol. **10**(1), 18 (2010)
6. Norris, S.L., Engelgau, M.M., Narayan, K.M.: Effectiveness of self-management training in type 2 diabetes: A systematic review of randomized controlled trials. Diab. Care **24**(3), 561–587 (2001)
7. Pal, K., et al.: Computer-based interventions to improve self-management in adults with type 2 diabetes: A systematic review and meta-analysis. Diab. Care **37**(6), 1759–1766 (2014)
8. Alharbi, N.S., et al.: Impact of information technology–based interventions for type 2 diabetes mellitus on glycemic control: A systematic review and meta-analysis. J. Med. Internet Res. **18**, 11 (2016)
9. Bickmore, T., Schulman, D., Yin, L.: Maintaining engagement in long-term interventions with relational agents. Appl. Artif. Intell. **24**(6), 648–666 (2010)
10. Bickmore, T.W., Mitchell, S.E., Jack, B.W., Paasche-Orlow, M.K., Pfeifer, L.M., O'Donnell, J.: Response to a relational agent by hospital patients with depressive symptoms. Interact. Comput. **22**(4), 289–298 (2010)
11. Bickmore, T.W., Gruber, A.: Relational agents in clinical psychiatry. Harvard Rev. Psychiatry **18**(2), 119–130 (2010)
12. Ring, L., Bickmore, T.W., Pedrelli, P.: An affectively aware virtual therapist for depression counseling. In: ACM SIGCHI Conference on Human Factors in Computing Systems (CHI) Workshop on Computing and Mental Health (2016)
13. Provoost, S., Lau, H.M., Ruwaard, J., Riper, H.: Embodied conversational agents in clinical psychology: A scoping review. J. Med. Internet Res. **19**(5), e151 (2017)
14. Zhang, Z., et al.: Maintaining continuity in longitudinal, multi-method health interventions using virtual agents: The case of breastfeeding promotion. In: Bickmore, T., Marsella, S., Sidner, C. (eds.) IVA 2014. LNCS (LNAI), vol. 8637, pp. 504–513. Springer, Cham (2014). https://doi.org/10.1007/978-3-319-09767-1_61

15. Bickmore, T.W., Caruso, L., Clough-Gorr, K.: Acceptance and usability of a relational agent interface by urban older adults, p. 1212 (2005)
16. Bickmore, T.W., Caruso, L., Clough-Gorr, K., Heeren, T.: 'It's just like you talk to a friend' relational agents for older adults. Interact. Comput. 17(6), pp. 711–735, Dez (2005)
17. Watson, A., Bickmore, T.W., Cange, A., Kulshreshtha, A., Kvedar, J.: An internet-based virtual coach to promote physical activity adherence in overweight adults: Randomized controlled trial. J. Med. Internet Res. 14(1), e1 (2012)
18. Bickmore, T.W., et al.: A randomized controlled trial of an automated exercise coach for older adults. J. Am. Geriatr. Soc. 61(10), 1676–1683 (2013)
19. King, A.C., et al.: Testing the comparative effects of physical activity advice by humans vs. computers in underserved populations: The COMPASS trial design, methods, and baseline characteristics. Contemp. Clin. Trials 61, 115–125 (2017)
20. Sillice, M.A., et al.: Using relational agents to promote exercise and sun protection: Assessment of participants' experiences with two interventions. J. Med. Internet Res. 20(2), e48 (2018)
21. ACSM: ACSM's Guidelines for Exercise Testing and Prescription, 10th Revised edn. Wolters Kluwer, Philadelphia (2017)
22. Bickmore, T.W., Puskar, K., Schlenk, E.A., Pfeifer, L.M., Sereika, S.M.: Maintaining reality: Relational agents for antipsychotic medication adherence. Interact. Comput. 22(4), 276–288 (2010)
23. Monkaresi, H., et al.: Intelligent diabetes lifestyle coach. In: Fifth International Workshop on Smart Healthcare and Wellness Applications (SmartHealth 2013), Adelaide, Australia (2013)
24. Thompson, D., Cullen, K.W., Redondo, M.J., Anderson, B.: Use of relational agents to improve family communication in type 1 diabetes: Methods. JMIR Res. Protoc. 5(3), e151 (2016)
25. INE: Sociedade da Informação e do Conhecimento – "Inquérito à Utilização de Tecnologias da Informação e da Comunicação pelas Famílias", Lisboa (2015)
26. Migneault, J.P., Farzanfar, R., Wright, J.A., Friedman, R.H.: How to write health dialog for a talking computer. J. Biomed. Inform. 39, 468–481 (2006)
27. Bickmore, T.W., Schulman, D., Sidner, C.: A reusable framework for health counseling dialogue systems based on a behavioral medicine. J. Biomed. Inform. 44, 183–197 (2011)
28. Michie, S., Atkins, L., West, R.: The Behaviour Change Wheel – A Guide to Designing Intervention. Silverback Publishing, London (2014)
29. Michie, S., et al.: The behavior change technique taxonomy (v1) of 93 hierarchically clustered techniques: Building an international consensus for the reporting of behavior change interventions. Ann. Behav. Med. 46, 81–95 (2013)
30. Cláudio, A.P., et al.: Virtual humans for training and assessment of self-medication consultation skills in pharmacy students. In: 2015 10th International Conference on Computer Science & Education (ICCSE). IEEE (2015)
31. Pastore, E., Rosa, L.D., Homem, I.D.: Relações de gênero e poder entre trabalhadores da área da saúde. In: Fazendo Gênero 8 - Corpo, Violência e Poder (2008)
32. Cabral, J.P., Cowan, B.R., Zibrek, K., McDonnell, R.: The influence of synthetic voice on the evaluation of a virtual character. In: Proc. Interspeech, pp. 229–233 (2017). https://doi.org/10.21437/interspeech.2017-325
33. Malanda, U.L., Welschen, L.M.C., Riphagen, I.I., Dekker, J.M., Nijpels, G., Bot, S.D.M.: Self-monitoring of blood glucose in patients with type 2 diabetes mellitus who are not using insulin. Cochrane Database Syst. Rev. 1(1) (2012). https://doi.org/10.1002/14651858. CD005060.pub3, Article No. CD005060

34. Farmer, A.J., et al.: Meta-analysis of individual patient data in randomised trials of self monitoring of blood glucose in people with non-insulin treated type 2 diabetes. BMJ **344**, e486 (2012)
35. Report on Self-Monitoring of Blood Glucose (SMBG) in Type 2 Diabetes Mellitus. Medicines Management Programme (2016). http://www.hse.ie/eng/services/publications/Clinical-Strategy-and-Programmes/Report-on-Self-Monitoring-of-Blood-Glucose-SMBG-in-Type-2-Diabetes-Mellitus.pdf
36. Risso, T., Furtado, C.: Rational use of blood glucose test strips for self-monitoring in patients with diabetes mellitus: Economic impact in the Portuguese healthcare system. Diabetes Res. Clin. Pract. **134**, 161–167 (2017)

Nursing Students Digital Competencies for the Self-management of Patients: Development of the DigiNurse Model's Interface

Pedro Parreira[1]([✉]) [iD], Paulo Santos Costa[2] [iD],
Anabela Salgueiro-Oliveira[1] [iD], Paulo Alexandre Ferreira[1],
Liliana B. Sousa[2] [iD], Inês A. Marques[2] [iD], Rafael Bernardes[2] [iD],
Raija Kokko[3], and João Graveto[1] [iD]

[1] Nursing School of Coimbra, 3046-851 Coimbra, Portugal
parreira@esenfc.pt
[2] The Health Sciences Research Unit: Nursing, 3000-232 Coimbra, Portugal
[3] Tampere University, 33520 Tampere, Finland

Abstract. Background: While the need for self-management support is increasing in the current aging European society, digital skills and competences in supporting self-management is not commonly a part of the nursing curriculum. In order to respond to this societal challenge, the Digital Nursing Model (DigiNurse) will be developed by an international consortium, offering a structured concept to be incorporated in the nursing curriculum. This project was financially supported through the Erasmus+ program, through the Key-Action "Cooperation for Innovation and the Exchange of Good Practices". The final goal is to develop a digital interface to be used by nursing students in the follow-up of patients with chronic diseases, guided by the key-principles of the Digi-Nurse Model. Objective: To reflect on the different theoretical contributions that supports the creation of digital interfaces to develop digital skills/competences in nursing students and professionals. Conclusion: The development of digital skills in nursing students is important for the follow-up of patients with chronic diseases. So, the analysis of different models will support the development of DigiNurse Model, whose implementation in educational and pedagogical models in nursing curricula can contribute to significant improvements in health care of patients with chronic illness.

Keywords: Digital · ICT · Nursing · Self-management · Technology

1 Background

A new approach in health care is needed to effectively face the increasing demands for tailor-made and patient-centered care. Currently, providing distance smarter care (online or digital) require a focus on disease prevention and early detection, as well as treatment compliance and management. Facing the worldwide aging of population and

© Springer Nature Switzerland AG 2019
J. García-Alonso and C. Fonseca (Eds.): IWoG 2018, CCIS 1016, pp. 249–256, 2019.
https://doi.org/10.1007/978-3-030-16028-9_22

associated chronic diseases, the main health challenge will be to provide more and better quality care within the same human resources.

In this context, successful sharing of electronic data, telecare and tele coaching require the development of an integrated care model, where patients/healthcare consumers are encouraged to be actively involved in their healthcare process. As such, a patient becomes co-pilot with the health care professionals in the management of his chronic illnesses and specific needs.

Recent technological developments have made possible a change from current care to an integrated health care. However, health care education institutions need to integrate the smart use of new technologies into their curriculum. By doing this, it will be ensured that the nursing students acquire digital competences, being future-proof and ambassadors of self-management support in health care.

However, in Europe, there is not a conceptual model for learning digital skills in nursing higher education institutions, nor any organized collaboration around the topic [1]. To address this issue, an international consortium composed by five nursing higher education from Portugal, Finland, Slovenia and Belgium is currently designing the framework of the DigiNurse Model. This challenge was recognized and financially supported through the Erasmus+ program, through the Key-Action "Cooperation for Innovation and the Exchange of Good Practices".

The DigiNurse model intended to be a generic model comprising organizational, educational and professional elements for the development of students' digital competences. The main purpose of this model is about digital coaching of patients, taking up an active role of nurses in the coordination of care for persons with complex and chronic care demands. The implementation of this model in higher education of nursing students will be preparing them for the outstanding revolution that is inevitable to happen in healthcare due to the aging population and associated chronic disabilities and their specificities in terms of health care. The digital skills will include tailor-made health promotion and education, monitoring data regarding health parameters, attending to decision protocols, setting life goals, supporting treatment compliance, assessing progress (follow-ups), and integrating advance care planning. The shared principle to this intervention in nursing students digital competencies is based on shared decision making, involving the health care professionals, caregivers, and patients. This will be possible through the development of a digital interface, used by nursing students.

The DigiNurse Model will guide the nursing students in their digital learning, specifically for a careful selection, observation and evaluation of teaching and learning methods. Active learning method will be integrated into this process and therefore nursing students will coach their patients in a way to remotely involve them in the assessment, implementation and evaluation of proposed activities.

The consortium aims to develop a logical, well-planned digital learning path for nursing students. This model will be generic and independent of teaching local or working culture. However, the development of digital educational interfaces in nursing is not an explored concept, being necessary to develop theoretical review of the main literature in this field.

Being this the focus of the study, we intended to analyze the existing theoretical contributions regarding the development of a digital coaching interface, identifying its main benefits, how to explore them, as well as to detecting strategies that can reduce the possibility of errors or mistakes. Attending to this, we will undertake a comprehensive approach of existing models that are commonly used in the conception of interfaces in similar scientific areas, identifying the dimensions that may be relevant to the DigiNurse Model's interface.

2   Contributions on Interface Usability

2.1   Narrative Review

To ensure adequate resources in health care and to further improve the level of care, care-delivery models need to be changed in a way that patients themselves become more involved in their own health care. In fact, the patient-centered care emerged in the early 50s, being recognized as a desirable attribute that respects patients' preferences, needs, and values by health care organizations, policy makers, regulators and researchers [2, 3]. Currently, patient-centered care is considered essential for high-quality healthcare systems [2]. In response to this demand, health coaching constitutes a natural fit and useful strategy in a way that nurses can help the patients to achieve their health and life goals [1], as an overall goal of the health care interventions.

Developing a coaching interface is a complex and time-consuming challenge, that requires four distinct phases: planning, implementing, evaluating and sustaining [1]. This process starts with a clear definition of scope, goals and intended outcomes. Then, during the development phase, tracking interface usability and assessment data are key-strategies to achieve a better product for the users' vision and values [1].

To attain this purpose, narrative reviews will be important to integrate different theoretical contributions that focus on the interface's level of usability and interactivity, allowing for critical reflection of all its components and being adapted to the digital skills and overall experience of its users.

2.2   Cognitive Walkthrough Method

As a theory-based method for evaluation of interfaces usability, the Cognitive Walkthrough Method (CWM) [4] is used to identify problems and generate proposals about their causes. Primarily, the CWM is proposed for application during the development process of interfaces, focusing in the user's cognitive processes and previous knowledge. This method measures the ease of learning, when the user explores or perform the task by a "trial and error" technique. According to Bligård and Osvalder [5], the CWM simulates the user's cognitive processes during a sequence of actions in performing a given task. By doing this, is possible to determine whether the user's background knowledge, together with hints from the interface, will lead to a correct sequence of goals and actions. This technique requires an evaluator or group of evaluators with sufficient knowledge because the quality of the results depends on how well the evaluators can place themselves in the situation as users [5]. The CWM involve a preparation stage, that requires the identification and definition of potential users and tasks, determining the correct sequence of actions in performing those tasks. Then, the analysis is a walkthrough conducted for the chosen tasks, and evaluators pose four questions for each stage in the sequence of action.

The following questions are used to simulate the user's cognitive process during the tasks execution: (a) will the user try and achieve the right outcome?; (b) will the user notice that the correct action is available to them?; (c) will the user associate the correct action with the outcome they expect to achieve?; and (d) if the correct action is performed, will the user see that progress is being made towards their intended outcome? [6]. These questions are answered affirmatively or negatively, and detailed reasons on the latter should be stated. Problems that arise are noted, along with the reason why the problems arose, based on assumptions made by the evaluators [6]. To finalize the CWM implementation, the follow-ups should be done, ensuring that proposals are given regarding possible modifications of the interface to eliminate or reduce the identified problems.

2.3   Unified Framework of Usability (TURF)

According to Zhang and Walji [7], the Unified Framework of Usability (TURF) describes, explains and predicts usability differences. This method objectively defines, evaluates, and measures usability in order to achieve designs with good usability. Once fully developed, TURF could also be used as a principle for developing Electronic Health Records usability guidelines and standards. Usability refers to how useful, usable, and satisfying a system is for the intended users. Specifically, it determines if the users accomplish the goals in performing certain sequences of tasks, constituting the three major dimensions under TURF: a system is usable if it is (i) easy to learn, (ii) efficient to use, and (iii) error-tolerant.

The first stage of applying TURF is user analysis, that provides user information necessary to conduct function, representation and task analyses. This includes age related skills, cultural background, personality, knowledge of computers, education background, cognitive functions, perceptual variations [7]. The second stage in TURF method is function analysis, that identifies the structure of the tasks that users will perform. According to [7], the work domain ontology should be invariant to work context, technology or cognitive processes to ensure their success. The third stage is representation analysis, which is the process of evaluating the appropriateness of the representations for a given task performed by a specific type of users. Different representations of a common abstract structure can generate different representational efficiencies, task difficulties, and behavioral outcomes. Subsequently, in phase four, task analysis identifies the task steps needed to carry out an operation by using a specific representation, the relations among those steps, and the nature of each one (mental or physical). By performing task analysis for the same operation in different user interfaces, user performance associated with different user interfaces can be compared in terms of execution time, number of steps, and mental effort (metrics of efficiency for usability).

In TURF, usability is defined as a human performance issue, considering usefulness as an important component of usability, along with the usableness and satisfaction dimensions. According to Zhang and Walji [7], usefulness is often more important than usableness for a product's success or failure.

3 Digital Interactive Interfaces Applied to Education

The development of technological resources, along with the expansion and need for (presential or remote) education, raised important challenges on elaborating dynamic strategies in training, education and pedagogy in several scientific areas [8]. In this sense, several theories and models of digital educational materials/instruments emerged.

According to Passos [8], the Digital Interactive Interfaces Applied to Education model (INTERAD) was developed based on research in the educational and interaction design areas, knowledge architecture and visual planning. Additionally, the author states that this contribution aims to provide an answer for the growing utilization of digital materials for pedagogic practices in order to direct health professionals on the use of interfaces that are adjusted to their courses.

To achieve this, the INTERAD model is composed by five modules: (i) comprehension, with the mapping of all existing information on the digital educational instruments that are planned to be used; (ii) preparation, which concerns the transformation of the information obtained in the previous module; (iii) experimentation, which happens when the practical part of the training is started, with the development of a structure for the materials or instruments; (iv) elaboration, which addresses the chosen type of interactivity, and where the wireframe is design and navigation is planned; and (v) presentation, the development of the materials/instruments having present the design of the visual identity and the interface's graphic project. Each module contains supporting information, goals, references, glossary of specific terms, and library for in- depth searches. Passos [8] states that is through the interface, that interaction occurs between the subject (student) and object (content), and it is desirable that the interactivity between both is well adjusted to the content and learning needs of the student. Therefore, the higher the level of interactivity of a digital educational material, the higher the quality/intuition the interface design should possess. Thus, the student-content interaction is better, giving meaning to the course of how to develop a methodology for digital interface design.

3.1 Promoting Action on Research Implementation in Health Services

The PARiHS (Promoting Action on Research Implementation in Health Services) framework is used as an organizational or conceptual framework intended to explain and predict whether or not the implementation of evidence in practice is successful. PARIHS was one of the first structures to make explicit the multidimensional and complex nature of research implementation into practice, highlighting the central importance of context [9]. This model can be characterized as an explanatory framework, originally developed in 1998, that has evolved over time based on analysis of concepts and exploratory research. According to Stetler, Damschroder, Helfrich and Hagedorn [10], PARiHS is a broadly cited conceptual framework that constructs three main and interrelating elements that influence the successful implementation of evidence-based practices: Evidence (E), Context (C), and Facilitation (F).

For Stetler et al. [10], evidence is codified and non-codified sources of knowledge, perceived by the multiple stakeholders involved, while context can be described as the quality of the environment in which the research is implemented. The facilitation component is a "technique by which one person makes things easier for others" (p. 3), by changing their attitudes, habits, skills, ways of thinking, and working [10]. PARiHS presents an intuitive appeal, providing a basic list of "to do tasks", flexibility in its application, and includes successful implementation as a desired outcome.

This model can be considered as a broad framework to guide the development of an interface focused on the implementation of interventions that effectively enable changes related to proposed model [10]. Specifically, it can be used to diagnose critical elements related to the implementation of an evidence based practice (E and C) and, thus, the development of an implementation strategy (F) to allow for successful and sustained changes. A PARiHS-based diagnostic analysis may additionally involve stakeholders in self-reflection on critical aspects of implementation and the related nature of the necessary change [10].

4 Contributions on User's Digital Competences and Technology Acceptance

4.1 Task Technology Fit Model

According to Hyun, Johnson, Stetson and Bakken [11], the Task Technology Fit model (TTF) argues that information technology is more likely to have a positive impact on individual performance and be used if those capabilities match the tasks the user must perform [12]. The same authors developed a measurement of task technology that consists of 8 factors: quality, localization, authorization, compatibility, ease of use/training, production time, system reliability and user relationship. Each factor is measured using two to ten questions on a seven points Likert scale, ranging from strong disagree to strongly agree. This measure acts as a predictor of performance and work effectiveness on the use of the system under investigation [12].

4.2 Technology Acceptance Model

Technology Acceptance Model (TAM) proposed by Davis, Bagozzi, and Warshaw [13] was initially focused on two fundamental dimensions to evaluate the acceptance of technology: (i) perceived utility; and (ii) perceived ease of use. This is one of the most used and powerful model to evaluate, explain or predict the acceptance of new technologies by possible users of the new technology to be implemented [14], being used in several contexts.

Recently, TAM has evolved into the Technology Readiness Acceptance Model (TRAM), incorporating the "Readiness" dimension (see Table 1).

Table 1. Dimensions of the technology readiness acceptance model (TRAM) - Adapted from Chang [14].

Dimension	Description
Perceived utility	The extent to which the person believes that their use will contribute to improving their performance [13]
Ease of perceived use	Degree in which the person believes that using the system will be free of effort [13]
Subjective norm	Perception of the individual about what most significant people will accept such behavior [15]
Technological readiness	Propensity to embrace and use new technology to respond to family and work needs [13]
Personal innovativeness in information technologies	Degree in which an individual demonstrates readiness to adopt new ideas [16]
Intention of Use and Current Use	The intention to use new technology influences its effective use [17]

5 Conclusions

The development of digital skills and competences in nursing students and professionals is determinant for the follow-up of patients who self-manage their own chronic diseases. However, the lack of implementation educational pedagogical models in this domain limits such approach. It is urgent to provide a structured form for incorporation the learning of the digital skills into the nursing curriculum.

Because technology acceptance is not a watertight reality, especially when applied to the process of health care self-management by patients with chronic diseases, it is important to be aware of the importance of different motivational, behavioral, economic, cultural and social realities that emerge as current challenges to be answered by conceptual models.

The scientific literature offers some models, theories, guidelines, procedures, methods and instruments that can be useful in the development, implementation and evaluation of new technologies. For example, the usability concept have been strongly associated to the acceptance of new technologies, which can bring indispensable contributions to strengthen the implementation of DigiNurse Model.

In this paper, we have described some major contributions on interface usability and interactivity assessment methods and procedures, as well as important conceptual models about digital interfaces development. These initial revision will guide and support the development of DigiNurse Model, that will be included in the nursing curricula of higher education institutions. We hope that this model can contribute to improve health care delivery through appropriate follow-up of patients with chronic illness.

References

1. Donner, G.J., Wheeler, M.M., Conseil international des infirmières: Coaching in Nursing: An Introduction. International Council of Nurses (2009)
2. Jayadevappa, R.: Patient centered care - a conceptual model and review of the state of the art. Open Health Serv. Policy J. **4**, 15–25 (2011). https://doi.org/10.2174/1874924001104010015
3. Greene, S.M., Tuzzio, L., Cherkin, D.: A framework for making patient-centered care front and center. Perm. J. **16**, 49–53 (2012). https://doi.org/10.1098/rsbl.2007.0630
4. Lewis, C., Wharton, C.: Cognitive walkthroughs. In: Helander, M., Landauer, T., Prabhu, P. (eds.) Handbook of Human-Computer Interaction, pp. 717–732. North-Holland, Amsterdam (1997)
5. Bligård, L.O., Osvalder, A.L.: Enhanced cognitive walkthrough: development of the cognitive walkthrough method to better predict, identify, and present usability problems. Adv. Hum.-Comput. Interact. **2013** (2013). https://doi.org/10.1155/2013/931698
6. Blackmon, M.H., Polson, P.G., Kitajima, M., Lewis, C.: Cognitive walkthrough for the web. In: Proceedings of the SIGCHI Conference on Human Factors in Computing Systems Changing Our World, Changing Ourselves – CHI 2002, p. 463. ACM Press, New York (2002)
7. Zhang, J., Walji, M.F.: TURF: toward a unified framework of EHR usability. J. Biomed. Inform. **44**, 1056–1067 (2011). https://doi.org/10.1016/j.jbi.2011.08.005
8. Passos, P.C.S.J.: Interad: uma metodologia para design de interface de materiais educacionais digitais (Master Thesis). Universidade Federal do Rio Grande do Sul (2011)
9. Harvey, G., Kitson, A.: PARIHS revisited: from heuristic to integrated framework for the successful implementation of knowledge into practice. Implement. Sci. **11**, 33 (2015). https://doi.org/10.1186/s13012-016-0398-2
10. Stetler, C.B., Damschroder, L.J., Helfrich, C.D., Hagedorn, H.J.: A guide for applying a revised version of the PARIHS framework for implementation. Implement. Sci. **6**, 99 (2011). https://doi.org/10.1186/1748-5908-6-99
11. Hyun, S., Johnson, S.B., Stetson, P.D., Bakken, S.: Development and evaluation of nursing user interface screens using multiple methods. J. Biomed. Inform. **42**, 1004–1012 (2009). https://doi.org/10.1016/j.jbi.2009.05.005
12. Goodhue, D.L., Thompson, R.L.: Task-technology fit and individual performance. MIS Q. **19**, 213 (1995). https://doi.org/10.2307/249689
13. Davis, F.D., Bagozzi, R.P., Warshaw, P.R.: User acceptance of computer technology: a comparison of two theoretical models. Manage. Sci. **35**, 982–1003 (1989). https://doi.org/10.1287/mnsc.35.8.982
14. Chang, C.P.: The technology acceptance model and its application in a telehealth program for the elderly with chronic illnesses. J. Nurs. **62**, 11–16 (2015). https://doi.org/10.6224/JN.62.3.11
15. Wu, I.-L., Chen, J.-L.: An extension of Trust and TAM model with TPB in the initial adoption of on-line tax: an empirical study. Int. J. Hum Comput Stud. **62**, 784–808 (2005). https://doi.org/10.1016/J.IJHCS.2005.03.003
16. Rogers, E.M.: Lessons for guidelines from the diffusion of innovations. Jt. Comm. J. Qual. Improv. **21**, 324–328 (1995). https://doi.org/10.1016/S1070-3241(16)30155-9
17. Legris, P., Ingham, J., Collerette, P.: Why do people use information technology? A critical review of the technology acceptance model. Inf. Manag. **40**, 191–204 (2003). https://doi.org/10.1016/S0378-7206(01)00143-4

Models and Politics of Cares of the Elderly in the Home

Rogério Ferrinho Ferreira^(✉) ⓘ, Ana Clara Nunes ⓘ,
and Ana Maria Canhestro ⓘ

Polytechnic Institute of Beja, Beja, Portugal
`ferrinho.ferreira@ipbeja.pt`

Abstract. Aging has been assumed as a challenge in the different areas of professional and political action. The aim of this study was to identify models and policies for elderly care at home. To that end, a integrative review of articles on the topic was published, retrospectively published until 2013. The results show three main axes that shape the models and policies of care for the elderly in a home context: (a) Despite government participation in the with regard to health and social support for elderly people in situations of dependency in the home, there is a need to expand such support, in particular to informal care-givers; (b) The need for greater coordination and integration of care, not only at the level of the health system, but between sectors, particularly at the level of social intervention; and (c) The tendency and convergence in most developed countries to broaden responses (home care) with the consequent permanence of the elderly in their places of residence for the maximum possible time, with recognized positive effects in terms of financial sustainability.

Keywords: Health policies · Home services · Elderly

1 Introduction

This study is part of the Project Interreg Spain-Portugal, the International Institute for Research and Innovation of Aging - 0445_4IE_4_P. It is linked to the Activity "Models and processes of care and public policies" and consists in the systematization of results of studies developed by the academy on this subject, from the collection carried out in scientific databases. Increased longevity associated with improved quality of life and technical and scientific advances present significant challenges for policies and services for the elderly. At the policy level, there is a greater increase in community care for the elderly. Health organizations and policy makers are increasingly supportive of older people staying and aging in their homes and community [1]. These policies are based on the principle of on-site aging, allowing older people to remain in their own homes and integrated into the community according to their preferences rather than residential care [1, 10].

Portugal is also tuned for policies that promote the maintenance of the elderly in their homes, with the increase of social and health responses that may minimize the difficulties and limitations that, with the advancement of time, arise.

© Springer Nature Switzerland AG 2019
J. García-Alonso and C. Fonseca (Eds.): IWoG 2018, CCIS 1016, pp. 257–268, 2019.
https://doi.org/10.1007/978-3-030-16028-9_23

However, in order to ensure that these policies can effectively represent an adequate and integral response for the elderly to stay in their homes in a dignified, safe and supportive manner or as a guarantee of their complete well-being, the need for complementarity with informal care, usually provided by family members.

It is highlighted that in the study of Boland et al. [1], most of the systematic reviews of the literature are favorable to the stay of the elderly in their home, with support. Informal caregivers, usually family and friends, have the role of trying to reconcile their daily activities with informal care for the elderly who remain in the community at home. Most of the care is provided by women, and through this, the gender issue is present in informal care for the elderly who remain at home [4].

In most developed countries, there are already programs and policies that allow the remuneration of family and friends as caregivers of the elderly. At the same time, we are witnessing a growing commitment by health services to the implementation of integrated care as a strategy to provide care for the elderly. It involves the use of a set of methods and models of financial, administrative, organizational, social and health services, in order to achieve greater alignment and collaboration in the provision of care for the elderly [3].

On the other hand, the evidence points to the increase in costs related to dependencies or multiple dependencies (in health and social intervention) to which the elderly, and especially the elderly, are voted. According to data from the OECD, their member countries increased the costs/expenditures of dependent elderly people between 2005 and 2011 to an annual rate of 4.8%, while their growth registered a rate of only 1.3%. These figures are all the more alarming because the forecasts point to rising costs for older people, so policies that promote effective responses to the needs of older people are needed, while ensuring the financial sustainability of the various countries [2].

It was the search for models and policies for the care of the elderly at home, which are examples of good practice, respecting the balance between costs and benefits that impelled us to the present investigation. As this is a current topic, the integrative review of literature has become an appropriate method to synthesize information from studies that address it, allowing the analysis of scientific evidence around the central question of this investigation. This study involved the definition of the objective, formulation of the research question, methodology, results and discussion and main conclusions.

2 Objective

Identify the models and politics of elderly cares at home.

3 Research Question

For the selection of articles and formulation of the research question, the PI [C] OD methodology was used, being the target population (P), the type of Intervention (I), the comparisons (C), the outcome - outcome (O) and type of study - design (D). The following question was elaborated to answer the objective outlined and that served as a guideline for this systematic review of the literature: What models and policies (Outcomes) of care (Intervention) to the elderly in the home (Population)?

4 Methodology

After the formulation of the question of departure, an exhaustive research was done on the subject under study. The EBSCOHOST database was selected and the databases ACADEMIC SEARCH COMPLETE, MEDLINE COMPLETE and CINHAL COMPLETE were selected, with the following descriptors: "Health policy", "Home care services" and "Elder*" With the Boolean operators "and". The descriptors were searched at EBSCO in the following order: [Health policy] and [Home care services] and [Elder *]. All descriptors were searched in full text and searched retrospectively until 2013. Inclusion and exclusion criteria were also defined and used during the research.

As inclusion criteria, articles with full-text quantitative and/or qualitative methodologies focused on the models and public policies of elderly care at home, from academic journals (analyzed by specialists) were favored, with references available and published between January 2013 and April 2018. In the exclusion criteria, all articles with ambiguous methodology, repeated in the various databases, without correlation with the object of study and with lower dates were considered to 2013. The selection of the studies involved the evaluation of the title and analysis of the abstract to verify that the articles met the inclusion and exclusion criteria. When the title and the abstract were not illuminating, the article was read in its entirety to minimize the loss of important studies for this systematic review.

150 articles were identified from the databases consulted. This evaluation was carried out in two phases: in the first phase there were 53 articles after reading the titles and in a second phase after reading the abstracts the potential interest for 10 articles was justified. Of these, 8 articles were selected due to the methodological quality analysis, after reading the article in full. In view of the eight articles selected, the critical analysis of methodological quality focused on the assessment of the levels of evidence of each article. We used the contributions of Melnyk and Fineout-Overholt [7] in order to identify the types of production of knowledge implicit in it. These authors considered the following levels of evidence:

- Level I – Systematic reviews (meta-analyzes, guidelines for clinical practice based on systematic reviews);
- Level II – Experimental studies;
- Level III – Nearly experimental studies;
- Level IV – Non-experimental studies;
- Level V – Program evaluation reports/literature reviews;
- Level VI – Opinions of authorities/consensus panels.

5 Results and Discussion

With the purpose of answering the question of departure, several articles were read, aiming the analysis of its content. The results obtained are summarized in Table 1.

Following the analysis carried out, three main categories emerged, supported by the indicators below systematized in Table 2.

Table 1. Results of bibliographic research

Authors/level evidence	Objective	Results
Kietzman, Benjamin and Mattias [4] Method: Quantitative and qualitative study Level of Evidence: IV Participants: 383 family caregivers and friends paid to provide personal care services for the disabled, elderly and eligible through In-Home Support Services Program California	Investigate the perceptions of caregivers about the options to take on the roles of paid caregivers	The results indicate that caregivers are well placed to provide culturally appropriate and responsive care to caregiver and caregiver preferences. In addition, the perception of choice in assuming the role of paid caregiver has implications for the caregiver's well-being. While the availability of public payments is useful for many caregivers, most describe reasons for care that are not related to financial reward
Neiterman, Vodchis and Bourgeault [9] Method: Qualitative study. Level of Evidence: IV Participants: Elderly (17) high risk patients with multiple chronic and family health conditions (19) who provided care to patients	Analyze how patients experience transitions to the community from hospitals, including problems of daily living and medical concerns	For the success of the transitions following discharge from hospital it is important: - preparation of housing, taking into account the organization of home care; - take into account the practical and emotional concerns of the elderly/family, considering the levels of health and social intervention
Vreugdenhil [10] Method: Case study. Level of Evidence: IV Participants: Intergenerational informal caregivers (12) of people with dementia	To analyze the elderly care policy in a community context	The study concludes that there is a need to review support for caregivers as a way to ensure an on-site aging in a sustainable way

(continued)

Table 1. (*continued*)

Authors/level evidence	Objective	Results
Janse et al. [3] Method: A quasi-experimental study with a control group. Level of Evidence: III Participants: Health and home care professionals involved in a network of home care for the elderly	Evaluate the integration processes that underlie the provision of integrated care for the frail elderly	Integrated intervention has significantly improved structural, social, and cultural integration, as well as agreement on goals, interests, power and resources, satisfaction with integration, adequacy and timeliness of care
Boland et al. [1] Method: Review of Literature without meta-analysis (synthesizes 19 systematic reviews) Level of Evidence: V	Assess the impact of home care versus alternative health care settings for the elderly	Evidence on the impact of home care compared to alternative care settings on the health of the elderly gives heterogeneous results. The impacts are positive in health for the elderly living in the community and receiving home support interventions. There is insufficient evidence to determine the health impact of elderly care recipients in alternative settings
Matus-López [6] Method: Documentary analysis and bibliographic review of the literature Level of Evidence: V (Inclusion of 17 academic articles and 2 books of recognized international prestige)	Identify aspects of convergence of financing models (public policies) and health and social responses for the elderly in a situation of dependency (Long-term care)	Three axes of convergence were identified in the design and development of public policies in most of the countries under analysis: - Universal and focused access (access to health and social services is universal but priority is given to those with the greatest health care needs) - Expansion of funding sources (taxes, contributions, private participation and joint ventures) based on individual contribution - Replacement of residential responses by community responses (home care and various and varied subsidies and financial supplements) that aim for the elderly to remain as long as possible in the places of residence

(*continued*)

Table 1. (*continued*)

Authors/level evidence	Objective	Results
Kuluski, Ho, Hans and Nelson [5] Method: Qualitative study Expert discussion groups Level of Evidence: IV Participants: 24 health and social care professionals	Investigate key components of care to support older people with multiple co-morbidities and social problems and their families in the community	The discussion and categories that have emerged result in a proposed framework for the design of interventions and programs for people with complex care needs: - Centrality of the person and family in the care process - Development of tools for global and comprehensive assessment of the real and potential needs of people with multiple problems - Integrated approaches to health and social areas
Mery, Wodchis and Laporte [8] Method: Quantitative (Longitudinal survey over 18 years) Level of Evidence: IV Participants: 7255 people aged 65 and over	- Distinguish 2 components of Home Care (CD): health care (CHA) and social care (CHA) - Evaluate the determinants to obtain from each type of home care - Investigate the interrelationship between the two types of care	- This study concludes by the importance of distinguishing between CDSa and CDSo (instead of approaching CD as a homogeneous service), which will have important political implications - The severity of dependency on ADLs, health status, family support, and financial status have all been found to be important determinants of the propensity to receive publicly funded health and social services - The use of public CDSa is complementary to the usufruct of public CDSo, which supports the thesis that after an elderly person accesses CD, the probability of receiving additional services is greater, increasing the inequalities between recipients and non-recipients of care in the same situation need for health care

Table 2. Synthesis of models and policies for elderly care at home

Categories	Indicators
Accountability and support in care for the elderly/family	- Responsibility of informal caregivers [4, 10]; - Public payment of informal caregivers [4, 10]; - Formal support services in home care (preparation of meals, cleaning of the home, assistance with daily activities, transportation, etc.) [9, 10]; - Right to flexibility at work (place, hours and hours) for informal caregivers [10]; - Right to compensate for care time for informal caregivers [10]; - Financing families to buy care and benefits for caregivers: [10]; - Centrality of the Person/Family in care [5];
Care integration	- Integrative care structures promote integrated care [3]; - Coordination and health care services in the home [1, 9]; - Preparation of the dwelling of the hospitalized person [9]; - Need to clearly distinguish between health CDs and social CDs [8]; - Multiple problems (from the social and health areas) require integrated responses [5]; - The need to develop global assessment instruments (health and social services) for highly complex situations [5];
Financing models (public and private policies)	Universal and focused access to health and social services [6]; - Expansion of funding sources (taxes, contributions, private participation and co-participation) [6]; - Replacement of residential responses by community responses [6]; - Determinants in access to home care [8]; - Financing models condition access to care [8]

Accountability and Support in Elderly/Family Care

Despite the limited information on the reasons that lead people to assume the roles of caregivers, we find that the process of role acquisition is related to recognition of the role of caregiver and, on the other hand, socially assumed as a family responsibility [4]. In addition, family caregivers and friends are seen as an experienced source of care for the elderly who remain at home.

The "informal caregiver responsibility" indicator is also present in Vreugdenhil's study [10], focusing on the Australian reality of elderly care, which uses the concept of "aging in place" to refer to older people with some level of have the possibility to remain in their own homes. The terminology of "sandwich generation" caregivers is also used for the children of the elderly who, in addition to assuming responsibility and the roles of informal caregivers of their parents, also take care of their family, involving partners/spouse, children and even grandchildren.

The indicator "public payment of informal caregivers" appears strongly in the study by Kietzman et al. [4], whose purpose was to analyze the reasons that determine family members and friends to take on the roles of paid caregivers, how they perceive that choice and how the reasons for care are related to the caregiver's well-being.

Regarding the importance of money, caregivers describe reasons unrelated to the monetary reward for caregiving, assuming that their motivations for caregiving are not primarily financial. However, the availability of public pay is seen as an aid to many caregivers, with implications for the well-being of the caregiver. It is also an incentive for caregivers to continue this important work, reconciling the satisfaction of the needs of the recipient, filling a sense of obligation and generating a necessary income for the caregiver's well-being [4].

This strategy should be framed with the assumption that care for the elderly and in situations of dependency in the home should reconcile the interests of the person who is cared for and the caregiver. The existence of public financing policies for home-based care, involving family and friends caretakers, is crucial in optimizing care [4].

Old-age care policies involve formal support through various home-based support services. It can involve assistance in preparing meals, cleaning the home, attending different daily activities, transporting the elderly, and other activities [9, 10]. The elderly can be supported through a range of formal home-based options, funded by government policies. Vreugdenhil's study [10] underscored the importance of co-responsibility of various family members as a way to reduce the overhead of the primary caregiver and the use of formal care services to support families.

Responsibility and support in caring for the elderly involves other strategies presented in the Vreugdenhil study [10]:

- Right to work flexibility (location, hours and hours) for informal caregivers;
- Right to compensation for the time of care for informal caregivers;
- Financing families to purchase care and benefits for caregivers.

These indicators are in line with the requirements that must be met by policy responses in the care of the elderly, from the perspective of informal care providers:

- Care services (quality and affordable);
- Time (right to reduce paid work without penalty and entitlement to compensation for length of service);
- Money (to buy care and benefits for caregivers).

On the other hand, the scientific evidence regarding health and social care for people with multiple care needs points to the challenge of the centrality of the person/family. In fact, the study by Kuluski et al. [5] concludes the need to involve, empower and empower people and their families for greater participation in care and decision-making. This situation requires the establishment of relationships of trust and therapeutic relationships between professionals (care providers) and users and families.

Care Integration

Integrative care structures, involving a multidisciplinary team, are fundamental in providing integrated care for the elderly with social and health problems, of great complexity and constantly changing [3]. Integration is a multidimensional concept, involving structural, social, cultural and strategic processes.

Structural processes concern the coordination of tasks, functions and activities and frequent and open communication. Social relations are crucial in building an environment of mutual understanding, trust, and respect. They are promoters of a collaborative work, which involves the acceptance and recognition of the roles and functions developed by the different professionals involved in the intervention to the elderly, with complementary work methods and approaches. Cultural integration occurs through the development of norms and values that are part of a culture shared by professionals involved in care for the elderly. Strategic integration presupposes a shared strategy, involving organizational structures and processes that are determinant in the governance and management of joint activities. In this case, it is necessary that the different professionals are aligned with the goals, interests, power and resources [3].

It should be noted that in the study by Janse et al. [3] and aiming to measure the impact of an integrated care intervention on the fragile elderly in the perception and satisfaction of the professionals with the integration processes, the results showed significant improvements in structural, cultural and social integration, in agreement on goals, interests, power and resources, and satisfaction with integration after the implementation of an integrated intervention aimed at the frail elderly. This study also confirmed that integrated care structures promote integration processes among professionals in a relatively short period of time.

The existence of coordination and home health care services is a decisive strategy for the elderly to stay at home, with support. This indicator is expressed in the studies of Neiterman et al. [9] and Boland et al. [1]. There is a growing number of home-based interventions and/or supports aimed at promoting their health and social independence in the community [1], although some elderly people anticipate their institutionalization by their own decision or by unforeseen changes in their life, such as the loss of a spouse or a disease situation [1].

It is also highlighted that in the systematic review of the literature developed by Boland et al. [1], there were no differences in outcomes between health care and rehabilitation at home and using conventional health and rehabilitation services. These inconclusive results may be related to the informed preferences, the individual needs of the elderly and the quality of the services available. In this case, these and other factors are conditioning and guiding your decision regarding staying at home or using alternative resources.

The indicator of "Preparing the dwelling of the hospitalized person" is present in the study of Neiterman et al. [9]. We analyzed the transition experiences of elderly adults from the hospital to the community, emerging short- and long-term challenges associated with these transitions. Short-term challenges include preparing the sick person's home and understanding the organization of care in their home. Long-term challenges emerge associated with practical and emotional concerns.

The transition of the person from the hospital to their home presupposes adaptation to daily life, involving cooking, dressing, bathing and other activities. Changes in personal life, changes in physical conditions, in the arrangement of life and in the organization of daily activities and home care can generate feelings of uncertainty and confusion, especially in situations where discharge was not adequately planned [9]. This process of transition from person to community makes it clear that personal networks and social support are crucial for the recovery of the person, allowing an adequate integration of health care with social support [9].

It is vital to improve the continuity of care during this transition process, making this process more stable for the elderly and their caregivers. This presupposes assessing post-discharge needs of food, equipment, transportation for health services, coordination and follow-up in health care and social care. It also presupposes the implementation of services that ensure an adequate integration of health care and social care in the transition from person to person [9]. Coordination of these services is crucial in the management of care and support to informal caregivers, health professionals and community services.

On the other hand, the development of tools that allow an overall and comprehensive assessment of the (real and potential) needs of people with multiple social and health problems is pointed out in the study by Kuluski et al. [5] as fundamental to integrated approaches to care.

Financing Models (Public and Private Policies)
In view of the social and demographic changes that have taken place in recent years, as the number of dependents, including older people with multiple dependencies has increased, one of the main challenges facing countries has been the definition of access to care as universalist or focused and, in case of decision by the focused system, define the variables determining access: the economic situation, the heritage or the severity of the disease the situation.

In the study by Matus-López [6], following the documentary analysis of models and public policies of care in 30 countries, it is concluded that, for the most part, access to health and social protection is universal.

However, universal access depends on some factors or components that translate into access advantages for those most in need or with greater levels of dependency. Thus, it is concluded by the focused universalism that consists of defining access to care/services as universal, but that gives priority to people with greater health needs. This concept allows the guarantor of Individual and Social Rights and, simultaneously, allows an adjustment to the resources according to the financial limitations and the priorities of attendance. Also in the study by Mery, Wodchis and Laporte [8], the conclusions indicate the state of health (situations of greater dependence) as determinant of the priority access to health and social responses. According to the same authors, these financing models promote inequality among citizens in the same situations, since accessing the CDSa is a strong predictor of access to additional services.

Another feature of convergence, in most of the countries under analysis, is the increase in the sources of financing of the systems with a greater individual contribution, either directly or indirectly (taxes, contributions, co-participations).

Finally, there is a clear trend towards broadening household responses to the detriment of institutional responses [6]. These three characteristics contribute to financial sustainability through cost containment and revenue growth.

6 Conclusion

The conclusions of our study point to three main axes that mark the Policies of Care for the elderly in the home:

- The need for greater participation and contribution of the State to the stay of the elderly in the home. This participation or contribution should be translated into a wide range of formal options for the direct care of the elderly and the informal caregiver (remuneration, labor flexibility, time), whose relevance in terms of participation in elderly care at home is unanimously recognized;
- The need for coordination and integration of care, not only at the level of the health system, but in between sectors, especially at the level of social intervention.

In Portugal, the Programs and Plans for the elderly, in general, or emanate from the Ministry of Health or the Ministry of Labor and Social Solidarity, confirming a large gap in the in between sectors and integration of care. However, the road to in between sectors has already started, namely with the creation of the National Network of Continuing Integrated Care within the Ministries of Health and Labor and Social Solidarity, which is not specifically targeted at the elderly but at the dependency, is a major response for dependency in the elderly.

Finally, we conclude by the tendency and convergence, in most developed countries, to increase community-based responses (home care) with the consequent residence of the elderly in their places of residence for the maximum possible time. Although it does not appear to be a primary reason, the continuity of the elderly in their homes has positive effects in terms of financial sustainability.

References

1. Boland, L., et al.: Impact of home care versus alternative locations of care on elder health outcomes: an overview of systematic reviews. BMC Geriatr. **17**(20) (2017). https://doi.org/10.1186/s12877-016-0395-y
2. Lipszyc, B., Sail, E., Xavier, A.: Long-term care: need, use and expenditure in the EU-27. European Commission. Economic Papers, No. 469 (2012)
3. Janse, B., Huijsman, R., Kuyper, R., Fabbricotti, I.: Do integrated care structures foster processes of integration? A quasi experimental study in frail elderly care from the professional perspective. Int. J. Qual. Health Care **28**(3), 376–383 (2016). https://doi.org/10.1093/intqhc/mzw045
4. Kietzman, K., Benjamin, A., Matthias, R.: Whose choice? Self-determination and the motivations of paid family and friend caregivers. J. Comp. Fam. Stud. **44**(4), 519–540 (2013). http://www.jstor.org/stable/23644636
5. Kuluski, K., Ho, J.W., Hans, P.K., Nelson, M.L.: Community care for people with complex care needs: bridging the gap between health and social care. Int. J. Integr. Care **17**(4), 2 (2017). https://doi.org/10.5334/ijic.2944
6. Matus-López, M.: Tendencias en las políticas de atención a la dependencia de ancianos y sus reformas. Cadernos de Saúde Pública **31**(12), 2475–2481 (2015). https://doi.org/10.1590/0102-311X00039315

7. Melnyk, B., Fineout-Overholt, E., Stetler, C., Allan, J.: Outcomes and implementation strategies from the first U.S. evidence-based practice leadership summit. Worldviews Evid.-Based Nurs. **2**(3), 113–121 (2005)
8. Mery, G., Wodchis, W.P., Laporte, A.: The determinants of the propensity to receive publicly funded home care services for the elderly in Canada: a panel two-stage residual inclusion approach. Health Econ. Rev. **6**, 8 (2016). https://doi.org/10.1186/s13561-016-0086-6
9. Neiterman, E., Vodchis, W., Bourgeault, I.: Experiences of older adults in transition from hospital to community. Canad. J. Aging/La revue canadienne du vieillissement **34**(1), 90–99 (2015). https://doi.org/10.1017/S0714980814000518
10. Vreugdenhil, A.: Ageing-in-place: frontline experiences of intergenerational family carers of people with dementia. Health Sociol. Rev. **23**(1), 43–52 (2014). https://doi.org/10.5172/hesm.2014.23.1.43

Effectiveness of an Educational Program to Enhance Self-care Skills After Acute Coronary Syndrome: A Quasi-Experimental Study

Lisa Gomes[1](✉) (iD) and Gorete Reis[2]

[1] Minho University, Campus de Gualtar, 4710-057 Braga, Portugal
lgomes@ese.uminho.pt
[2] Évora University, Largo do Senhor da Pobreza, 7000-811 Évora, Portugal

Abstract. Background: The aim of this study is to determine the effectiveness of an educational program to enhance self-care skills in patients after an acute coronary syndrome

Methods: A quasi-experimental pretest-posttest design was used in the study. A rehabilitation nurse provided an educational program (PEpSCA-CARE) to the intervention group (n = 32), and the control group (n = 35) received the conventional nursing pre-discharge care. The data was collected using the Therapeutic Self-Care Scale (TSCS) in four dimensions: medications, symptoms, activities of daily living and health status management, applied before hospital discharge and one month after hospital discharge to both groups. Patients were recruited from an intensive cardiovascular care unit during 2016.

Results: The results showed statistically significant differences between both groups (p < 0.001). The intervention group tended to improve their self-care skills while the control group had opposite trends, self-care skills decreased.

Conclusions: According to the findings of the study, a systematized and structured educational program, is effective in developing self-care skills in patients after an acute coronary syndrome.

Keywords: Self-care skills · Educational program · Acute coronary syndrome

1 Background

Over the years in Portugal declining mortality and birth rates, increasing life expectancy and modifying health/disease patterns, explain the high prevalence of chronic diseases and the increasing levels of functional disability among the population. Chronic disease management requires a level of demand for permanent care and has a priority dimension in healthcare [1].

Cardiovascular Diseases are chronic diseases with the highest morbidity and mortality rate worldwide [2]. The high number of hospital admissions for Acute Coronary Syndrome and the low adherence to the Cardiac Rehabilitation (CR) constitute an opportunity for nurses to develop interventions aimed to encourage patients to take an active role in their own health care. Self-care is viewed as a process underlying

© Springer Nature Switzerland AG 2019
J. García-Alonso and C. Fonseca (Eds.): IWoG 2018, CCIS 1016, pp. 269–279, 2019.
https://doi.org/10.1007/978-3-030-16028-9_24

the performance of health-related activities. The process involves the recognition of changes in a health condition that require remediation and the selection of an engagement in activities to address these changes [3].

Acute Coronary Syndromes (ACS) represents a life-threatening manifestation of atherosclerosis. It is usually caused by acute thrombosis induced by a ruptured or eroded atherosclerotic coronary plaque, with or without concomitant vasoconstriction, causing a rapid and critical reduction in blood flow [4].

ACS have been described as an extremely traumatic cardiac event and the consequences influence physical and psychosocial well-being over a significant period of time [5]. Considering that this is a chronic disease and therefore will accompany the patient throughout life, in recent year's research studies seek to understand the implications that the diagnosis, progression, and consequences of the disease have on patients and family members.

National and international associations, such as the American Association of Cardiovascular and Pulmonary Rehabilitation [6] as well as the European Association of Cardiovascular Prevention and Rehabilitation [7], recommend CR as a secondary prevention strategy. The World Health Organization defines CR as the "sum of activities required to influence favorably the underlying cause of the disease, as well as to provide the best possible physical, mental and social conditions, so that the patients may, by their own efforts, preserve or resume when lost, as normal a place as possible in the community" [8]. CR aims to reduce mortality, morbidity, and disability promotes healthy behaviors and improves quality of life. Several studies also show that CR reduces the number of hospitalizations and consequently reduces costs for the Health System [9, 10].

Despite these recommendations, the number of patients participating in cardiac rehabilitation programs is extremely low, only one-third of coronary patients have access this programs in Europe [11]. In Portugal, according to the National Coordination for Cardiovascular Diseases, the main reasons for CR underutilization are economic (financial difficulties), organizational (low medical referral rate), as well as lack of dissemination, patient's motivation, few CR clinics and poor geographical distribution of this clinics [12].

Considering that the 30 days following hospital discharge after a cardiac event is crucial for the ongoing health of ACS patients because of the high levels of stress, rehospitalization (18.5%) and mortality (12.5%) and it is a critical psychological period in accepting the need for lifestyle changes [13], nurse interventions during hospitalization should include promoting self-care and improving quality of life through non-pharmacological recommendations, evaluation of the signs/symptoms, stimulation of healthy habits/lifestyle, and education about the disease and the use of medicines [14].

The importance of the therapeutic regimen to control coronary disease and the consequent risks of non-adherence, make it necessary the development of strategies that promote a greater adherence to the prescribed treatment. These facts determine the importance of educational programs that enable the development of self-care skills, taking into consideration that the educational process is gradual, systematized, personalized and complemented by professionals. This requires that the patients have access to information and understand the importance of modifying their lifestyle to increase daily function.

To study the above-mentioned issues, we provided an educational program to patients following an ACS. Therefore, we sought to test the following **hypothesis:** patients that attended an educational program as a nurse intervention develop self-care skills compared to patients that did not attend the program.

2 Methods

2.1 Study Design

The effectiveness of an educational program to enhance self-care skills in patients after an acute coronary syndrome for up to 1 month after hospital discharge was explored. The study used a nonequivalent, control group, pretest-posttest design due to the impossibility of group randomization. It is not possible to guarantee other common characteristics like the age and sex because of the unpredictability of acute illness episodes. Also, considering the organization of the ICCU, the participants in the intervention group were in the same ward as the non-participants, that is, if randomization was the choice, the participants of the control group would also attend the educational intervention.

2.2 Study Participants

The participants were adult/elderly patients diagnosed with ACS (acute myocardial infarction/unstable angina pectoris), hospitalized at an ICCU in the northern region of Portugal, speak and understand Portuguese, had preserved cognitive and verbal ability and agreed to participate in the study.

Throughout 2016, during 1-week period participants were included in the intervention group and the following week the participants were included in the control group and so on until reaching the required number of participants for our study. In the first phase, data collection was performed in the hospital, 1 month after discharge all participants were contacted by telephone.

2.3 Educational Program (PepSCA-CARE)

The educational process is necessary for the acquisition of knowledge and development of self-care skills. The objective of this educational program is to aware patients of the disease, the importance of changing lifestyles and controlling modifiable risk factors so they post-ACS patients (PEpSCA-CARE) was created to promote the development of self-care skills. It is intended that the actions to be implemented in this context contribute to a greater participation in the social, economic and cultural life of the communities and to guarantee a better quality of life.

In order to obtain meaningful learning for the development of skills, the implementation of the program was carried out through educational sessions built in a structured and systematic method. The training plan involved three educational areas, considering that at the end of the educational program the patient would be able to: (i) know the risks of heart disease (cognitive area); (ii) understanding that by modifying their behavior, their quality of life increases (affective area) and, in the psychomotor area (iii) knowing how to control the signs and symptoms of heart disease and knowing how to perform their most instrumental self-care [15, 16].

The PePSCA-CARE consists of 4 educational sessions, with the following pedagogical strategies: (i) information and transmission of knowledge about the situation through interviews with the nurse rehabilitation specialist; (ii) transmission of specific knowledge through the use of an educational video; (iii) verification of the information retained and clarification of doubts, using a checklist/pamphlet and (iv) verification of the knowledge retained and information about self-care performance, using telephone for follow-up interview.

The first session is individual and performed at the Intensive Coronary Care Unit (ICCU) 12 to 24 h after hospitalization and depending on the hemodynamic stability of the patient. An interview was conducted by the nurse rehabilitation specialist and as a didactic resource, we opted for the individual visualization of a video with the following themes and contents: How does the heart function? What is coronary heart disease? Diagnosis of coronary disease; Therapeutic Management; Modifiable Risk Factors and Healthy Lifestyle.

The second session was a group and held the following day, and aims to identify the patient's knowledge regarding the content exposed in the video and clarification of doubts. We chose to use this strategy since the beliefs about the disease as well as the personal experience also stem from the social experience [17]. Loring and Holman, explain that social persuasion can improve the perception of self-efficacy [18].

During its accomplishment, it fosters the sharing of doubts, ideas, and experiences. The third session was held on the day of hospital discharge and a checklist with the contents of the video was applied. Considering that the checklist has the following purposes: (i) organize and systematize the information so that the nurse can identify difficulties and (ii) serve as a leaflet for patient guidance when the patient has doubts at home.

The fourth and last session is performed, one month after discharge and aims to monitor the patient and reinforce the information.

Due to the geographical dispersion of the area of affluence of the hospital, this session is carried out by telephone. Telephone monitoring is seen as a good way of exchanging information, providing health education and counseling, recognizing complications, ensuring peace of mind, and providing quality post-treatment services. During this monitoring, nurses can detect abnormal conditions and implement effective actions to prevent complications.

3 Measurement

The Therapeutic Self-Care Scale (TSCS), was developed to assess self-care ability in acute-care settings. This scale assesses a patient's ability to perform four dimensions of self-care activities: taking medication as prescribed by the physician; identify and manage symptoms; to carry out activities of daily living and manage changes in health status [19]. The maximum score is 60 points and corresponds to a high level of performance in therapeutic self-care.

The original version of the instrument by Doran et al. was translated, validated and adapted to the Portuguese population by Cardoso et al. [19] and shows very good internal consistency (Cronbach's $\alpha = 0.979$), relative to the internal consistency of the original study (Cronbach's $\alpha = 0.93$). In the current study, Cronbach's $\alpha = 0.94$ at the first moment and Cronbach's $\alpha = 0.96$ in the second moment.

3.1 Data Collection Procedure

Initial data for the pretest were collected between May and November 2016. The elements of both groups provided written consent for study participation. The cognitive status of the patients was evaluated through the Mini-Mental Status Examination and those with cognitive deficit were excluded from the program. Participants from the intervention group started the educational program 12 to 24 h after hospitalization. The rehabilitation nurse starts the educational program explaining what is going to happen, and the patient begins the visualization of the educational video in the ICCU. Each patient had a television so they could stop watching whenever they felt tired or could repeat if something wasn't so clear.

The study had 2 distinct moments that correspond to the admission in the ICCU - pre-intervention educational evaluation and one month after hospital discharge from - post-intervention evaluation.

Patients from both groups, who agreed to join the study, were advised that they would receive a telephone follow-up from a nurse one month after hospital discharge.

3.2 Data Analysis

For data treatment, we used descriptive and inferential statistical techniques. Statistical analysis was performed using the Statistical Package for Social Science (SPSS) software, version 23 of 2016.

The statistical techniques applied were frequency (absolute and relative), measures of central tendency (arithmetic mean and median), measures of dispersion or variability (minimum value, maximum value and standard deviation), coefficients (Cronbach's and Spearman's alpha) and tests (Chi-square test, Fisher's exact test, Mann-Whitney U test, Wilcoxon test, Spearman's correlation coefficient significance test and Shapiro-Wilk test as a normality test).

For all tests, the value of 0.05 was set as the limit of significance, that is, the null hypothesis was rejected when the probability of type I error (probability of rejection of the null hypothesis when it was true) was lower than the set value, when $p < 0.05$, that is, $p < 5\%$.

4 Results

The results show that most of the elements of both groups had a diagnosis of acute myocardial infarction, with percentages of 90.6% and 88.6%, respectively in the intervention and control groups.

All subjects from both groups underwent invasive medical procedures, and in the majority of cases (78.1% and 85.7%), a percutaneous coronary intervention was performed.

Regarding therapeutic self-care skills, the results allow us to verify that in the first moment of evaluation the participants of the intervention group obtained values between 54 and 60 points, with an average result of 58.31 ± 1.20 points. Half of the members of this group had values equal to or greater than 58.00 points and the frequency distribution was significantly different from a normal distribution ($p < 0.001$).

Comparing the two groups, using the Mann-Whitney U test, we concluded that there are statistically significant differences ($p < 0.001$) and the values of the central tendency measures allow us to affirm that at the first moment of evaluation, the elements of the experimental group showed a better capacity for therapeutic self-care than those in the control group.

In the second moment, all the elements of the experimental group obtained results equal to 60.00 points (maximum value of the scale of evaluation of the therapeutic self-care). Consequently, the mean value was 60.00 ± 0.00 points, the median presented the same value and the frequency distribution could not be considered normal ($p = 0.000$). In the control group, the results were between 21 and 58 points, with the mean value being 38.77 ± 7.74 points. It was verified that half of the elements of this group presented values equal or superior to 39.00 points and the distribution of frequencies reveals characteristics similar to those of a normal distribution ($p = 0.883$). The Mann-Whitney U test revealed significant differences between the two groups ($p < 0.001$) and comparison of the values of the central tendency measures revealed that the participants in the intervention group showed better therapeutic self-care than those in the control group.

Using the Wilcoxon test in order to compare the two groups between each evaluation moment, we verified statistically significant differences in both cases ($p < 0.001$) and the comparison of the mean and median values suggests that, between the first and the second evaluation, the elements of the intervention group tended to improve their therapeutic self-care skills while in the control group the tendency was opposite, that is, self-care skills decreased (Table 1).

Table 1. Therapeutic self-care results

Group	Intervention	Control	p
Variable			
Therapeutic self-care (1st moment)	58.31	43.54	<0.001
x̄	58.00	43.00	
Md	1.20	6.57	
s	54	31	
x_{min}	60	60	
x_{max}	<0.001	0.299	
p			

(*continued*)

Table 1. (*continued*)

Group Variable	Intervention	Control	p
Therapeutic self-care (2nd moment)	60.00	38.77	<0.001
$\bar{x}$	60.00	39.00	
Md	0.00	7.74	
s	60	21	
x_{min}	60	58	
x_{max}	0.000	0.883	
p			
p	<0.001	<0.001	

During hospitalization, it is possible to provide the patient with the basic knowledge so they can have the opportunity to make their own decisions regarding health care and to achieve physical condition that allows independence and autonomy once at home [20].

4.1 Hypothesis Testing

The data in this study corroborates that CR is associated with improvement of health status perception within cardiac patients, reinforcing their self-confidence and allowing a more complete family, social and professional reintegration, [21]. Fernandes [22] study also indicates that patients with more knowledge about the disease after the intervention, continue to gain after two months, resulting in a greater benefit from the intervention in terms of anxiety, decreased perception symptoms, concern about the disease, and the importance of emotional response. It adds that health professionals who promote educational interventions should pay particular attention to promoting knowledge about the disease and treatment.

These behavioral changes are addressed through educational interventions aimed at the patient and family/caregivers through educational sessions with information, clarification, and discussion of secondary prevention issues and accompanied by the didactic material such as pamphlets and audiovisual media [16]. In the present study, we emphasize the importance of using the didactic material because the data obtained regarding the patient's perception about the most important issue they learned at the hospital, the participants of the intervention group referred that it was the contents exposed in the video.

5 Discussion

CR should start at the hospital and preferably still will patient is in the ICCU [23]. At this stage, the patient is particularly available to change behaviors and understands the need to change his behaviors and adhere to a complex therapeutic regimen. During hospitalization, it is possible to provide the patient with the basic self-care knowledge to allow independence and autonomy that is required after hospital discharge [20].

Many of the participants of both groups, 78.1% intervention group, and 91.4% control group, had no medical indication to attend CR after discharge. Peters and Keeley's study [24] suggest advanced age, female gender, comorbidities such as heart failure, diabetes mellitus or stroke, low socioeconomic status, the absence of health insurance, or subsystem of medical assistance and distance/accessibility between home and the rehabilitation center, predictors of non-referral. Although this study does not identify the causes of non-referral to attend a CR, we emphasize that these results reinforce the importance of Phase I CR implementation in all ICCU and Cardiology Care Units and associating them with an educational nurse intervention program. It is a rethinking of the path to be taken to include the largest number of patients and to develop and test strategies to improve the overall rehabilitation of the cardiac patient. However, if the first step is not given in the hospital context, all other strategies for developing self-care skills and modeling adherence to therapeutic regimens become difficult to implement.

The study by Kadda et al. [25] about nursing education after a cardiac event, concluded that many studies have highlighted the value of nursing support in CR. Nurses and educational programs are associated with a reduction in complications rate, a decrease in anxiety levels and rehospitalization. In addition, nursing interventions aimed at adhering to healthy lifestyles effectively influence cardiac risk factors and can improve patient's prognosis. Although the results support the benefits of educational interventions, through increased knowledge and behavior change, another systematic review of the literature, warns of the need for studies on educational interventions more explicitly characterized in order to be reproduced and evaluated [26].

Often patients fear complications and rehospitalizations because of self-imposed limitation of their daily living activities. Consequently, there is dependence on personal care and daily tasks as well as emotional lability associated with sadness and depression which can lead to family and social isolation. As a consequence, there is a progressive reduction of functional capacity and quality of life that requires a multi-disciplinary approach to complete rehabilitation [27].

Dickson et al. [28] explain that for better self-care management patients need vigilance and action. In our study, 65.6% of participants of the intervention group said they did not have any health professional to provide assistance and 88.6% was the percentage of response within the participants of the control group responded. These data also support the need for nurse vigilance so patients can maintain developing self-care skills for better adherence to treatment plan and self-care management such as the ability to recognize and respond appropriately to the presence of signs and symptoms. Also in our study, most of the participants in the intervention group (68.8%) said they had a cardiology consultation since discharged, 65.7% of the participants of the control group reply that they did not have a cardiology consultation. Patients need follow-up for an encouragement to continue in developing self-care skills and maintain a healthy lifestyle and adherence to the therapeutic regimen [23].

6 Conclusions

The results of this study indicate that the implementation of PEpSCA-CARE in ICCU can improve patient rehabilitation. Although only valid for this specific context, the results show that an educational program as a nurse intervention can make a significant difference in the patient's self-care skills. The educational program contributes to addressing unmet self-care needs, especially for patients that do not have access to CR after discharge. The overall goal of any educational program designed to promote healthcare is based on the prevention of complications and in the improvement of the quality of life [29].

Interventions aimed at developing self-care skills were fundamental so that the patients were able to manage their therapeutic regimen and adapt to their new health condition. However, there is a need for greater awareness and investment in educational nurse interventions and new online tools to facilitate an interactive communication between nurse and patient after hospital discharge so that the care provided is of an effective quality.

References

1. Grady, P.A., Gough, L.L.: Self-management: a comprehensive approach to management of chronic conditions. Am. J. Publ. Health **104**(8), e25–e31 (2014). https://doi.org/10.2105/AJPH.2014.302041
2. WHO: Noncommunicable Diseases Progress Monitor, 2017. World Health Organization, Geneva. Licence: CC BY-NC-SA 3.0 IGO (2017)
3. Sidani, S.: Self-care. In: Doran, D.M. (ed.) Nursing Outcomes: The State of the Science, 2nd edn, pp. 79–130. Jones & Bartlett, Sudbury (2011)
4. Drakopoulou, M., Toutouzas, K., Tousoulis, D.: Chapter 2.5 – Acute coronary syndromes. In: Tousoulis, D. (ed.) Coronary Artery Disease, pp. 201–233. Academic Press (2018)
5. Chauvet-Gelinier, J.-C., Bonin, B.: Stress, anxiety and depression in heart disease patients: a major challenge for cardiac rehabilitation. Ann. Phys. Rehabil. Med. **60**(1), 6–12 (2017). https://doi.org/10.1016/j.rehab.2016.09.002
6. Balady, G.J., et al.: Referral, enrollment, and delivery of cardiac rehabilitation/secondary prevention programs at clinical centers and beyond: a presidential advisory from the American Heart Association. Circulation **124**(25), 2951–2960 (2011). https://doi.org/10.1161/CIR.0b013e31823b21e2
7. Piepoli, M.F., et al.: 2016 European Guidelines on cardiovascular disease prevention in clinical practice: the sixth joint task force of the European Society of cardiology and other societies on cardiovascular disease prevention in clinical practice (constituted by representatives of 10 societies and by invited experts) developed with the special contribution of the European Association for Cardiovascular Prevention & Rehabilitation (EACPR). Eur. Heart J. **37**(29), 2315–2381 (2016). https://doi.org/10.1093/eurheartj/ehw106
8. World Health Organization: Needs and Action Priorities in Cardiac Rehabilitation and Secondary Prevention in Patients with Coronary Heart Disease. WHO Regional Office for Europe, Geneva (1993)

9. Magalhães, S., et al.: Efeitos a longo prazo de um programa de reabilitação cardíaca no controlo dos fatores de risco cardiovasculares. Rev. Port. Cardiol. **32**(3), 191–199 (2013). https://doi.org/10.1016/j.repc.2012.08.005
10. Foster, J.G., Lewis, S.F., Hennekens, C.H.: Editorial commentary: cardiac rehabilitation: major benefits and minor risks. Trends Cardiovasc. Med. **27**(6), 426–427 (2017). https://doi.org/10.1016/j.tcm.2017.03.001
11. Bjarnason-Wehrens, B., et al.: Cardiac rehabilitation in Europe: results from the European cardiac rehabilitation inventory survey. Eur. J. Cardiovasc. Prev. Rehabil. **17**(4), 410–418 (2010). https://doi.org/10.1097/HJR.0b013e328334f42d
12. Coordenação Nacional para as Doenças Cardiovasculares, 2009. Reabilitação Cardíaca: Realidade Nacional e Recomendações Clínicas. http://www2.portaldasaude.pt/NR/rdonlyres/466A7B26-7BB4-48D9-9DC1-FBAE234AA579/0/ReabilitacaoCardiaca.pdf
13. Chen, H.Y., et al.: Decade-long trends in 30-day rehospitalization rates after acute myocardial infarction. J. Am. Heart Assoc. **4**(11), e002291 (2015). https://doi.org/10.1161/JAHA.115.002291
14. Boisvert, S., Proulx-Belhumeur, A., Gonçalves, N., Doré, M., Francoeur, J., Gallani, M.C.: An integrative literature review on nursing interventions aimed at increasing self-care among heart failure patients. Revista Latino-Americana de Enfermagem **23**(4), 753–768 (2015). https://doi.org/10.1590/0104-1169.0370.2612
15. Adams, N.E.: Bloom's taxonomy of cognitive learning objectives. J. Med. Libr. Assoc. JMLA **103**(3), 152–153 (2015). https://doi.org/10.3163/1536-5050.103.3.010
16. Rice, H., Say, R., Betihavas, V.: The effect of nurse-led education on hospitalisation, readmission, quality of life and cost in adults with heart failure: a systematic review. Patient Educ. Couns. **101**(3), 363–374 (2018). https://doi.org/10.1016/j.pec.2017.10.002
17. Sousa, M.R., Martins, T., Pereira, F.: O refletir das práticas dos enfermeiros na abordagem à pessoa com doença crónica. Revista de Enfermagem Referência **6**, 55–63 (2015)
18. Holman, H., Lorig, K.: Patient self-management: a key to effectiveness and efficiency in care of chronic disease. Public Health Rep. **119**(3), 239–243 (2004). https://doi.org/10.1016/j.phr.2004.04.002
19. Cardoso, A., Queiros, P., Ribeiro, C., Amaral, A.: Cultural adaptation and psychometric properties of the portuguese version of the therapeutic self-care scale. Int. J. Caring Sci. **7**(2), 426 (2014)
20. Mampuya, W.M.: Cardiac rehabilitation past, present and future: an overview. Cardiovasc. Diagn. Ther. **2**(1), 38–49 (2012). https://doi.org/10.3978/j.issn.2223-3652.2012.01.02
21. Rocha, E., Nogueira, P.: As doenças cardiovasculares em Portugal e na região Mediterrânica: uma perspetiva epidemiológic. Revista Factores de Risco **36**, 35–44 (2015)
22. Fernandes, A.: Avaliação da eficácia de um programa de intervenção psicológica breve em pacientes pós-síndrome coronária aguda. (PhD), Universidade do Minho, Braga (2012)
23. Abreu, A., et al.: Mandatory criteria for cardiac rehabilitation programs: 2018 guidelines from the Portuguese society of cardiology. Rev. Port. Cardiol. **37**(5), 363–373 (2018). https://doi.org/10.1016/j.repc.2018.02.006
24. Peters, A.E., Keeley, E.C.: Trends and predictors of participation in cardiac rehabilitation following acute myocardial infarction: data from the behavioral risk factor surveillance system. J. Am. Heart Assoc. **7**(1) (2017). https://doi.org/10.1161/jaha.117.007664
25. Kadda, O., Marvaki, C., Panagiotakos, D.: The role of nursing education after a cardiac event. Health Sci. J. **6**(4), 634 (2012)
26. de Melo Ghisi, G.L., da Silva Chaves, G.S., Britto, R.R., Oh, P.: Health literacy and coronary artery disease: a systematic review. Patient Educ. Couns. **101**(2), 177–184 (2018). https://doi.org/10.1016/j.pec.2017.09.002

27. Ades, P.A., et al.: Cardiac rehabilitation exercise and self care for chronic heart failure. JACC Heart Fail. 1(6), 540–547 (2013). https://doi.org/10.1016/j.jchf.2013.09.002

28. Dickson, V.V., Nocella, J., Yoon, H.-W., Hammer, M., Melkus, G.D., Chyun, D.: Cardiovascular disease self-care interventions. Nurs. Res. and Pract. 2013, Article ID 407608 (2013). https://doi.org/10.1155/2013/407608

29. Megari, K.: Quality of life in chronic disease patients. Health Psychol. Res. 1(3), e27 (2013). https://doi.org/10.4081/hpr.2013.e2

Health Interventions to Support Caregivers of Elderly People

Sensitive Indicators to Rehabilitation Nursing Care in a Rehabilitation Program for People in the Surgical Process, Based on the Health Quality Model

Vânia Nascimento[1,2(✉)], César Fonseca[2], Maria Céu Marques[2], and Abílio Costa[3]

[1] ULSLA, Santiago do Cacém, Portugal
vaniardn@hotmail.com
[2] Évora University, Investigator POCTEP 0445_4IE_4_P, Évora, Portugal
[3] HGO, Almada, Portugal

Abstract. Continued improvement in care is one of the primary objectives of Rehabilitation Nursing. With the current medical-surgical evolution, the Rehabilitation Nurse faces new challenges related to the recovery, enhancement and maintenance of the functionality and capacity of the person in the surgical process. The identification of the indicators that are sensitive to the care of Rehabilitation Nursing, presents in the intervention plans carried out, allow us to measure the quality of the care provided and guarantee the excellence of the care performed. **Objective:** To identify sensible indicators for Rehabilitation Nursing care, presents in the Rehabilitation programs executed to the person in the surgical process, based on the health quality model. **Methods:** A systematic review of the literature was carried out through the EBSCO host (MEDLINE with Full Text, CINAHL Plus with Full Text and MedicLatina), using the PI [C] O method. **Results:** 49 indicators were identified, with emphasis on: "Percentage of clients to whom rehabilitation plan and/or rehabilitation program has been implemented to maximize functional capabilities"; "Percentage of clients with potential to improve the walking ability" and "Percentage of clients with risk of muscle stiffness who were monitored for the range of joint motion through the goniometer". **Conclusion:** The surgical patient, in the various areas of intervention (vascular, neurosurgical, orthopedic), presents health gains with the implementation of Rehabilitation programs, with 49 indicators that are sensitive to Rehabilitation Nursing care in the programs executed.

Keywords: Nursing · Rehabilitation ·
Sensitive indicators to the care of rehabilitation nursing · Surgical process

1 Introduction

The medical-surgical evolution contributed to better clinical results and, consequently, a greater survival in potentially fatal and/or incapacitating diseases, such as neoplasias and diseases of the circulatory system, implying new needs in the area of Rehabilitation of these people, consequent to the reduction of their autonomy [1, 2].

© Springer Nature Switzerland AG 2019
J. García-Alonso and C. Fonseca (Eds.): IWoG 2018, CCIS 1016, pp. 283–294, 2019.
https://doi.org/10.1007/978-3-030-16028-9_25

Each year, more than 187 million surgeries are performed worldwide [1]. In Portugal, in 2016, more than 2552 surgeries were performed per day [3]. Surgical treatment can, sometimes, be the only method to avoid disability and preserve life, and each year, it is estimated that surgeries are performed for 63 million people suffering from traumatic injuries and 31 million people with malignant tumors [1, 4].

The surgical process begins at the moment of surgical indication and is divided into three phases: preoperative, intraoperative and postoperative. The first phase ends when the patient arrives at the operating room, the second phase when the patient arrives at the post anesthetic recovery room, and the third phase begins when the patient leaves the operating room and lasts until their recovery is complete [6]. This event has repercussions at various levels and can be a reason for incapacity, both for the restrictions required, and for the complications that may result from their realization. It has been documented that 3 to 22% of surgeries have associated major complications [5], of which 7 million patients undergoing surgery per year will have major complications. The surgical process needs a biopsychosocial cultural monitoring, because it is a stressful process that always implies adaptation to a new reality, for the client and their family [7].

It's Rehabilitation Nurse (RN) competency to develop and implement intervention plans aimed at promoting people's capacities and helping them to adapt to the processes of health/illness transition, accompanying the person at all stages of their life cycle, in the various contexts of the practice of care, including the surgical process, where promotes and maximizes the person's functionality and promotes the reintegration into society [8].

The intervention of the RN will have visibility in the health gains of the person, when prevents the postsurgical complications, "increase respiratory and motor functional capacity, (…) (increase the) capacity of response to the effort and ability to perform the ADL (…) that interferes with the quality of life" [9].

As reported by OE (2010), the need to objectively demonstrate these gains emerges, thus guaranteeing the quality of nursing care and the effectiveness of the individualized interventions implemented, with a view to the excellence of care provided [8]. Thus, the indicators that constitute "specific markers of the health status of the populations, capable of translating the unique contribution of the professional practice of nurses to health gains of the population" appear. With specific indicators, we intend to measure the sensitive results to Nursing care, which can be defined as nursing care that focuses on the needs of individuals or groups, and that focus on factors such as experience, vast knowledge and organization and that will have repercussions on functional status, safety and client satisfaction [11].

These indicators are distributed in three dimensions, according to Donabedian, who focused his research on quality in health care, developing a model that relates three concepts (dimensions): Structure, Process and Results. The "Structure" refers to the space where health services are provided, human, material and organizational resources, the "Process" evaluates care and interpersonal relationships and the "Results" refers to the provided care consequences [13].

This study is integrated into the project development: "Structured Proposal for Rehabilitation Nursing Intervention: Sensitive Gains to Nursing Rehabilitation Care for the Person with Deficit in Self-care and in the Surgical Process" in the context of the

Master's Degree in Rehabilitation Nursing, which showed interest in defining which indicators are sensitive to the Rehabilitation Nursing care found in the Rehabilitation programs for people in the surgical process, based on the health quality model, that allows measure the gains with the interventions carried out by RN's.

2 Method

A systematic review of the literature was carried out, as Bachion and Pereira (2006) points out, translates into a review of studies through a systematic approach, with a clearly defined methodology, presenting as a way of developing the evidence that support for "evidence-based decision-making" [13].

We used the formulation of question PI[C]O: What indicators (Results) are sensitive to Rehabilitation Nursing care (Intervention) in a Rehabilitation program (Intervention) in people in the surgical process (Population).

The research was carried out in September 2018, through the database EBSCOHost - Research Databases. From this scientific database it was possible to access the following databases: CINAHL, MEDLINE, Cochrane Database of Systematic Reviews, Nursing & Allied Health Collection: Comprehensive and MedicLatina, with the descriptors: "nursing", "rehabilitation nursing", "rehabilitation", "surgery" and "neurosurgery", with the boolean descriptors "and" and "or".

The descriptors were introduced into the database previously referred to in the following order [(Nursing)] AND [(rehabilitation) or (rehabilitation nursing)] AND [(surgery) or (neurosurgery)]. Inclusion criteria were: full text in the English language and publications in the last 8 years (2010–2018). Participants included only adults, preferably in surgical process, articles where Rehabilitation programs were applied in different surgical contexts and with conclusions that presented indicators that are sensitive to Rehabilitation care. Repeated articles and articles prior to 2010 were excluded.

The preliminary selection of articles was carried out by reading the title and abstracts. Subsequently, the articles were read in order to answer the question PI[C]O previously established.

The methodological quality of the articles were determined through a critical analysis of the articles, thus, the level of evidence presented was used, according to Melnyk and Fineout-Overhold (2010), seven levels of evidence were identified: level I (Systematic Reviews of Literature or Meta-Analysis), level II (Controlled Randomized Studies), level III (Radomization-controlled study), level IV (Case-control study or Cohort study), level V (Systematic review of qualitative or descriptive studies), level VI (Qualitative or descriptive study) and level VII (Opinion or consensus) [14] and Briggs methodological quality evaluation, integrating articles that met more than 50% of quality criteria according to JBI - QARI Critical Appraisal Tools and JBI - MAStARI Critical Apprai-salt Tools [15]. All articles were analyzed by two authors. This way 9 products were found.

The following flowchart explains the path taken to determine the articles found (Flowchart 1):

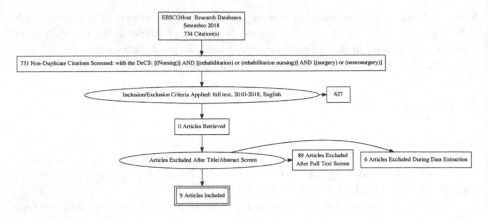

Flowchart 1. Articles selection (Adapted from PRISMA Flow Diagram Generator [16]).

3   Results

Table 1 summarizes the articles results.

Table 1. Article summary.

Title/authors/level of evidence	Goals	Results/Conclusions
Authors: Bruch, F. *et al.* [17] **Methodology:** Qualitative **Level of evidence:** VI **Participants:** A 51-year-old man recovering from an incomplete spinal cord injury submitted to discectomy and cervical laminectomy.	Describe the interdisciplinary rehabilitation of a tetraplegic.	- Gains in patient autonomy in different self-care settings. - Members of the Rehabilitation team of various specialties can play synergistic roles when working together within the context of a comprehensive and regularly updated management plan.
Authors: Crotty, M.; Killington, M.; Walker, R. [18] **Methodology:** Controlled Randomized Study. **Level of evidence:** II **Participants:** 28 patients, nursing home residents, submitted to hip arthroplasty, their families and nursing home team.	Understand the path of nursing home residents after hip fracture and perceptions about the rehabilitation program implemented.	- Dissatisfaction of the Patient family and the nursing team of the nursing home regarding the postoperative care at the hospital level; - Poor transmission of information after discharge; - Difficulties in managing the emotions and pain of residents undergoing surgery and initiating mobilizations.

(continued)

Table 1. (*continued*)

Title/authors/level of evidence	Goals	Results/Conclusions
Authors: Benedicic, M.; Kos, B.; Kos, N. [19] **Methodology:** Qualitative **Level of evidence:** VI	The importance of early rehabilitation in patients submitted to brain tumor neurosurgery.	- With individualized early rehabilitation, it is often possible to achieve independence in patient mobility and daily tasks before leaving the hospital. - A more accurate assessment of the functional status of patients should be performed after completion of oncologic therapy to stratify patients who should be referred for Rehabilitation. - The odds of a good functional outcome in patients with malignant brain tumors can be increased with good early rehabilitation treatment.
Authors: Bahouth et al. [20] **Methodology:** Qualitative **Level of evidence:** VI **Participant:** 55 year old patient with intracerebral hemorrhage.	Describe the hemodynamic responses and ICP during progressive mobility interventions performed in a patient with two external ventricular drains.	- The early progressive mobilization assisted by device was safe in this patient with hemorrhagic stroke, when accompanied by an interdisciplinary team of qualified health professionals. - Further studies are needed to obtain information on hemodynamic and neurophysiological responses associated to early mobilization in acute stroke to identify subsets of patients to benefit from this intervention.
Authors: Aiba *et al.* [21] **Methodology:** Case-control study **Level of evidence:** IV **Participants:** 91 (intervention group) + 91 (control group) over 65 years old, intervened by HSDC between 2001 and 2008.	To assess the efficacy and adverse effects of early postoperative mobilization in elderly patients with chronic subdural hemorrhage.	- Early mobilization after craniotomy with a drainage system prevents postoperative complications without increasing the risk of relapse in patients with chronic sub-dural hematoma aged 65 years or older.

(*continued*)

Table 1. (*continued*)

Title/authors/level of evidence	Goals	Results/Conclusions
Authors: Ekstrom *et al.* [22] **Methodology:** Controlled Randomized Study. Recruited patients over a 12-month period with an intervention group treated with an individualized postoperative rehabilitation program and a control group treated in a traditional manner, according to hospital routines. The final evaluation was performed 4 months after surgery. **Level of evidence:** II **Participants:** patients with hip fracture over 65 years: 285 clients (intervention group) + 218 (control group)	Investigating whether patient empowerment coupled with an individually designed postoperative Rehabilitation program can reduce hospital stay time and whether patients have a better chance of retaking their previous life.	- The mean hospital stay was 4 days less in the intervention group than in the control group. - 90% of clients in the intervention group resumed their previous life compared to 80% in the control group. - Client empowerment by trained nursing staff with an individualized Rehabilitation program can be beneficial in helping clients have a shorter hospital stay and resume their previous lifestyle.
Authors: Cruz et al. [23] **Methodology:** Non-Randomized Controlled Study. Implementation of a rehabilitation program that includes exercises to restore strength and joint mobility and improve the functional capacity of the users. **Level of evidence:** III **Participants:** 78 users with total knee prosthesis over 60 years old.	To compare home rehabilitation with standard hospital rehabilitation in terms of improvement of knee joint mobility, recovery of strength and muscle function in users after total knee replacement.	- After the intervention, both groups showed significant improvements in pain (visual analogue scale), range of flexion-extension movement and muscle strength, disability (Barthel and WOMAC indexes), balance and walk. - This study reveals that Rehabilitation programs at home or at the hospital are equally effective.
Authors: Chen, C. *et al.* [24] **Methodology:** Randomized controlled trial. A routine care program (including 1 to 2 rehabilitation sessions), a subacute care program (geriatric consultation, ongoing rehabilitation and discharge planning) and a comprehensive care program (subacute care + health: control of symptoms of depression, nutrition and prevention of falls).	To compare the effects of an interdisciplinary comprehensive care program with subacute and usual care programs on the health-related quality of life of elderly patients with hip fractures.	- Comprehensive care group participants improved physical function, general health, and mental health relative to the usual care group. - The subacute care group improved physical and social function relative to the usual care group. - The effects of intervention for comprehensive and subacute care have increased over time.

(*continued*)

Table 1. (*continued*)

Title/authors/level of evidence	Goals	Results/Conclusions
Level of evidence: II **Participants:** 299 elderly patients with hip fractures were randomized into three groups: subacute care (n = 101), comprehensive care (n = 99) and usual care (n = 99).		- Comprehensive care programs and subacute care can improve the health outcomes of elderly people with hip fracture.
Authors: Cavill *et al.* [25] **Methodology:** A randomized controlled trial. Rehabilitation was performed twice per week for at least three and at most four weeks prior to surgery, one hour each. **Level of evidence:** II **Participants:** 74 users undergoing arthroplasty.	To investigate the effect of pre-rehabilitation on quality of life and function in patients with total knee arthroplasty and total hip arthroplasty.	- The increase of pre-treatment to usual care improved significantly the range of knee flexion movement in the postoperative period; - There were no significant improvements in the function or benefits of quality of life.

4 Discussion

After analyzing the studies, 49 indicators were identified that are sensitive to the care of Rehabilitation Nursing to the person in the surgical process, present in Rehabilitation programs.

Table 2 shows the indicators [26] identified, dividing them according to the Donabedian model proposal in Structure, Process and Results [31].

Table 2. Sensitive indicators to Rehabilitation Nursing care identified.

Type	Indicator
Structure	- Percentage of clients with risk of **joint stiffness** who were monitored the range of joint movement through the goniometer [23–25]. - Percentage of clients who were provided with an auxiliary device to **stand up** [18–20]. - Percentage of clients in whom scale was applied to assess **body balance** [23]. - Percentage of clients to whom scale was applied for assessment of muscle strength [17, 23] (**Muscle Movement**).

(continued)

Table 2. (*continued*)

Type	Indicator
Process	- Percentage of clients to whom rehabilitation plan and / or program has been implemented to maximize functional capabilities [17–25] (**Health promotion**). - Percentage of clients with potential to improve knowledge about adaptive **walking** technique [17, 18, 21, 24, 25]. - Percentage of clients with potential to improve **walking** ability [17, 18, 21, 22, 24, 25]. - Percentage of clients with potential to improve knowledge about **walk** with walker [23]. - Percentage of clients with potential to improve knowledge about **self-care: eating** auxiliary devices [19]. - Percentage of clients with potential to improve ability to use **self-care: eating** auxiliary devices [19]. - Percentage of clients with potential to improve knowledge about adaptation techniques for **self-care: going to the toilet** [24]. - Percentage of clients with potential to improve knowledge about adaptation techniques for **self-care: clothing** [19, 24]. - Percentage of clients with potential to improve ability to use adaptive technique for **self-care: clothing** [19, 24]. - Percentage of clients with potential to improve knowledge about adaptation technique to **stand up** [19, 25]. - Percentage of clients with the potential to improve knowledge about auxiliary device to **stand up** [19]. - Percentage of clients with potential to improve ability to use auxiliary device to **stand up** [19]. - Percentage of clients with potential to improve ability to use adaptive technique to **stand up** [18, 26]. - Percentage of clients with potential for better knowledge about adaptation technique to **transfer** [17, 24]. - Percentage of clients with potential to improve ability to use adaptive technique to **transfer** themselves [17, 24]. - Percentage of clients who had been used a scale to assess **spasticity** [17]. - Percentage of clients with potential to improve knowledge about muscle and joint exercise technique [17]. (**Spasticity**) - Percentage of clients with potential to improve knowledge about **body balance** technique [23, 24]. - Percentage of clients with potential to improve ability to use **body balancing** technique [23, 24]. - Percentage of clients with potential to improve knowledge about muscle and joint exercise techniques [17, 18, 23–25]. (**Muscle Movement**) - Percentage of clients with potential to improve ability to perform muscle and joint exercise techniques [17, 19, 23–25]. (**Muscle Movement**)

(*continued*)

Table 2. (*continued*)

Type	Indicator
Results	- **Patient satisfaction** index with rehabilitation nursing care [24, 26].
	- Satisfaction of care providers index (..) with rehabilitation nursing care provided to the patient [18]. (**Patient Satisfaction**)
	- Effectiveness rate in the prevention of **joint stiffness** [20, 23].
	- Gains in ability to perform muscle and joint exercises techniques [28, 24]. (**Joint stiffness**)
	- Gains in knowledge about adaptive **walking** technique [17, 25].
	- Gains in **walking** ability [17, 18, 21, 23–25].
	- Gains in knowledge about adaptation techniques for **self-care: going to the toilet** [24].
	- Gains in knowledge about adaptive technique for **self-care: clothing** [17, 24].
	- Gains in ability to use the technique of adaptation to the **self-care: clothing** [17, 24].
	- Gains in the ability to use the adaptation technique for **self-care: moving in a wheelchair** [17].
	- Resolution rate of **standing up** committed [17, 21].
	- Gains in knowledge about adaptive technique for **standing up** [17, 25].
	- Gains in ability to use the adaptation technique to **stand up** [17, 19, 25].
	- Gains in ability to use adaptation technique to change the body **position** [23].
	- Gains in knowledge about adaptive technique to **transfer** [17, 23, 24].
	- Gains in ability to use the adaptive technique to **transfer** [17, 24].
	- Gains in knowledge about muscle and joint exercise technique [17]. (**Spasticity**)
	- Gains in ability to perform muscle and joint exercise techniques [17]. (**Spasticity**)
	- Gains in knowledge about **body balance** technique [23, 24].
	- Gains in ability to use **body balancing** technique [23, 24].
	- Gains in improvement of **muscle movement** [17, 23–25].
	- Gains in knowledge about muscle and joint exercise technique [17, 23, 25]. (**Muscle Movement**)
	- Gains in ability to perform muscle and joint exercise technique [17, 23, 25]. (**Muscle Movement**)

Os bilhetes de identidade de cada Indicador sensível aos cuidados de Enfermagem de Reabilitação encontram-se a negrito.

The following indicators are highlighted in the different dimensions: "Percentage of clients with risk of joint stiffness who were monitored for joint movement amplitude through the goniometer" and "Percentage of clients who were offered auxiliary stand-up device" in the Structural dimension; "Percentage of clients to whom rehabilitation plan and/or program has been implemented to maximize functional capabilities" and "Percentage of clients with potential to improve walking capacity", in the Process dimension and "Gains in ability to walk" and "Gains in improvement of muscle movement" in the Results dimension.

Most of the indicators are related to the Results dimension, thus showing the repercussions of the planned and executed interventions.

The indicator "Percentage of clients to whom rehabilitation plan and/or program has been implemented to maximize functional capabilities" has been found in all studies, meeting RN's specific competencies, which maximizes the person functionality, in order to develop their capabilities [8].

5 Conclusions

Excellence in care can only be guaranteed when results are measured and objective. The surgical patient, in the various areas of intervention (vascular, neuro-surgical, orthopedic), presents health gains with the implementation of Rehabilitation programs, with 49 indicators that are sensitive to Rehabilitation Nursing care in the programs executed.

It is necessary to carry out more studies that focus on the structural dimension, since all dimensions are interconnected, and it is necessary to perceive the repercussions of each one on the quality of care provided.

References

1. World Health Organization (WHO): World Health Statistics 2017: Monitoring Health for the SDGs. World Health Organization (2017). https://doi.org/10.1017/CBO9781107415324.004
2. Ministério da Saúde: Rede Nacional de Especialidade Hospitalar e de Referenciação Neurocirurgica (2017). https://www.sns.gov.pt/wp-content/uploads/2017/09/RRH-Neurocirurgia-Aprovada-a-6-setembro-2017.pdf
3. Instituto Nacional de Estatística (INE): Cirurgias (exceto pequenas cirurgias) por dia (nº) nos hospitais por Localização geográfica (NUTS – 2013). Instituto Nacional de Estatística (2017). https://www.ine.pt/xportal/xmain?xpid=INE&xpgid=ine_indicadores&indOcorr Cod=0008030&contexto=bd&selTab=tab2
4. Dindo, D., Demartines, N., Clavien, P.: Classification of surgical complications: a new proposal with evaluation in a cohort of 6336 patients and results of a survey. Ann. Surg. (2004). https://www.ncbi.nlm.nih.gov/pmc/articles/PMC1360123/
5. Gibbs, N.: Safety of anesthesia in Australia. A review of anaesthesia mortality 2000–2002. In: Australian and New Zealand College of Anaesthetists, Melbourne (2006). http://www.anzca.edu.au/resources/college-publications/a-review-of-anaesthesia-related-mortality-1997-199
6. Monahan, F.: A enfermagem perioperatória. In: Enfermagem Médico-Cirúrgica: Perspectivas de Saúde e Doença, p. 245. Lusodidata, Loures (2010)
7. Juan, K.: O impacto da cirurgia e os aspectos psicológicos do paciente: uma revisão. Psicol. Hosp. 5(1), 48–59 (2007). http://pepsic.bvsalud.org/scielo.php?script=sci_arttext&pid=S1677-74092007000100004
8. Ordem dos Enfermeiros (OE): Regulamento das competências específicas do enfermeiro especialista em Enfermagem de Reabilitação (2010). https://www.ordemenfermeiros.pt/arquivo/legislacao/Documents/LegislacaoOE/RegulamentoCompetenciasReabilitacao_aprovadoAG20Nov2010.pdf
9. Malcato, M.: A pessoa submetida a cirúrgia cardiotorácica. In: Cuidados de Enfermagem de Reabilitação à pessoa ao longo da vida, pp. 515–523. Lusodidacta, Loures (2016)

10. OE: Resumo Mínimo de Dados e Core de Indicadores de Enfermagem para o Repositório Central de Dados da Saúde (2007) http://www.esenfcvpoa.eu/wp-content/uploads/2012/03/RMDE.pdf
11. Doran, D., et al.: An empirical test of nursing role effectiveness model. J. Adv. Nurs. **30**(1), 29–39 (2002). https://doi.org/10.1046/j.1365-2648.2002.02143.x
12. McDonald, K., et al.: Closing the quality gap: a critical analysis of quality improvement strategies. In: Agency for Healthcare Research and Quality, Rockville, vol. 7 (2007). https://www.ncbi.nlm.nih.gov/books/NBK44015/
13. Bachion, M., Pereira, A.: Atualidades em revisão sistemática de literatura, critérios de força e grau de recomendação de evidência. Rev. Gaúcha Enferm. **27**(4), 491–498 (2006). https://seer.ufrgs.br/index.php/RevistaGauchadeEnfermagem/article/view/4633/2548. Accessed in 2009/2018
14. Melnyk, B., Fineout-Overholt, E., Stetler, C., Allan, J.: Outcomes and implementation strategies from the first U.S. evidence-based practice leadership summit. Worldviews Evid. Based Nurs. **2**(3), 113–121 (2005)
15. Briggs, J.: Joanna Briggs Institute (2018). http://joannabriggs.org/research/critical-appraisal-tools.html
16. PRISMA Flow Diagram Generator. http://prisma.thetacollaborative.ca
17. Bruch, F., et al.: Interdisciplinary rehabilitation for a patient with incomplete cervical spinal cord injury and multimorbidity. Medicine **96**(34) (2017). http://web.a.ebscohost.com/ehost/detail/detail?vid=4&sid=2a20aa9a-398e-405c-b2b8ab507d1763b6%40ssionmgr4008&bdata=Jmxhbmc9cHQtYnImc2l0ZT11aG9zdC1saXZl#AN=124940379&db=ccm
18. Crotty, M., Killington, M., Walker, R.: The chaotic journey: recovering from hip fracture in a nursing home. Arch. Gerontol. Geriatr. **67**, 106–112 (2016). http://web.b.ebscohost.com/ehost/detail/detail?vid=4&sid=76cfdc85-0aa0-492d-b5c6-ce64966ff02c%40sessionmgr103&bdata=Jmxhbmc9cHQtYnImc2l0ZT11aG9zdC1saXZl#AN=27483995&db=mdc
19. Benedicic, M., Kos, B., Kos, N.: Early medical rehabilitation after neurosurgical treatment of malignant brain tumors in Slovenia. Radiol. Oncol. **50**(2), 139–144 (2016). http://web.a.ebscohost.com/ehost/detail/detail?vid=6&sid=2a20aa9a-398e-405c-b2b8ab507d1763b6%40sessionmgr4008&bdata=Jmxhbmc9cHQtYnImc2l0ZT11aG9zdC1saXZl#AN=115049443&db=ccm
20. Bahouth, M.N., et al.: Physiological effects of early incremental mobilization on a patient with acute intracerebral and intraventricular hemorrhage requiring dual external ventricular drainage. Neurocritical Care **27**(1), 115–119 (2017). http://web.a.ebscohost.com/ehost/detail/detail?vid=9&sid=2a20aa9a-398e-405c-b2b8-ab507d1763b6%40sessionmgr4008&bdata=Jmxhbmc9cHQtYnImc2l0ZT11aG9zdC1saXZl#AN=28243999&db=mdc
21. Aiba, T., et al.: Efficacy and safety of postoperative early mobilization for chronic subdural hematoma in elderly patients. Acta Neurochir. **152**(7), 1171–1174 (2010). http://web.a.ebscohost.com/ehost/detail/detail?vid=11&sid=2a20aa9a-398e-405c-b2b8-ab507d1763b6%40sessionmgr4008&bdata=Jmxhbmc9cHQtYnImc2l0ZT11aG9zdC1saXZl#AN=20336332&db=mdc
22. Ekstrom, W., et al.: Power to the patient: care tracks and empowerment a recipe for improving rehabilitation for hip fracture patients. Scand. J. Caring Sci. **29**(3), 462–469 (2015). http://web.a.ebscohost.com/ehost/detail/detail?vid=13&sid=2a20aa9a-398e-405c-b2b8-ab507d1763b6%40sessionmgr4008&bdata=Jmxhbmc9cHQtYnImc2l0ZT11aG9zdC1saXZl#AN=24953232&db=mdc

23. Pérez-de la Cruz, S., et al.: Home-based versus hospital-based rehabilitation program after total knee replacement. Biomed. Res. Int. **2015**, 1–9 (2015). http://web.a.ebscohost.com/ ehost/detail/detail?vid=15&sid=2a20aa9a-398e-405c-b2b8-ab507d1763b6%40sessionmgr 4008&bdata=Jmxhbmc9cHQtYnImc2l0ZT1laG9zdC1saXZl#AN=109273968&db=ccm

24. Chen, C., et al.: Comprehensive and subacute care interventions improve health-related quality of life for older patients after surgery for hip fracture: a randomised controlled trial. Int. J. Nurs. Stud. **50**(8), 1013–1024 (2013). http://web.a.ebscohost.com/ehost/detail/detail? vid=17&sid=2a20aa9a-398e-405c-b2b8-ab507d1763b6%40sessionmgr4008&bdata=Jmxhbb mc9cHQtYnImc2l0ZT1laG9zdC1saXZl#AN=23245454&db=mdc

25. Cavill, S., et al.: The effect of prehabilitation on the range of motion and functional outcomes in patients following the total knee or hip arthroplasty: a pilot randomized trial. Physiother. Theory Prat. **12**(4), 262–270 (2016). http://web.a.ebscohost.com/ehost/detail/detail?vid= 5&sid=07874f83-ca12-4242-a73f-e9ffcf8831da%40sessionmgr4007&bdata=Jmxhbmc9c HQtYnImc2l0ZT1laG9zdC1saXZl#AN=27050325&db=mdc. Accessed Sep 2018

26. OE (Mesa do Colégio da Especialidade de Enfermagem de Reabilitação da Ordem dos Enfermeiros Mandato 2011-2015 e 2016-2019): Bilhetes de identidade dos indicadores que integram o core de indicadores por categoria de enunciados descritivos dos Padrões de Qualidade dos Cuidados de Enfermagem de Reabilitação. OE (2018). https://www. ordemenfermeiros.pt/media/5443/enfermagemreabilitacao.pdf

Violence Against the Elderly: Social Representations of Portuguese and Brazilian Caregivers

Felismina Mendes[1(✉)] ⓘ, Tatiana Mestre[1] ⓘ, Elaine Santana[2] ⓘ,
Luciana Reis[2] ⓘ, and Manuel Lopes[1] ⓘ

[1] Department of Nursing, University of Évora, Évora, Portugal
fm@uevora.pt
[2] Postgraduate Programme in Memory: Language and Society,
State University of Southwest of Bahia, Vitória da Conquista, Brazil

Abstract. The increase in life expectancy and elderly people in society, coupled with changes in family structure, have highlighted the importance of formal
and informal caregivers of elderly people. **Objective:** To analyse the social
representations of violence against the elderly, of two groups of formal and
informal caregivers. **Methods:** Exploratory, quantitative and qualitative
research, supported by the theoretical-methodological reference of the Social
Representations Theory and in the context of this, the Central Core Theory. The
sample was participated in by 81 formal caregivers from the project "Aging in
Safety in the Alentejo - Understanding to Act, of the University of Évora" and
20 informal caregivers from the project "Qualification of caregivers and aspects
related to the quality of life of the elderly people dependent on primary and
tertiary care: Implementation and protocol evaluation, of the State University of
Southwest of Bahia". We used the Free Word Association Technique. The data
was analysed by prototypical analysis based on two matrices by the software
IRAMUTEQ (Interface de R pour les Analyses Multidimensionnelles de Textes
et de Questionnaires) 0.7 alpha 2. **Results:** In Portugal, the elements "bad,
mistreatment, I will be, sad, anger, patience, physical, injustice, irritation and
meanness" stood out in the central core. In Brazil the mention of "hitting" was
emphasized. **Conclusions:** In both Portugal and Brazil, physical violence takes
on particular significance in the social representations of caregivers, rather than
verbal and psychological violence, which is not present in the central core of
social representations of violence against the elderly in either of the countries.

Keywords: Aging · Elderly people · Caregivers · Violence

1 Introduction

1.1 Sociodemographic Characterisation

In view of the changes in health conditions and birth rates of the population, as a result
of socioeconomic development, there was a general increase in average life expectancy.

© Springer Nature Switzerland AG 2019
J. García-Alonso and C. Fonseca (Eds.): IWoG 2018, CCIS 1016, pp. 295–306, 2019.
https://doi.org/10.1007/978-3-030-16028-9_26

Currently, one of the major social challenges is the growth of the number of elderly people worldwide (Brito et al. 2018).

Research on aging became more prominent in the 1950s when the process of demographic change occurred in Europe and the United States (Castro et al. 2013). However, in developing countries, such as Brazil, this problem began to become more visible later in the mid-1980s (Prado and Sayd 2006; Silveira et al. 2018).

In Portugal, the average life expectancy has increased in recent decades, with 80.8 years in 2016 - 83.4 years for women and 77.7 years for men (Pordata 2018). In 2017, Portugal had a Longevity Index of 53.2% and an Aging Index of 153.2%. In the same year, the Alentejo region had an Aging Index of 197.0%, much higher than the 153.2% that was verified in the whole country (Portada 2018).

In Brazil, the aging population has maintained the trend observed in recent years, with a growth of 18% since 2012, reaching 30.2 million elderly people in the country in 2017 (IBGE 2015). In the State of Bahia, the National Survey by Continuous Sampling of Households, revealed a figure of 1.9 million elderly people, corresponding to 12.6% of the population (IBGE 2015).

1.2   The Vulnerability of the Elderly: Risk Factor for Violence

The implications of the phenomenon of the aging population have revealed a major impact on society, mainly affecting the public spheres of health and social security. The elderly population is that which uses the health services most, mainly hospital admissions, besides the constant need for continuous care (Veras and Oliveira 2018). In addition to the cognitive and physical losses of aging, there are the problems related to socio-cultural conditions and incomes. These factors lead to greater vulnerability in these individuals who increasingly need the support of third parties to carry out their daily activities (Mariano et al. 2015).

Given this reality, the caregiver becomes an agent of great importance in the routine of the elderly person. A caregiver can be defined as formal or informal. A formal caregiver is one who performs the care as a professional activity, receiving payment for it, while the informal caregiver performs the care in a non-professional way, and is often provided by relatives, friends or neighbours (Vieira et al. 2011; Batista et al. 2014).

Research on the problem of functionality demonstrates the association between age and dependence, which places the elderly person in a state of greater vulnerability (OPSS 2015; Barbosa et al. 2017; Mariano et al. 2015). According to Ayres et al. (2012), vulnerability in the health field is associated with the elements of the aging process and disease, both at an individual level, as well as socially and operationally. Decreased functionality of elderly people leads to increased risk of vulnerability, which simultaneously exposes elderly people to a greater risk of violence (Apratto 2010; Oliveira et al. 2012). Second Report of the World Health Organization (2002, p. 2) "violence constitutes one of the main public health problems in the world" and can be understood as any isolated or repetitive act that entails physical, sexual or psychological harm, including situations of neglect, exploitation, suffering or distress.

This topic has remained hidden for a long time, but in view of the new population profile, it needs to be extensively explored, mainly from approaches that seek to reach the subjectivities involved in a context influenced by moral and cultural conceptions. Thus, the Social Representations Theory is a theoretical tool that helps to better understand this sociocultural and public health phenomenon.

1.3 Social Representations

Authors such as (Danic 2006; Porto 2006; Junqueira 2005) think that the concept of social representations arose from the foundation of sociology as a discipline. At the end of the nineteenth century, in 1898, Durkheim revealed in his research that social representations show social nature by revealing that in their interpretation there exists a physical world and a social world and that these show the influence of society on the individual (Danic 2006). In 1961, Moscovici, a social psychologist, gave a new approach to the Social Representations Theory, as a particular form of acquiring knowledge and communicating acquired knowledge, from the perceptions that individuals produce and give meaning to everyday life (Moscovici 2007).

Taking the collective representations previously proposed by Durkheim as his starting point, Moscovici sought to analyse collective thoughts based on the premise that sociological aspects are unifying, while psychological processes operate in integrity and coherence. Moscovici's proposal does not invalidate collective representations but adds phenomena to the field, developing a social psychology that demonstrates both social and psychological perspectives as imperatives to achieve social phenomena (Moscovici 2007; Duveen 2007; Sá 1996).

The social representations generate and dictate behaviours, conceptualise the stimuli, at the same time, that give meanings to the answers (Sá 2002). For Moscovici (2007), this judgment demonstrates the relevance in understanding the theory, because when he mentions the collective he is, in fact, referring to the individuals who construct meanings for his reality, and this is how the social representation of a given object is born.

The representations "restore the collective consciousness and shape it by explaining objects and events in such a way that they become accessible to everyone and coincide with our immediate interests" (Moscovici 2007, 52).

All representations have the universal function of making something unfamiliar familiar, and for these two processes are used, called anchoring and objectification. Anchoring is the means by which we seek to classify, name or even find a place for something that seems unfamiliar to us. Objectification is an imaginary and structuring operation that gives a specific form/character to the materialising knowledge. It means to reproduce a concept through an image (Moscovici 2007).

According to Abric (2001), the representations can be understood through their content and organisation. The content is important, but it cannot be disregarded that there is a hierarchy of elements, an organisation structure. This approach is presented in the Central Core Theory where representations have a central core related to historical and ideological conditions. The representations present in the central core are those that are resistant to change because they have a common basis shared by the individuals. Whereas, the representations present in the periphery constitute the interface between concrete reality and the central system (Sá 1996).

2 Methodology

An exploratory investigation was carried out, with a qualitative and quantitative approach, which has the Social Representations (SR) theory, adjacent to the central core theory, as the theoretical-methodological reference.

For the conception of the instrument, the Free Speech Association Technique (TALP) was used, adapted for research in social representations by Di Giacomo (1981), where each caregiver was asked to say five words about violence against the elderly.

The objective of this investigation was to analyse and compare the Social Representations of violence against the elderly, of two groups of caregivers in Portugal and Brazil.

In Portugal, the sample included the voluntary participation of 81 formal caregivers of ten Residential Care Homes for Seniors (ERPI), in the Evora district. The inclusion criteria were: being employed at the institution for more than one year; full time; working directly with the elderly people. The data collection took place from March to May 2018, in those institutions.

In Brazil, the sample included the voluntary participation of 20 informal caregivers, coming from Bahia, more concretely from the city of Vitória da Conquista. Data was collected from January to February 2018. The inclusion criteria were: over 18 years old; being an informal caregiver of an elderly person; and living with them.

All the ethical procedures of human research were followed. Thus, all the authorisations required for the study were requested, as well as informed consent of the professionals. All conditions of anonymity and confidentiality of the responses obtained were also guaranteed. The Portuguese project was approved by the Ethics Committee of the Health and Welfare Area of the University of Evora under number 16012 of 05/19/2016, while the Brazilian project was approved by the Research Ethics Committee of the State University of the Southwest of Bahia under number 1.875.418 of 08/15/2016.

The data analysis related to the automatic classification of lexical hierarchical groupings associated to the social representations of violence against the elderly was carried out by the software IRAMUTEQ (*Interface de R pour les Analyses Multidimensionnelles de Textes et de Questionnaires*) version 0.7 alpha 2, created by Ratinaud (2009). This software allowed the matrices of the lexical units to be explored, where in the context of the studies the prototypical analysis was carried out.

The words mentioned were entered into an Excel database, composed of the variables: caregiver identification, age, sex, profession, amount of time in the job in the institution/in the provision of informal care, words mentioned and their rank. The rank signifies the order in which the words were mentioned.

3 Results

3.1 Characterisation of the Portuguese Sample

81 caregivers aged 26–68 participated in the study. It was confirmed that 2 caregivers were male and 79 female.

The dominant professions expressed by the sample were: 47 direct action assistants, 11 general service assistants (13.58%). It should be noted that the direct action assistants have a representativity of 58.02% of the sample. The remaining professions were: from the food division, senior technicians from the social and nursing area.

Representatively, 62.95% of the caregivers have between 1 and 10 years of professional experience in the job, 25.92% have between 11 and 20 years of professional experience in the job and 11.1% of caregivers present between 21 and 32 years of experience in the job.

3.2 Characterisation of the Brazilian Sample

In the study carried out in Brazil, 20 informal caregivers, aged between 18 and 60, participated in the study, 16 of which were female and 4 were male.

In relation to the professions exercised by the caregivers, it was confirmed that the greatest representation was in 6 maids, followed by 3 general services assistants. With an equal number of each, there were 2 students, 2 nursing technicians and 2 independent workers. The remaining sample consists of 1 artisan, 1 administrative assistant, 1 kitchen assistant and 1 teacher.

In relation to the practice of care, 8 of these caregivers have between one and three years' experience; 6 caregivers have more than ten years' experience; 2 of the caregivers have between four and six years' experience; and only 4 caregivers have less than one year's experience.

3.3 Prototypical Analysis of Portugal

Through the data obtained in the single frequency and in the multiple frequency, $f \geq 4.25$ and $f < 4.25$ was established as a cohort bridge, in order to determine the minimum frequency to be considered for constitution of the prototypical analysis, together with the diagram of the four social representations of violence against the elderly, expressed in Table 1. Prototypical analysis is a simple and efficient technique developed exclusively for the study of social representations in order to identify the representational structure based on the frequency criteria and order of word mentions from the Free Speech Association Technique (Abric 2003a).

The four quadrant diagram (Table 1) is composed of elements separated according to frequency and order of mention. This plan is made up of four quadrants: the central core; the first peripheral zone; the second peripheral zone and the contrast elements. The upper quadrant group (first quadrant) consists of the central elements, with a higher frequency and a lower mean order of mention, indicating the words that have a high frequency, that is, the words that were most quickly mentioned by the caregivers in the first order (Abric 2003b), when compared with the remaining quadrants (Torres and Camargo 2014). Thus, they become like the probable indicators of the central core of the social representation. In the specific case of our investigation, the constituents "bad", "mistreatment", "I will be", "sad", "anger", "patience", "physical", "injustice", "irritation", "meanness".

Regarding the upper right quadrant (second quadrant) that point to the elements of the first periphery, the following mentions are highlighted: "respect", "family", "abandonment", "attention", "psychological", "defenceless", "affection". They are the words that have a high frequency, but which had a higher average order, which means they were not immediately mentioned by the caregivers (Camargo and Justo 2013).

In the lower left quadrant (third quadrant), the contrast zone contains elements that were quickly mentioned, but often below the given cohort point (Camargo and Justo 2013). In the case of our investigation, in this quadrant words like "crime", "heart", "horrible", "must not do", "cruelty", "stupidity", "aggressiveness", "sadness", "frustration", "environment" were found.

In the lower right quadrant is the second peripheral zone, i.e. the most active ones, where words such as "shouting", "verbal", "they do not think", "I do not like", "hitting", "horror", "care", "work", "I think about my parents", "institutions", "support", "tiredness", "talk", "humanity", "training", "words", "rage", "inhumane", "compression", "frustration". These are the words that have a low frequency, but which have a higher mean order of mention, which means that they were the words most quickly mentioned by the caregivers compared to the right quadrant (first quadrant).

According to Sá (1996) there are several methods of data collection concerning the elements of the central core of a social representation. In this study we chose the method of identification of central mentions supported in the Free Word Association Technique. This method is based on two basic quantitative criteria: the frequency of mentions and the average order of mentions. The combination of these two criteria reveals the possible central elements of a social representation, in this case in the social representation of violence against the elderly.

Table 1. Prototypical analysis of the SR of Violence against the elderly of the formal caregivers of Portugal Source: Prepared by the Authors (2018)

Average order of mention ≤ 2.45			Average order of mention > 2.45		
≥ 4.25	*Central core*			*First peripheral zone*	
	Words	*f*	*OME*	*Words*	*f*	*OME*
	Bad	11	2.3	Respect	12	3
	Mistreatment	11	1.5	Family	8	2.9
	I will be	10	2.3	Abandonment	6	2.5
	Sad	7	2	Attention	6	3
	Anger	7	2.4	Psychological	6	2.5
	Patience	7	2.3	Defenceless	5	4
	Physical	7	2.3	Affection	5	3.2
	Injustice	6	1.8			
	Irritation	5	2			
	Meanness	5	2.4			

(*continued*)

Table 1. (*continued*)

Average order of mention ≤ 2.45			Average order of mention > 2.45		
f < 4.25	*Elements of contrast*		*Second peripheral zone*		
	Crime	4	1.5	Shouting	4	3
	Heart	4	1.8	Verbal	4	2.5
	Horrible	4	2.2	They do not think	4	2.5
	Must not do	4	1.5	I do not like	3	2.7
	Cruelty	3	2.3	Hitting	3	2.7
	Stupidity	2	1	Horror	2	4
	Aggressiveness	2	1	Care	2	5
	Sadness	2	1	Work	2	3.5
	Frustration	2	1	I think about my parents	2	2.5
	Environment	2	1	Institutions	2	4
				Support	2	3
				Tiredness	2	2.5
				Talk	2	4
				Humanity	2	4
				Training	2	2.5
				Words	2	2.5
				Rage	2	2.5
				Inhumane	2	2.5
				Understanding	2	2.5
				Frustration	2	2.5

3.4 Prototypical Analysis of Brazil

Also through the data in Brazil, we obtained the single frequency and the multiple frequency, where f ≥ 5.25 and f < 5.25 was established as a cohort bridge, in order to determine the minimum frequency to be considered for constitution of the prototypical analysis, together with the diagram of the four quadrants of the social representations of violence against the elderly, expressed in Table 2.

Thus, they become like the probable indicators of the central core of the social representation. In the specific case of this investigation is the mention "hitting" in the upper left quadrant (first quadrant). Regarding the right upper quadrant (second quadrant) it indicates the elements of the first periphery, where words such as "verbal" and "not caring" are observed. In the lower left quadrant, in the contrast zone, words such as "money", "attention", "ridicule", "hygiene", "responsibility" and "psychological" are found. In the lower right quadrant is the second peripheral zone where words such as "not feeding", "abandonment" and "respect" appear.

Table 2. Prototypical analysis of the SR of the Violence against the elderly of the informal caregivers of Brazil Source: Prepared by the Authors (2018)

Average order of mention ≤ 2.3				Average order of mention > 2.3		
≥ 5.25	*Central core*			*First peripheral zone*		
	Words	*f*	*OME*	*Words*	*f*	*OME*
	Hitting	15	1.9	Verbal	12	2.9
				Not caring	8	2.6
f < 5.25	*Elements of contrast*			*Second peripheral zone*		
	Money	4	2.2	Not feeding	5	2.4
	Attention	3	1	Abandonment	4	3.5
	Ridicule	3	1.7	Respect	3	2.7
	Hygiene	2	1.5			
	Responsibility	2	1			
	Psychological	2	2			

4   Discussion

4.1   Discussion of Results from Portugal

The structural approach to social representations was chosen as a guideline for methodological procedures, aiming at identifying the structure and organisation of the contents of social representations. This structure is constituted by hierarchical elements, organised into two systems: central and peripheral.

According to our prototypical analysis, more specifically that expressed in the central core, (first quadrant) the mentions that stand out are "bad", "mistreatment", "I will be". It is revealed that "mistreatment" is a concept similar to the concept of violence advocated by several authors such as Dias (2010), Duarte and Barbosa (2011). The mention "I will be" represents the feeling regarding concerns with personal perspectives, as if there was a projection of what the future holds.

In the first periphery (second quadrant), the mentions: "respect", "family" and "abandonment" are in line with the WHO concept (2014, p. 78), which includes various types of violence. "Abandonment (...) refers to actions that compromise dignity and respect." The mention "family" is explained by the APAV (2010) when it reveals and frames the family association with violence, stressing that (...) the elderly person is one of the most fragile members (...) in the family hierarchy, (...) rarely occupying top place, where such determining powers like finances, organisation, leadership, influences and decisions are concentrated (...)" (p. 54). The APAV (2010) further points out that when institutionalised the elderly person may be at high risk of violence, especially when they are abandoned by relatives in an institution.

In the third quadrant, the contrast zone contains words like: "crime". "Aging is associated with the phenomenon of crime and violence committed against the elderly" (APAV 2010, p. 41). This Association shows that the concepts of physical, psychological, sexual violence, neglect, financial violence and abandonment, are crimes under

Portuguese legislation. This representation expresses the meaning of the Portuguese legislation regarding violence against the elderly.

In the second periphery (fourth quadrant) are the words "shouting" and "verbal". To Luoma et al. (2011), psychological violence includes verbal and non-verbal emotional violence, which can be defined as active or passive. These are actions that aim to inflict mental suffering or distress on an elderly person. In this sense it is possible to add "shouting", as a practice of psychological violence.

4.2 Discussion of Results from Brazil

In the Brazilian investigation, the centrality of the mentions is in the central core (first quadrant), in the term "beat", which is a practice of physical violence. According to the UN (2002) and the *Manual de enfrentamento à violência contra a pessoa idosa* (Handbook for combating violence against the elderly) (Brazil, 2013), physical violence refers to the use of physical force to force the elderly or to cause physical pain and injury, among other punishments. The most visible violence is usually through pinching, slapping, shoving, or even aggression with knives or firearms.

In turn, the mentions found in the first periphery (second quadrant) constitute the types of violence. The "verbal" element is associated with verbal violence, such as threats and humiliation, which are classified as psychological violence. The term "not caring" refers to neglect.

In the second periphery (fourth quadrant) the "not feeding" and "abandonment" mentions were also associated with neglect. According to Minayo (2006), this is based on the refusal or omission of the necessary care.

In relation to the elements of contrast (third quadrant), the term "money" has been referenced, which is incorporated in financial violence, which is recognised as the improper use or use without consent of the elderly person's material assets. This is a type of violence that has been growing in Brazil, representing 40.1% of the reports of violence against the elderly population (Brazil, 2013). The terms "attention", "ridicule", "hygiene" and "responsibility" refer to the issue of neglect, and although it is a frequent type of violence, it is not always identified as such. Also, the "psychological" mention referred to as the last element of contrast corresponds to psychological violence, which may be exercised in a verbal or non-verbal way (Gondim 2011).

4.3 Discussion of Results from Portugal and Brazil

Through the prototypical analysis carried out in both studies, there are some similarities mainly at the central core level. As we can see in Table 2, the word "hitting" is present, then in Table 1, the formal caregivers when referring to violence against the elderly mention "physical" as one of the main words. Thus, it is possible to conclude that in both Portugal and Brazil physical violence is of great prominence. This can be justified because it is the type of violence that most often leaves visible marks. Or rather, it becomes a facilitator so that this is a social representation common to most individuals, from both countries. Also in the study conducted by Leite et al. (2008) on social representations carried out with informal Brazilian caregivers, they said that violence against the elderly is concentrated around "physical aggression, such as hitting and pushing" (p. 217).

In the first peripheral zone of Table 2, the word "verbal" is expressed, a word that is also present in the second peripheral zone of Table 1, which means that it was mentioned more by Brazilian caregivers than by Portuguese caregivers. In comparison, in Table 2, in the second peripheral zone there are typically the mentions "abandonment" and "respect", but in Table 1, these are in the first peripheral zone.

As in Table 2, also in Table 1 are the words "psychological". However, while this is found in the contrast elements of Table 2, Table 1 is present in the first peripheral zone, as is the case regarding the mention "attention". As verbal and psychological violence and neglect have already been mentioned, they end up being less visible, or rather, they will be less noticeable by not being taken into account as the social representation of violence against the elderly (Leite et al. 2008).

5 Conclusion

The social representations mentioned by the caregivers are consistent with concepts already validated by epistemological and methodological bases. These social representations derive from the negative representations of the practice of caring for the elderly, which is prevalent in today's society. Violence against elderly people is based on disrespectful behaviour and humiliation and depictions of violence reflect, in essence, the prevailing social attitude towards aging.

In the conclusion of the investigation in Portugal and Brazil it was verified that Physical Violence is of great prominence in both countries. The basis of this representation happens to be the type of violence that leaves visible marks. Verbal, psychological violence and neglect, due to being less visible, are less valued for the definition of the representations, as can be seen from the fact that they are not present in any central core of the social representations of violence against the elderly.

It is therefore considered important to replicate this study in more regions of both countries, so that it can be understood, according to the Social Representations Theory, whether there are significant differences regarding the community and institutional context where caregivers develop their caring practices.

References

Abric, J.: Abordagem estrutural das representações sociais: desenvolvimentos recentes. In: Campos, P., Loureiro, M. (eds.) Representações sociais e práticas educativas. UCG, Goiânia (2003a)

Abric, J.: La recherche du noyau central et de la zone muette des représentations sociales. In: Abric, J. (ed.) Méthodes d'étude des représentations sociales. Érès, Ramonville-Saint Agne (2003b)

Apratto, P.: A violência doméstica contra idosos nas áreas de abrangência do Programa Saúde da Família de Niterói (RJ, Brasil). Ciênc. Saúde Coletiva 15(6), 2983–2995 (2010)

Associação Portuguesa de Apoio à Vítima.: Manual Títono - Apoio a Pessoas Idosas Vítimas de Crime e de Violência (2010). http://www.apav.pt/pdf/Titono_PT.pdf. Accessed 8 Oct 2018

Ayres, J., Calazams, G., Saletti Filho, H., França Júnior, I.: Risco, vulnerabilidade e práticas de prevenção e promoção da saúde. In: Akerman, M., Campos, G., Carvalho, Y., Drumond Jr., M., Minayo, M. (eds.) Tratado de Saúde Coletiva, 2nd edn., pp. 375–416. Hucitec, São Paulo (2012)

Barbosa, K., Costa, K., Pontes, M., Batista, P., Oliveira, F., Fernandes, M.: Envelhecimento e vulnerabilidade individual: um panorama dos idosos vinculados à estratégia saúde da família. Texto Contexto Enferm. **26**(2), e2700015 (2017)

Batista, M., Almeida, M., Lancman, S.: Cuidadores formais de idosos: contextualização histórica no cenário brasileiro. Rev. Bras. Geriatr. Gerontol. **17**(4), 879–885 (2014)

Brito, A., Belloni, E., Castro, A., Camargo, B., Giacomozzi, A.: Representações sociais do cuidado e da velhice no Brasil e Itália. Psic. Teor. Pesq. **34**, 3455 (2018)

Camargo, B., Justo, A.: IRAMUTEQ: um software gratuito para análise de dados textuais. Temas Psicol. **21**(2), 513–518 (2013)

Castro, A., Guilam, M., Sousa, E., Marcondes, W.: Violência na velhice: abordagens em periódicos nacionais indexados. Ciênc. Saúde Coletiva **18**(5), 1283–1292 (2013)

Danic, I.: La notion de représentation pour les sociologues. Premier aperçu (2006)

Davison, E., McCabe, M., Visser, S., Hudgson, C., Buchanan, G., George, K.: Controlled trial of dementia training with a peer support group for aged care staff. Int. J. Geriatr. Psychiatry **22**, 868–873 (2007)

Di Giacomo, J.: Aspects méthodologiques de l'analyse des réprésentations sociales. Cah. Psychol. Cogn. Curr. Psychol. Cogn. **1**, 397–422 (1981)

Dias, I.: Violência doméstica e justiça: respostas e desafios. Soc. Rev. Fac. Let. Univ. Porto **20**, 245–262 (2010)

Duarte, N., Barbosa, C.: Manual do Envelhecimento Ativo. In: Ribeiro, O., Paúl, C. (eds.) Envelhecimento Ativo, 1st edn. Lidel, Lisboa (2011)

Instituto Brasileiro de Geografia e Estatística. Pesquisa Nacional por Amostra de Domicílios: síntese de indicadores 2013. Coordenação de Trabalho e Rendimento, Rio de Janeiro, 2 edn., 296 p. (2015)

Junqueira, L.: A noção de representação social na sociologia contemporânea. Estudos Soc. **18**(19), 145–161 (2005)

Leite, M., Hildebrandt, L., dos Santos, A.: Maus-tratos a idosos no domicílio: concepção de familiares. Rev. Bras. Geriatr. Gerontol. **11**(2), 209–221 (2008)

Luoma, M., et al.: Prevalence study of abuse and violence against older women: Results of a multicultural survey conducted in Austria, Belgium, Finland, Lithuania and Portugal. THL, Department of Health and Welfare, Helsinki, Finland (2011)

Mariano, P., Baldissera, V., Martins, J., Carreira, L.: Nursing work organization in long-stay institutions for the elderly: relationship to pleasure and suffering at work. Texto Contexto Enferm. **24**(3), 756–765 (2015)

Observatório Português dos Sistemas de Saúde. Acesso aos cuidados de saúde. Um direito em risco? Relatório de Primavera (2015). http://www.opss.pt/sites/opss.pt/files/RelatorioPrimavera2015.pdf

Oliveira, M., Gomes, A., Amaral, C., Santos, L.: Características dos idosos vítimas de violência doméstica no Distrito Federal. Rev. Bras. Geriatr. Gerontol. **15**(3), 555–566 (2012)

Organização Mundial De Saúde: Relatório Mundial sobre a Prevenção da Violência 2014. Núcleo de Estudos da Violência (Trad.), São Paulo (2014)

PORDATA Fundação Francisco Manuel dos Santos, Esperança de vida à nascença: total e por sexo. Portugal. Europa. Municípios. https://www.pordata.pt/Portugal/Esperan%C3%A7a+de +vida+%C3%A0+nascen%C3%A7a+total+e+por+sexo+(base+tri%C3%A9nio+a+partir+de +2001)-418. Accessed 8 Oct 2018

PORDATA, Fundação Francisco Manuel dos Santos, Indicadores de Envelhecimento. https://www.pordata.pt/Portugal/Indicadores+de+envelhecimento-526. Accessed 8 Oct 2018

PORDATA, Fundação Francisco Manuel dos Santos, Indicadores de Envelhecimento. https://www.pordata.pt/Municipios/%C3%8Dndice+de+envelhecimento-458. Accessed 8 Oct 2018

Porto, M.: Crenças, valores e representações sociais da violência. Sociologias **8**(16), 250–273 (2006)

Prado, S., Sayd, J.: A gerontologia como campo do conhecimento científico: conceito, interesses e projeto político. Cien. Saude Colet. **11**(2), 91–501 (2006)

Ratinaud, P.: IRAMUTEQ: Interface de R pour les Analyses Multidimensionnelles de Textes et de Questionnaires [Computer software] (2009). http://www.iramuteq.org. Accessed 8 Oct 2018

Sá, C.: Núcleo Central das Representações Sociais, 2nd edn. Vozes, Petrópolis (1996)

Silveira, E., Vieira, L., Souza, J.: Elevada prevalência de obesidade abdominal em idosos e associação com diabetes, hipertensão e doenças respiratórias. Ciênc. Saúde Coletiva **23**(3), 903–912 (2018)

Torres, T., Camargo, B.: Redes associativas e representações sociais do envelhecimento e rejuvenescimento para diferentes grupos etários. In: Lopes, M., Mendes, F., Silva, A. (eds.) Envelhecimento: Estudos e Perspetivas. Martinari, São Paulo (2014)

Veras, R., Oliveira, M.: Envelhecer no Brasil: a construção de um modelo de cuidado. Ciênc. Saúde Coletiva **23**(6), 1929–1936 (2018)

Vieira, C., Fialho, A., Freitas, C., Jorge, M.: Práticas do cuidador informal do idoso no domicílio. Rev. Bras. Enferm. **64**(3), 570–579 (2011)

World Health Organization: Informe mundial sobre la violencia y la salud (2002)

From No Man's Land to Places. The Lived Territory in Nursing Homes

Ângela Simões[1,2,3](✉) (iD) and Paula Sapeta[1,3]

[1] Escola Superior de Saúde Dr. Lopes Dias,
Instituto Politécnico de Castelo Branco, Castelo Branco, Portugal
angela.simoes@gmail.com, paulasapeta@ipcb.pt
[2] Hospital Amato Lusitano, Unidade Local de Saúde de Castelo Branco,
Castelo Branco, Portugal
[3] Age.Comm - Interdisciplinary Research Unit on Building Functional Ageing
Communities, Castelo Branco, Portugal

Abstract. In an ideal situation, the elderly live in their natural environment, such as their own home or that of their relatives and is free to decide on the various aspects of their daily life in a safe environment. The decline or loss of the independence level, autonomy, social support, adverse economic conditions, loss of the dominant role within the family and loneliness are some of the causal factors that may modify this ideal situation. If action on these causal factors is insufficient or not possible, admission to a nursing home may occur as a temporary or permanent solution. After the establishment of the exchange situation, the elderly start a path of acceptance of the circumstances of living as a user of a nursing home, which becomes their home.

This article intends to present some of the results obtained during a Grounded Theory research on the Promotion and Preservation of Dignity in the context of care in nursing homes, carried out in the context of the PhD in Nursing of the University of Lisbon.

From the initial analysis of the data, it was noticed that residentes will try to maintain a daily life close to the one before admission, molding it to existing rules and standards, establishing a relation of use with time and space, in which relationship emerge the appropriation of social experiences and build daily life. Territoriality will allow the elderly to reinvent themselves and preserve themselves simultaneously.

Keywords: Nursing homes · Space · Territoriality · Grounded Theory

1 Introduction

Although there is no doubt that there is a progressive increase in the number of elderly people in the population structure, it is important to recognize that the constitution of old age as a social problem, that is, the subject of social policy measures, is far from being

Â. S. L. Simões and A. P. A. G. Sapeta are integrated researchers at Age.Comm - Interdisciplinary Research Unit on Building Functional Ageing Communities

© Springer Nature Switzerland AG 2019
J. García-Alonso and C. Fonseca (Eds.): IWoG 2018, CCIS 1016, pp. 307–318, 2019.
https://doi.org/10.1007/978-3-030-16028-9_27

the mere result of the growth in the number of elderly people, suggests by the notion of demographic aging [1]. The progressive aging of the population; geographical mobility, coupled with changes in family structure, the death of the elderly's spouse and consequently the difficulty in living alone; the insecurity and the fear that something happens and that no one is around to help him; the deterioration of the housing conditions, making the house unsuitable for the needs; the increased vulnerability and fragility of the elderly and the fact that care services are insufficient to guarantee the maintenance of the elderly at home are the main factors of institutionalization. The loss of autonomy and functionality are associated with these factors; worsening of health status; the conflict in family relations; the disagreement of interests, the inefficiency of their network of interactions; isolation; the precariousness of economic and housing conditions; the absence of solidarity networks and loneliness [2].

Costa [3] points out that from the psychological point of view many of the elderly who require institutionalization do so because of the need to seek alternative links in a different relationship of protection, shelter and support, in order to live the rest of their days in safety.

In the emergence of asylum space, its function was not to promote the recovery of the individual resident and to encourage their return to the wider social life. It was a custodial institution, a guardian of elderly individuals, offering only "enough care" to the people who are in their last days of life [4]. From the time of the first shelters and later the asylums, old age gained a "place", a geographical place, and at the same time a symbolic one, for the asylum of old people was and continues to be a place deeply loaded with meanings. With the emergence of the asylum, old age gains a "place," but at the same time symbolically loses its place in life [5].

In the scientific literature on nursing homes there is a tendency to follow mainly the ideas of Goffman (1974) or Townsend (1964). These works inspired a series of investigations in the 1960s and 1970s on inherently depersonalizing institutional care that reduced the identity of residents to mere passive care recipientes.

However, a number of papers have challenged Goffman and Townsend's perspective on the influence of residents on the day-to-day practice of institutions by opposing the idea that life within the nursing home is a uniform process that limits the way in which residents can establish themselves as people.

In the present study, the attempt of the residents to maintain or restore normality prior to admission to the home is well known. When this new normality is accepted, this new place of residence can then be seen as a home.

It is noticed that the residents establish a relation of use with the time and the space, being in this relation that emerge the appropriation of the social experiences and where they construct the daily lifes. Pais [6] defined quotidian as a linear, progressive, repetitive and routine time, which is simultaneously a time of unforeseen senses, breaks, and new discoveries.

What is of social importance is not space, which is "[...] a form which in itself produces no effect" but the "social experiences that flow from it and transform it from an emptiness into something with a sociological meaning" [7, p. 21].

Certeau [8] mentions that "a place is the order" (whatever it is) according to which elements are distributed in the relations of coexistence. In addition to a place, the asylum acquires a space as well. The space is produced by the practices of the place, and is constituted of a system of signs, presents itself as a symbol of shelter of the elderly, and is where the actions occur.

The asylum space gains an identity, because the elderly relate to each other and at the same time identify with space, getting used to, and creating affinities with it.

2 Methods

Within the interpretative paradigm, Grounded Theory was adopted as methodology. Data were collected through participant observation and interviews in a nursing home with approximately 350 residents distributed in three residential structures in the county of Castelo Branco, Portugal, for 21 months (2013/2015). Through theoretical sampling, elderly residents, nurses and nursing aids participated. The constant comparative analysis of the data occurred simultaneously with data collection supported by NVivo 10® and NVivo 11® software.

The results will be presented and discussed simultaneously, in a theoretical way, illustrated with quotations from participants that will appear in italics highlighted in the text.

3 The Space

In the Nursing Home the resident is not in his house, but also is not in the house of others and thus finds himself on land that is no one's. According to Augé [9] we are facing "non-places" that are configured as no-man's land. According to Simmel [7] when we speak of non-places we speak of "constructed spaces" as opposed to places that correspond to "lived spaces". The "lived spaces" correspond to the "anthropological place" defined by Augé [9], an identity, relational and historical place. To the anthropological places of Augé [9] correspond the "space of the places" referred by Castells [10], spaces to which individuals inhabit and link their history.

A true place is a particular space that is clothed with meaning by individuals or a group. Therefore, the basic meaning of a place does not come from its location, but rather from the experiential relationship that is established between individuals and space, thus forming itself as a building center of human existence.

According to Relph [11], the place must be regarded, above all, as a center of meanings, appearing as an inseparable part of human existence and argues that "being human is living in a world surrounded by significant places: being human is having and knowing his place" (p. 1). The place, in this perspective, is seen as a product of the intersubjective experience between the individual and the world, endowed with symbolic and affective value by those who belong to it and feel they belong.

Relph [12] points out that at a more complex level, places are centres of attention that bring together objects, activities and meanings and bring together elements that give it a particular quality, which is distinct from other places, and it is this very capacity for meeting, effected through of authentic attitudes, which confer to an indeterminate space a certain degree of "place".

The meanings of places are not static, they are built up from a dynamic process in which they are continually constructed, deconstructed and endowed with new meanings. Finally, places do not necessarily have the same meaning for all people [13, 14], acting differently in thoughts, feelings, mood, social interactions and physic well-being.

Macedo et al. [15] reported that associated with the studies on the place, concepts such as identity and attachment arise. From the conceptual point of view, attachment to the place emerges as an important component in the constitution of the Self, contributes to its development and maintenance, being useful in understanding the emotional relationships that establish between the person and the environment [16].

When an person comes to an institution, he may undergo a process of "mortification of the self," a concept introduced by Goffman [17], which refers to a suppression of the "self-conception" and the "apparent culture" that are formed in family and civil life. These "attacks on the self" are more felt as greater the "stripping away" of their role by imposing barriers in contact with the external world are, the "framing" by the imposition of rules of conduct, the "dispossession of goods" that makes lose their set of identity and personal safety, and "contaminating exposure." The observation of daily life made it possible to highlight the possible resistance of the elderly to the rigid disciplines and mortifications of the Self as well as the micro-negotiations of meanings that materialize in space, most of the time invisible from the point of view of macro-institutional analysis. Through the visibility of small changes, the power for the constitution of individualizing places is evident, but also collective and generating new sociabilities.

It was noticed in the interviews that despite the valuation of cleaning, ambient temperature, odors and noise, personal dignity goes beyond the available amenities and certain characteristics such as space, modern devices, among others. For example, one of the participants shared the room with another resident and was later transferred to a new, private and very spacious room. He said that having her own room was pleasant, but it did not reinforce her personal dignity. Another resident said that she thought that having her own toilet would be crucial until the day she stopped being able to move alone. They point out that other aspects, like the details in space that reflect their own identity, are much more relevant, as expressed in this interview excerpt:

"… my room is smaller and there are bigger ones, and at the time [admission] I was told that when there was a bigger one to change there, but I do not want to change because mine has a window on the street and the others in general they have a balcony … and I want my little one with the window to the street, so I see the catedral, I see the castle, I see all this […] and now it does not make a big difference, because I'm going to the street and I walk in the street, or in my car, or on foot, as I fancy … but in a while I do not know if I can go to the street […] and if I can not walk and go to the street and all this […] I go to the window and see the cars passing and things in the street […] if i move to another I just see the balcony and nothing else. So the window to the street is so important." E3

Residents are allowed to furnish and decorate their room with photographs, furniture and personal objects they were familiar with and which represent their unique universe. The rooms are filled with frames with family photographs, sacred images and objects with important significance. "These objects establish the bridge with pieces of life left behind and, for this reason, they are of great importance and symbolism for the elderly" [18, p. 130]. In creating territory, the elderly want to create and enhance the environment.

The care team described how these personal objects can contribute to support the identity, continuation of the Self of the elderly and increase the feeling of being at home and how their absence are an indication of the difficulties in the trajectory, as expressed in field diary:

> As we walk the corridors, I and the nurse on duty, we are called by a resident and we enter into her room [...] when we go out she comments with me: "I do not know if you noticed the room of this gentleman, it is empty. There are no photographs, no personal objects, nothing, even the clothes are still in the suitcase next to the bed. This means that for him the nursing home is not yet definitive. He have not yet become fully aware of being here, of starting to make her life here ... it happens sometimes". I wonder if he will do it. He shrugs and replies "Eventually ... but we have to help (smiles)". (Field diary 5).

4   Building Territories

Residents quickly perceive the existence of territories in a space-time structure. Existing territories to be shaped and territories available to be appropriate. Altman [19] states that primary, secondary and public territories differ in two dimensions. The first refers to the length of time spent on the permanence of ownership of a territory. The second is the centrality of a territory, referring to its psychological importance, incorporating the level of control that individuals have over access to territory and the behaviors that occur.

Cefeteria and common rooms are considered as secondary territory. Semipublic or semiprivate spaces are governed by more or less formally defined rules on the right of access and use. In the cafeteria the seats are marked. In the common room occupants exercise authority over places, but they are not always the same people occupying them at the same time.

Corridors and balconies are public territory. Accessible to all residents.

In addition to the places whose access ends up being reserved for specific groups, Goffman also gives attention to those that each individual tries to claim for himself, where he seeks to expand his facilities a little, rediscover some independence and affirm tacitly recognized rights that he does not have to share with any other individual, unless he want and express it explicitly. They are the "personal territories" or refuges, where the individual feels more protected and can elevate his level of satisfaction, to escape to the subjection to rules on which he exerts no influence.

The bedroom is considered primary territory. It is a geographic space regularly occupied by the resident and usually controlled by the occupant. This type of territory ensures the privacy function and can be customized. The identity of the owner is so strongly evident that the intrusion or intrusion can be felt as an aggression. Primary territories are, therefore, interpersonal supports essential to the processes of border control and personal identity.

In this study it was evident the reference to the bedroom as a primary or primary territory, especially in cases where there is a single room. The room was also considered a "safe haven" and seen as a place where participants can find "solitude," "peace," "a sanctuary," a place of shelter and recovery "where memories are kept."

"Sometimes I spend the whole afternoon here watching the photos ... remembering ... you know, from different times that no longer exist." E1

Cohen-Mansfield et al. [20] also found varying views on single and shared rooms. One patient in a three bedroom stated that he felt safe because he was never alone. Others did not like sharing rooms, because they were upset by seeing the suffering of others, or wanted greater privacy. There were also varying views on levels of noise. One patient disliked the noise from other peoples' radios, and from staff talking loudly. However, several others liked the fact that the unit was lively and not too quiet.

It has been realized that the qualities of a territory are not inherent to the place or object, but result from the interactions between the person and the place or object. For those who do not have the privilege of accessing a single room, other objects can be a refuge, such as a bedside table or cabinet, where photographs, sacred images, or small props are available. The bedside tables do not correspond to a mere piece of furniture with drawers and doors. They act as places to live, where objects, images and pieces of other spaces are stored. Thus, the bedside tables are "corners" of the world that shelter memories and past experiences.

Residents who share a room, personal territory can be reduced to the point of being no more than a bag, from which the resident never separates. Another example of personal territory, in the sense given by Goffman [17], that is, of space, however small, on which residents seek to exercise their control, is evident in the fact that practically all the elderly women in the nursing home take a certain chair or highchair in the living room. Some of them even demarcate their seats, put some personal object on it so that no one dares sit there and if, by chance, such a situation occurs, the intruder is immediately warned and constrained to return the place to its "owner".

This appropriation of space in secondary territories is expressed in this annotated dialogue in the field diary:

Investigator (I): "Why do you sit there?"
Resident (R): "Because this is my place."
I: "But you could sit there (pointing to an empty armchair)"
A: "Well, I could, nobody forbade me, but this is my place, I have my things here (points to the blanket and cushion)"
I: "What if one day you come and someone is sitting there?"
He looks at me in silence and replies, "They will not sit down, I know that [...] yesterday the son of that lady came to visit and sat down. When I arrived she immediately told him to get up. You know, there are things that are like that [...] but I do not get upset [...] if someone is here, I'll go for a walk and come later. I do not si in another chair. This is mine"
I: "But why do you sit there, is it better?"
A: "Look, neither worse, nor better, from that one (points) you see the television better, but when I came they were already occupied ... and look, this is mine and that is hers (points) and that's it."

Fischer [21] points out that in many situations the personal spaces are symbolic extensions of the body itself, as well as the appropriation of the objects in them. In its conception, the more controlled the institutional space is, the more rudimentary the spaces of refuge, and in some cases may be reduced to the place where the individual arranges his personal objects, directly linked to his body space.

The objects that accompany the elderly throughout life serve as an identity bond, and are what Bosi [22] calls biographical objects. Small objects, most of the time, old, but loaded with meanings and affectivities.

Regardless of where the primary or personal territory is constructed, it is necessary to construct what Goffman [17] calls the "nest". In Fischer's interpretation [21, p. 149], in these spaces individuals seek to develop a "psychological niche". Refuges reflect the need to organize "spaces of isolation".

They say that it has been difficult to get used to the space of the home, to the songs and nooks, public and private and to realize the small size of their life.

> "When we enter here it deceives […]. It looks like a mansion, but then we see that the largesse is not so much. I have a room with a roommate and my life fits all here. Everything I have is here." E7

The results of this study are similar to the territoriality descriptions identified by Altman [19]. Territories exist to meet physical and social needs, are temporary or permanent, controlled, marked or personalized, and potentially defended by occupiers or owners. In turn, territoriality comprises a specific set of behavioral, affective, and cognitive tendencies and is formed by ties of affinity with space and/or individuals who appropriate it. Thus, the concept of territoriality is imbued with other aspects such as, for example, the identity and the relational processes between subject-subject, subject-space.

For Sahr [23] territory is not a product, but an "expression", a cultural creation of society and that has a certain form, "face", a certain "physiognomy". The territory is territorialized between the significance of the concept of existence of the same and the subjectivity that each individual makes about it. That is why territory is a concept and also a territory of action, being a partner of the actors that inhabit it [23]. In this sense, the territory would be the part of the space with which a person identifies himself and maintains intimacy, and in which he lives and maintains ties of identity [24].

For Sachs [25] territory is the product of the territorialization of means and rhythms. Territory, therefore, is not just a "thing", it is a set of objects, but above all, action, rhythm and repetitive motion. Territory can not be decoupled: space is wandering, it is living, it is acting, and territory is rooted. Territory is the expression of a lived behavior. Territoriality happens when there is in the nursing home the significance and at the same time the subjectivity of people which interact.

Thus the nursing home as institution is territorialized because it has the concept of existence that was built by society and the subjectivity of the elderly. For some elderly the is a space of refuge, of identification, of pleasure in being there, but for others it is a space of non-identification, refusal, repulsion. In the territory there are the subjectivities, the symbolism, the culture. The territory gains symbolism from its use, is the "territory used" or "territory of daily life."

From no man's land, nursing home moves to places and finally to territories.

5 Social Place

If a resident fells inconvenienced in one of the secondary or public territories, he may not attend it if he is physically independent:

"I'm sorry that the living room on the first floor, which is the largest, is occupied by those people. They are constantly complaining, always speaking bad things about others and I do not go to these places, I do not like them." E2

There was a range of views on the desired level of social interaction. Engle, Fox-Hill and Graney (1998) and Ternestedt and Franklin (2006) also states that some patients wished to remain socially active, continuing to mix with others as long as possible [26, 27]. However, not all patients wanted to mix with others, and some preferred to remain in their own rooms. This idea is also shared by Froggatts [28] and Franklin, Ternestedt and Nordenfelt [29].

The observation and interviews indicate that there are hierarchies among the residents that dictate the occupation of the territories.

"There are little groups in here, I don't know if you noticed? Ah, there is. There are leaders here … I will not individualize, but there are people that when they get up the others get up too, when they argue the others also argue, it turns out to be funny (laughs) they look like school girls (laughs)." E2

This hierarchy influences the flow of conversation in the dinning room tables and in the occupation of territory and sometimes is a source of conflict.

"That little girl thinks she's the greatest because she has a lot of stuff that her daughter brings her, a lot of folk embroidered blouses with shiny things and she does not want any of us to look better than her […] and she's also very authoritarian. One day, by force, she wanted Ms Y to get up from the couch so she could sit on it and I was sitting in my chair and something was inside me, until I got up and went down to her and told her: Now tell me, what have more right to sit in the chair than this lady who is there? Be quiet. Look, she would turn to me and say: look at the doctor, she came two days ago and she wants to boss around, we who have been here for so long and she wants to boss us… You know, they are the ones who have been here for a long time, they think they boss us, but they are very deceived with me … that little one, I don't like …" E5

This claim of space is in agreement with several studies that show that people who share rooms, particularly rooms without a clearly defined territory for each individual, are more territorial in claiming space, be it in a section of the hallway or a chair in the living room. In other words, when people do not have enough privacy and personal territory provided through the physical environment, they create their own social and psychological privacy by limiting their interactions with other people. The boundaries in physical space though symbolic, according to "unwritten rules" should be treated with respect by other people.

The "unwritten rules" refer to culture-specific codes established and known only by the residents. Power seems, first of all, to derive from antiquity in place following the "company" which causes some seniors to prefer a bedroom with tree beds, which they call "dormitory", to a double room, that is, to share the room with another person is what they try to avoid. This aspect had already been approached by Paúl [30] when she said that: "[…] this system of large collective rooms was preferable … the rooms of two persons usually have one that arrives first and one that comes later. The latter will share a private space with another that she does not know and that dominates the territory" (p. 343).

Belonging to a place is part of an imagistic-discursive construction that is carried out, daily, through strategies and symbols that weave the plot of power. On the relation between physical space and social space, Bourdieu [31] tells us that the physical space occupied by a given individual locates it in the social space and places it relationally in a given social position, that is, the physical space structures reproduce the structures of social space.

It should be noted that Goffman's observations regarding the control that is expressed through the use of the spaces coincide with Fischer's reflections on the social psychology of the environment. In fact, this author bases the idea that all institutional space is a space under control, which obeys a set of rules of surveillance and that has to be analyzed as the expression of a power structure, as a space of molding the conduct.

There are elderly people who take advantage of unused spaces in the home and with permission occupy these spaces and decorate them with personal objects. Largely compatible with these data are the spaces that Goffman designates as "spaces free of control" and Fischer as "interstitial" spaces defined as fluid spaces which, due to their poor contours defined, leave to those who occupy them the possibility of defining their use or function, allowing them to be the object of individual investment in order to safeguard a significant life and preserve the integrity and dignity of their "self" unforeseen by the organization.

Of the several interviewees, most stressed the desire to be alone. Through the construction of a refuge, singularization is sought, even if it is accompanied by isolation. The refuge reflects the need to organize "spaces of isolation" or "places of solitude" as referred by Goffman, and this distance is a means to protect against the widespread invasion that the individual feels when residing in a nursing home.

People living in homes are forced to share an enclosed and limited space. Everything is known, either through comments, conversations or chunks of conversation that are heard, or even through the observation of the daily life of the nursing home. They can observe the habits of others, is routines, the way they interact with others including is own family when they visit them.

"I like all the residentes that are here, I give myself to everyone but my dear, I am not a person to walk [...] this stays between us ... talking to that, them talking to the other (lowers her voice) because I know what it costs [...] I know what it is to talk to a, b and c! (speak louder). Because you know very well, people do not know each other, do they? And sometimes they say this and that and that one...There are two, but then one will say to another, and this repeats itself, which I have already seen and I do not like it." E1

It has been observed that mainly the independent elderly tend to isolate themselves and establish superficial relationships within the nursing home, not to engage in interpersonal relationships with other residents.

Living in a nursing home means that all life and intimacy are exposed to the looks and comments of others. This relation of neighborhood, of promiscuity, as Goffman would imply, reinforces the protection of oneself, a determination of the distance between the elderly, avoiding to share with others what one feels and what one lives, in an effort of protection of self, for fear that everything may be the object of gossip. This exacerbates the isolation of the elderly and the superficiality of relationships.

Graeff [32] called this conduct of isolation as "spaces of intimacy": "[...] the intimate forum, guided by silence and solitude, ends up being a privileged moment of tranquility. To guard against situations of sociability and playful moments creates a time of suspension, of prudence in the application of the models of self-control. Instead of being systematically placed in the flow of exchanges and sociability, seclusion and silence become ... a moment of affirmation of intimacy" (p. 13)

During this study, the notion of surveillance and security was encapsulated by the term "Watched freedom". For most of the elderly, these "boundaries" of the territory are quite flexible, but not fully permeable. For professionals, recognizing vulnerability (or potential vulnerability) while promoting trust and freedom is an important and complex balancing act.

The elderly state that the "boundaries" and "borders" of the home provide a protected environment and help isolate them from possible abuse.

"... and I tell you without problems, I'm afraid to be alone. We live in a very bad world, I do not know where we're going to end, every day we hear about assaults, deaths, and I feel safe here, seriously, I'm not afraid that something bad happens to me." E2

"There is the closed door ... yes, yes ... but I, as a user, like to get there and be closed, looks great, because security starts at the door ... and today more than ever, (hits on the table) ... there at that corner is a individual who hit yoy and takes something that we have ... and if it's just hit we're lucky (laughs). Today as you know it is sadness ... the world is like this ..." E4

6   Conclusion

Most residents began to formally connect with home life at their own pace by creating territory and devoting time to meaningful activities. They gradually begin to accept this new daily life and no longer focus their attention exclusively on the nursing home as an institution and the losses associated with admission are no longer the main concern. This is the result of the passage of time and normality that has been reestablished and begin to glimpse and appreciate the gains of living in a nursing home. The feeling of belonging to the space in which one lives, of conceiving space as the locus of practices, where the complex web of sociability is rooted, is that it grants this space the character of territory. The appropriation of a certain space is constituted from the moment in which the individual or group represents it for himself and for the others.

Space can be conceptualized as the "product of interrelations" and as a "sphere of the possibility of the existence of multiplicity", which can always be under construction and therefore unfinished [33]. For the nursing home space, each old person brings their Person, their own history, their trajectory, and these trajectories intersect, connect and disconnect themselves. Space becomes a social dimension in the sense of involvement within multiplicity. It is a sphere of continuous production and a reconfiguration of heterogeneity in which the home space finally makes sense. It is in this interaction between physical space, human space and subjectivity that spaces are perceived and understood [33].

The nursing home functions as a space that includes the old individual rejected, forgotten, abandoned, but on the other hand, this same place is seen by society as the place of the excluded. In this contradiction between the space of inclusion and exclusion, we were to find in the space inside the Home, men and women, in their private or collective world, united with the "his" in the attribution of meanings to the territories they inhabit, in the permanent construction of places.

The results of this study once again reinforce the need for institutions and professionals to be aware of the existence of "built spaces" and "living spaces", spaces within the home space, considered refuges, sanctuaries, shelters … Only by allowing the freedom necessary to "create" places can the nursing home be considered a home.

References

1. Lenoir, R.: L'invention du troisième âge. Constitution du champ des agents de gestion de la vieillesse. Actes Rech. Sci. Soc. **26**(27), 57–82 (1979)
2. Pimentel, L.: O Lugar Do Idoso Na Família: Contextos e Trajectórias, 2nd edn. Quarteto, Coimbra (2005)
3. Costa, G.: Tríplice visão do envelhecimento: longevidade, qualidade de vida e aspectos biopsicossociais da velhice. Rev. Soc. Bras. Atividade Motora Adaptada **8**(1), 27–39 (2003). SOBAMA
4. Davim, R., Torres, G., Dantas, S., Lima, V.: Estudo com idosos de instituições asilares no município de Natal/RN: características socioeconômicas e de saúde. Rev. Lat. Am. Enferm. **12**(3), 518–524 (2004)
5. Groisman, D.: Asilos de velhos: passado e presente. Estudos interdisciplinares sobre o envelhecimento. Porto Alegre **2**, 67–87 (1999)
6. Pais, J.: Paradigmas sociológicos na análise da vida quotidiana. Anál. Soc. **XXII**(90), 7–57 (1986)
7. Simmel, G.: Fidelidade e gratidão e outros textos. Relógio d'Água, Lisboa (2004). (1908)
8. Certeau, M.: A Invenção do Cotidiano: Artes de Fazer. Vozes, Petrópolis (2002)
9. Augé, M.: Não lugares: introdução a uma antropologia da sobremodernidade, 1ª edição francesa (1992). 90 Graus, Lisboa (2005)
10. Castells, M.: A sociedade em rede, vol. 1. Fundação Calouste Gulbenkian, Lisboa (2002)
11. Relph, E.: Place and Placelessness. Pion Books, London (1976). https://openlibrary.org/books/OL4954978M/Place_and_placelessness. Accessed 24 Aug 2015
12. Relph, E.: Reflexões Sobre a Emergência, Aspectos e Essência de Lugar. In: Marandola Jr., E., Holzer, W., Oliveira, L. (Orgs.) Qual o espaço do lugar? Geografia, epistemologia, fenomenologia, pp. 17–32. Perspectiva, São Paulo (2012)
13. Gustafson, P.: Meanings of place: everyday experience and theoretical conceptualzations. J. Environ. Psychol. **21**, 5–16 (2001)
14. Purcell, A., Peron, E., Berto, R.: Why do preferences differ between scene types? Environ. Behav. **33**, 93–106 (2001)
15. Macedo, D., Oliveira, C., Günther, I., Alves, S., Nóbrega, T.: O lugar do afeto, o afeto pelo lugar: o que dizem os idosos? Psicol. Teor. Pesq. **24**(4), 441–449 (2008)
16. Speller, G.: A importância da vinculação aos lugares. In: Soczka, L. (Org.) Contextos humanos e Psicologia Ambiental, pp. 133–167. Fundação Calouste Gulbenkian, Lisboa (2005)
17. Goffman, E.: Manicômios, Prisões e Conventos. Editora Perspectiva, São Paulo (1974)

18. Guedes, J.: Viver num Lar de Idosos. Identidade em risco ou Identidade riscada. Editora Coisas de Ler, Lisboa (2012)
19. Altman, I.: The Environment and Social Behavior. Brooks/Cole, Monterey (1975)
20. Cohen-Mansfield, J., Thein, K., Dakheel-Ali, M., Marx, M.: Engaging nursing home residents with dementia in activities: the effects of modeling, presentation order, time of day, and setting characteristics. Aging Mental Health **14**, 471–480 (2010)
21. Fischer, G.: Psicologia Social do Ambiente. Instituto Piaget, Lisboa (1994)
22. Bosi, E.: O Tempo Vivo da Memória: Ensaios de Psicologia Social. Ateliê Editorial, São Paulo (2003)
23. Sahr, C.: A problemática "espaço/território" a partir de geograficidades existenciais (2008). http://www.observatoriogeograficoamericalatina.org.mx/egal12/Geografiasocioeconomica/Geopolitica/24.pdf. Accessed 4 Dec 2015
24. Costa, R.: O mito da desterritorialização: do "fim dos territórios" à multiterritorialidade, 3rd edn. Bertrand Brasil, Rio de Janeiro (2007)
25. Sachs, I.: Espaços, Tempos e Estratégias de Desenvolvimento. Edições Vértice, São Paulo (1986)
26. Ternestedt, B., Franklin, L.: Ways of relating to death: views of older people resident in nursing homes. Int. J. Palliat. Nurs. **12**, 334–340 (2006)
27. Engle, V., Fox-hill, E., Graney, M.: The experience of living-dying in a nursing home: self-reports of black and white older adults. J. Am. Geriatr. Soc. **46**, 1091–1096 (1998)
28. Hall, S., Kolliakou, A., Petkova, H., Froggatt, K., Higginson, I.: Interventions for improving palliative care for older people living in nursing care homes (review). Cochrane Collab. **16** (3), 1–31 (2011)
29. Franklin, L., Ternestedt, B., Nordenfelt, L.: Views on dignity of elderly nursing home residents. Nurs. Ethics **13**(2), 130–146 (2006)
30. Paúl, M.C.: Percursos pela velhice: Uma perspectiva ecológica em psicogerontologia. Tese de Doutoramento. Universidade do Porto. Instituto de Ciências Biomédicas de Abel Salazar (1991). http://repositorio.ispa.pt/handle/10400.12/1668. Accessed 24 Nov 2014
31. Bourdieu, P.: A Miséria Do Mundo. Vozes, Petrópolis (1997)
32. Graeff, L.: Instituições totais e a questão asilar: uma abordagem compreensiva. Estud. Interdiscip. Sobre Envelhec. **11**, 9–27 (2007)
33. Massey, D.: Um sentido global do lugar. In: Arantes, A.A. (org.) O espaço da diferença, pp. 176–185. Papirus, Campinas (2000)

Biological and Socio-Demographic Predictors of Elderly Quality of Life Living in the Community in Baixo-Alentejo, Portugal

Margarida Goes[1] , Manuel José Lopes[2] ,
Henrique Oliveira[3(✉)] , César Fonseca[2] , and David Mendes[2]

[1] Escola Superior de Saúde, Instituto Politécnico de Beja, Beja, Portugal
[2] Escola Superior de Enfermagem de São João de Deus,
Universidade de Évora, Évora, Portugal
[3] Instituto de Telecomunicações, IST Torre Norte - Piso 10,
Av. Rovisco Pais, Lisbon, Portugal
hjmo@lx.it.pt

Abstract. Objectives: To identify the biological and socio-demographic factors considered as predictors of the Quality of Life of elderly people residing in an aged and predominantly rural community in Portugal, namely the Baixo-Alentejo.

Methods: Cross-sectional and descriptive study, with a random sample of 351 elderly residing in the community, stratified by gender and age group, with data collection performed by health professionals in people's homes, using the WHOQOL-BREF instrument. In addition to a brief description of the general characteristics of the sample, a linear regression model by blocks was performed, in order to investigate about the biological and sociodemographic factors considered as predictors of Quality of life.

Results: Highest percentage of women in the sample. Decreased Quality of Life in all domains as well as in the General Health Facet as age progresses. Higher average Quality of Life score obtained for the Social Relationships domain and smaller to the Physical Health one. Higher Quality of Life scores obtained for males compared to females. Education considered as one of the most significant predictors of Quality of Life, whose score increases with higher education levels.

Discussion: Regarding the biological factors, age appears to be a significant predictor in the Physical Health and Environment domains, while the gender seems to be a significant predictor in the Physical Health and Psychological ones. In respect to the sociodemographic factors, the marital status appeared to be a significant predictor in Psychological and Social Relationships domains, but education was the only factor identified as a statistically significant predictor in all domains of Quality of Life.

Keywords: Aging · Nursing · Quality of Life

© Springer Nature Switzerland AG 2019
J. García-Alonso and C. Fonseca (Eds.): IWoG 2018, CCIS 1016, pp. 319–326, 2019.
https://doi.org/10.1007/978-3-030-16028-9_28

1 Introduction

The population aging is usually characterized by some indicators, notably by the aging index, defined by the relationship between the elderly population (persons with 65 years of age or older) and the young population (persons younger than 15 years old). Portugal is the European Union country that features one of the highest rates of population aging (153.2 elderly per 100 young) [1], and the national estimates indicate that the value of this index will more than double until 2080 (317 elderly for every 100 young) [2].

The region of Baixo Alentejo (RBA), the geographic area within the scope of this paper, chosen as it shows predominantly rural areas and it is also identified as one of the most aged in the country, presents considerable aging indexes of 144.1, 183.9 and 285.5 elderly per 100 young, respectively to the following types of areas: predominantly urban area; medium-sized urban area; predominantly rural area [3].

The human aging is characterized by being a complex phenomenon, due to the various physical health, psychological, social and environmental changes that affects directly people's Quality of Life (QoL) as they age. On the other hand, aging is also characterized as heterogeneous, since it is experienced differently from person to person. Therefore, taking into account that there is a lack of studies on the subject in Portugal, it stands out as extremely relevant to investigate the biological and sociodemographic factors that interfere in the QoL of persons with 65 years or older residing in RBA, since the results will led to the development of an important empirical basis to help the identification, planning and monitoring of interventions, especially in the field of health services.

The World Health Organization Quality of Life group (WHOQOL), formally created by the World Health Organization (WHO), led to development of a WHOQOL-100 instrument used for QoL assessment, aiming to *"sensitize health care professionals to look beyond diseases, disabilities and symptoms"* [4]. However, to minimize the time spend to apply it, a shortened version of it was also developed, namely the WHOQOL-BREF. This short version is composed of 26 questions and covers four domains: Physical Health; Psychological; Social Relationships; and Environment, as well as a General Health Facet (GHF) that includes: (i) how a person himself assesses its QoL; (ii) and to what extent a person himself is satisfied with is health. The WHOQOL-BREF stands out for being a self-administered questionnaire, adapted to the Portuguese population [5], which preserves the 24 facets of WHOQOL-100, and since it is transcultural it can be applied to persons in different contexts. Additionally, the WHOQOL-BREF stands out for being generic, thus allowing the evaluation of a range of aspects of people's lives (including those whose age is greater than or equal to 65 years old), even when they present different health conditions [5]. On the other hand, it was also the most widely instrument used that revealed better applicability in 91.7% of 48 scientific studies included in a bibliometric research on the assessment of QoL [6].

Therefore, the main objective of this study is to investigate the relationship between biological (age and gender) and sociodemographic (marital status, and education) factors with the QoL, taking into account the concept developed by the WHO and covering the four domains encompassed by the WHOQOL-BREF, in order to identify the factors that are the best predictors of QoL of the elderly living in RBA.

2   Methods

The present research, approved by the Ethics Committee of the Local Health Unit of Baixo Alentejo (Unidade Local de Saúde do Baixo Alentejo - ULSBA) was classified as: observational, as the researcher measured the QoL but did not intervene; descriptive, as it aimed to describe the QoL of a community; and cross-sectional, as QoL data were obtained through a questionnaire (instrument) at a certain point in time [7].

This study involved the population with 65 years old or more residing in the RBA (a region comprising thirteen municipalities). The sample size was calculated in accordance with the formulation as advocated by the WHO [8]. The following inclusion criteria were adopted, cumulatively: (i) be 65 years old or older; (ii) be interested in participating in the study; (iii) residing in the RBA in their own home or at the home of a family or friends; (iv) be able to make its own decisions, even if the person is sick or hospitalized. The final sample (randomly chosen), stratified by gender (male and female) and age group (65 to 74 years, 75 to 84 years, 85 or more years) totaled 351 persons, those who signed the informed consent form and answered correctly to the questionnaire. A confidence level of 95% and a margin of error of 5% were considered during the statistical calculations.

The questionnaire applied was the WHOQOL-BREF, after requesting for the necessary authorization for its use to the authors of the Portuguese version [9]. Data were collected between February 2016 and May 2017 at the individuals' homes by teams of health professionals from ULSBA. The scores in the four domains and in the GHF were calculated on a scale from 0 to 100. IBM SPSS Statistics version 23 Armonk, NY, was the software used to perform all the statistical procedures.

The initial stage of the statistical analysis (descriptive statistics) consisted on the description of the biological and sociodemographic variables included in the study, using relative frequencies (gender, age group, marital status and education level), along with measures of central tendency and dispersion (age, the scores of four QoL domains and GHF). The reliability of the construct (questionnaire) was evaluated using the *Cronbach's alpha* (α). The *Student's t-test* was used to test for differences in the mean QoL domain scores and in the GHF regarding gender, after invoking the central limit theorem (CLT) and verified that the distributions are not strongly asymmetric [10]. Finally, a linear regression model using blocks was calculated for each QoL domain (first block including the biological variables - gender and age, and a second block comprising the sociodemographic ones - education and marital status) to identify the biological and the sociodemographic variables predictive of elderly's QoL [10].

3   Results

The study sample showed a higher proportion of females (53.6%) than males (46.4%), as can be seen by the analysis of the values listed in Table 1. The age group of older persons (85 years old and over) is the one that presented the lowest proportion (23.9%), when compared to the two remaining age groups, both very identical in proportion.

Table 1. Biological and socio-demographics characteristics of the 351 respondents residing in the RBA.

Biological and socio-demographics factors	Number of samples (n)	Percent (%)
Gender		
Male	163	46.4
Female	188	53.6
Age group		
65–74	132	37.6
75–84	135	38.5
85 and higher	84	23.9
Marital status		
Single/Divorced/Separated	31	8.8
Married/Living as Married	206	58.7
Widowed	114	32.5
Educational level		
Does not know how to read or write	104	29.6
Knows how to read and/or write	59	16.8
1st–4th grade	165	47.0
More education	23	6.6

Concerning the marital status, the six categories presented in WHOQOL-BREF have been reduced to three, due to the very lower absolute frequencies observed in some categories (less than or equal to 5 in the categories "Living as Married", "Divorced" and "Separated"), with the majority of the respondents being married (58.7%). A considerable proportion of the sample is composed of widowers (32.5%, where the proportion of females in this category is 76.3%, while for males is 23.7%).

Regarding education, the eight categories listed in the WHOQOL-BREF were reduced to only four, due to the very lower absolute frequency observed in the categories related to an higher level of education, with almost half of the respondents (46.4% = 29.6% + 16.8%) mentioning that never went to school and 29.6% of the study sample (57.8% female and 42.2% male) were considered as illiterate.

The reliability of the construct was measured by the *Cronbach's alpha* (α - *coefficient of reliability*) which was classified as "Good" for the Physical Health ($\alpha = 0.871$) and Psychological ($\alpha = 0.852$) domains, "Reasonable" for the Environment domain ($\alpha = 0.770$) and General Facet ($\alpha = 0.762$), "Weak" for the Social Relations domain ($\alpha = 0.604$), but "Very good" ($\alpha = 0.934$) when analyzing all 26 items (questions) of the questionnaire [11].

The significance of mean score variation in the four QoL domains as well as in the GHF, as a function of gender, was assessed using the *Student's t-test* for two independent samples. The results listed in Table 2 suggest that there is statistical evidence to state that mean scores of QoL are significantly different between males and females, but only for the Physical Health and Psychological domains (considering $p < 0.05$) and for the General Facet (considering $p < 0.10$), tending to be higher for males when compared to females.

Table 2. Results of *Student's t-test* to determine if the QoL mean scores between males and females are significantly different from each other.

Variables and statistical tests	QoL domains				GHF
	Physical health	Psychological	Social relationships	Environment	
M	56.3	59.8	61.0	59.1	51.4
SD	19.54	16.95	13.92	13.16	20.84
Gender:					
Male	*M* = 60.7 *SD* = 19.89	*M* = 62.7 *SD* = 17.11	*M* = 61.8 *SD* = 19.89	*M* = 60.1 *SD* = 13.62	*M* = 53.5 *SD* = 21.26
Female	*M* = 52.6 *SD* = 18.48	*M* = 57.3 *SD* = 16.47	*M* = 60.2 *SD* = 14.05	*M* = 58.3 *SD* = 12.72	*M* = 49.6 *SD* = 20.35
Student's t-test	*t* = 3.937 (*p* < 0.001)	*t* = 2.976 (*p* = 0.003)	*t* = 1.056 (*p* = 0.291)	*t* = 1.232 (*p* = 0.219)	*t* = 1.731 (*p* = 0.084)

The predictive biological and sociodemographic factors in the various domains of the WHOQOL-BREF were identified through multiple block linear regression models [10] whose results are listed in Table 3, with Block 1 representing the biological variables (age and gender) and Block 2 the sociodemographic ones (marital status and education level). Regarding the Physical Health, age, gender and education were statistically significant predictors in this domain. In the Psychological domain, gender, education level and marital status were also identified as significant predictors. In the case of the Social Relations domain, age and gender were not statistically significant predictors of QoL, which is why the respective linear regression model only comprises only one block although both marital status and education level variables are significant predictors. Finally, age and education level were significant predictors in the Environment domain. The variances explained by the four models ranged from 17.1% (which was case of the Psychological domain) to 10.4% (which was case of the Social Relations domain).

Table 3. Parameters of the linear regression models using blocks of variables, showing only those considered as statistical significant.

QoL domains			Standardized coefficients (β)	BLRM - R^2 (*p*)
Physical health	Block 1	Age	−0.156*	0.157 (*p* < 0.001)
		Gender	0.197*	
	Block 2	Knows how to read and/or write	0.133**	
		1st–4th grade	0.219*	
		More education	0.229*	
Psychological	Block 1	Gender	0.112**	0.171 (*p* < 0.001)
	Block 2	1st–4th grade	0.265*	
		More education	0.278*	
		Married/Living as Married	0.153*	

(*continued*)

Table 3. (continued)

QoL domains			Standardized coefficients (β)	BLRM - R^2 (p)
Social relationships	Block 1	–	–	0.104 (p < 0.001)
	Block 2	1st–4th grade	0.214*	
		More education	0.250*	
		Married/Living as Married	0.114**	
Environment	Block 1	Age	−0.161*	0.129 (p < 0.001)
	Block 2	Knows how to read and/or write	0.127**	
		1st–4th grade	0.256*	
		More education	0.229*	

* p < 0.01
** p < 0.05

4 Discussion

The QoL of each person is related to the sociodemographic context and the biological, cultural and environmental characteristics of the setting in which they live, which was observed in the present study. For instance the sample revealed that almost half of the respondents (46.4%) never went into a school and almost one third (29.6%) were considered as illiterate, a characteristics that is commonly found in some rural areas of the World [12], as in the case of RBA, notably a predominant rural area in the middle South of Portugal. On the other hand, the sample considered followed the trend portrayed in the scientific literature considered within the scope of this paper, with a predominance of females [13–15], particularly in the of oldest age group, a phenomenon known as the "feminization of the aging" [16].

Regarding gender, the results seem to suggest that men showed better QoL in all domains compared to women, whose difference is considered statistically significant only for the Physical Health and Psychological domains. This difference may probably be related to a greater tendency of women for physical and mental problems, as compared to men, showing a greater difficulty in accepting their aging and thus probably resulting in a more negative evaluation of QoL, as observed in some research works [5, 13, 16]. Other studies reported that long-lived women present greater limitations and greater loss of functional capacity, due to higher prevalence of some illnesses, such as chronic pain, rheumatic disease, osteoporosis, osteoarthritis, depression, among others, with impairment in QoL in the two domains mentioned [17].

In relation to the four domains covered by the WHOQOL-BREF, the highest average of QoL score was obtained for the Social Relationships domain, whose result may be related to the fact that in rural areas (like the RBA, notably predominantly rural) the visiting or neighbors, or the presence or relatives that live nearby, may have a stronger positive effect on subjective well-being of the elderly residing in those types of areas [18]. The lowest QoL was reached for the Physical Health domain, which may be related to the increasing overall burden of diseases as the person ages, thus resulting in a decline in health [19]. Regarding the respective standard deviation of the answers, the highest value was obtained for the Physical Health domain (a greater dispersion in the answers obtained for this domain), with the lowest been observed for the Environment domain (revealing a less dispersion of the observed answers).

Regarding the biological and sociodemographic factors predictors of QoL, the results obtained by the linear regression models using blocks, results seem to suggest that QoL increases significantly with education in all domains, with gender in Physical Health and Psychological, and marital status in Psychological and Social Relationships domains. Regarding the age, QoL seems to decrease significantly in the Physical and Environmental domains as people grow older. The results obtained here are somewhat in harmony with those obtained by other authors [20].

5 Conclusions

Regarding the biological factors, age appears to be a significant predictor in the Physical Health and Environment domains, while the gender seems to be a significant predictor in the Physical Health and Psychological ones. In respect to the sociode-mographic factors, the marital status appeared to be a significant predictor in Psychological and Social Relationships domains, but education was the only factor identified as a statistically significant predictor in all domains of Quality of Life. The authors suggest that the findings of this may help the identification, planning and monitoring of interventions, especially in the field of health services focusing elderly persons living in rural areas like the RBA.

Acknowledgements. This work was supported by 4 IE project (0045-4 IE-4-P) funded by the Interreg V-A España-Portugal (POCTEP) 2014-2020 program.

Compliance with Ethical Standards

Conflict of Interest: The authors declare that they have no conflict of interest.

Ethical Approval: The research ethics committee of the Unidade Local de Saúde of Baixo Alentejo (ULSBA) approved the study protocol including study design, interview questionnaires, and informed consent.

Informed Consent: Informed consent was obtained from all the 351 participants.

References

1. PORDATA Homepage. https://www.pordata.pt/en/Europe/Ageing+index-1609. Accessed 12 Apr 2018
2. INE Homepage "Projections of resident population in Portugal". https://www.ine.pt/xportal/xmain?xpid=INE&xpgid=ine_destaques&DESTAQUESdest_boui=277695619&DESTAQUESmodo=2&xlang=en. Accessed 12 Apr 2018

3. INE Homepage. https://www.ine.pt/clientFiles/WkZJKJAmW3dyY43UAN6B7-aY_57871. xls. Accessed 12 Apr 2018
4. WHO Quality of Life Assessment Group.: What quality of life?/The WHOQOL Group. World Health Forum 17(4), 354–356 (1996)
5. Canavarro, M., et al: WHOQOL disponível para Portugal: Desenvolvimento dos instrumentos de Avaliação da Qualidade de Vida da Organização Mundial de Saúde (WHOQOL-100 e WHOQOL-BREF). In: Canavarro, M.C., Serra, A.V. (eds.) Qualidade de vida e saúde: Uma abordagem na perspectiva da Organização Mundial de Saúde, pp. 171–190. Fundação Calouste Gulbenkian, Lisboa (2010)
6. Angelim, R., et al.: Análise da Qualidade de Vida por meio do WHOQOL: Análise bibliométrica da produção de Enfermagem. Revista Baiana de Enfermagem 29(4), 400–410 (2015)
7. Bonita, R., Beaglehole, R., Kjellström, T.: Epidemiologia básica, 2nd edn. Livraria Santos Editora Comércio e Importação, São Paulo (2010)
8. Lemeshow, S., et al.: Adequacy of Sample Size in Health Studies. http://apps.who.int/iris/ bitstream/10665/41607/1/0471925179_eng.pdf. Accessed 12 Apr 2018
9. Canavarro, M., et al.: WHOQOL-BREF (Versão em Português de Portugal do Instrumento Abreviado de Avaliação da Qualidade de Vida da Organização Mundial de Saúde). http:// www.fpce.uc.pt/saude/WHOQOL_Bref.html. Accessed 10 Mar 2016
10. Marôco, J.: Análise Estatística com o SPSS Statistics, 7th edn. Report Number, Lisbon (2018)
11. Pestana, M., Gageiro, J.: Análise de Dados para Ciências Sociais, 6th edn. Edições SÍLABO, Lisboa (2014)
12. Ferrell, S., Howley, A.: Adult literacy in rural areas. J. Read. 34(5), 368–372 (1991). http:// www.jstor.org/stable/40032077. Accessed 2018/04/12
13. Rodrigues, L., et al.: Quality of life of elderly people of the community and associated factors. J. Nurs. UFPE 11(3), 1430–1483 (2017). https://periodicos.ufpe.br/revistas/ revistaenfermagem/article/view/13985. Accessed 12 Apr 2018
14. Paiva, M., Pegorari, M., Nascimento, J., Santos, A.: Fatores associados à qualidade de vida de idosos comunitários. Ciência & Saúde Coletiva 21(11), 3347–3356 (2016)
15. Nicodemo, D., Godoi, M.: Juventude dos anos 60–70 e envelhecimento: estudo de casos sobre. Revista Ciência em Extensão 6(1), 40–53 (2010)
16. Pereira, R., et al.: Contribuição dos domínios físico, social, psicológico e ambiental para a qualidade de vida global de idosos. Revista de Psiquiatria do Rio Grande do Sul 28(1), 27–38 (2006)
17. Lopes, M., et al.: Evaluation of elderly persons' functionality and care needs. Revista Latino-Americana de Enfermagem 21(Spec.), 52–60 (2013)
18. Carta, M., et al.: Quality of life and urban/rural living: preliminary results of a community survey in Italy. Clin. Pract. Epidemiol. Mental Health CP EMH 8(2012), 169–174 (2018)
19. World Health Organization Homepage "Global Health Observatory (GHO) data". http:// www.who.int/gho/mortality_burden_disease/en/
20. Gameiro, G., et al.: Factores Sociais e Demográficos de variabilidade da Qualidade de Vida na população geral. In: Canavarro, M.C., Serra, A.V. (eds.) Qualidade de vida e saúde: Uma abordagem na perspectiva da Organização Mundial de Saúde, pp. 251–268. Fundação Calouste Gulbenkian, Lisboa (2010)

The Relationship Between Burnout and the Risk of Violence Against Institutionalised Elderly People: The Case of Formal Care

Felismina Mendes[(⊠)] and Joana Alegria Pereira

Department of Nursing, University of Évora, Évora, Portugal
fm@uevora.pt

Abstract. The work overload of the formal caregiver of the elderly is frequent and can cause health problems, both psychological and physical. One is Burnout, a phenomenon which is already considered a public health problem, which mainly affects caregivers (both formal and informal) [1]. This study aimed to analyse how the Burnout of caregivers of the elderly may be related to the risk of violence against institutionalised elderly people. 82 formal caregivers participated, from institutions that receive elderly people, temporarily or permanently, and that collaborated with the project Aging in Safety in the Alentejo - Understanding to Act, of the University of Évora. The Copenhagen Burnout Inventory (CBI) and the Caregiver Abuse Screen (CASE) were applied, and a quantitative approach was applied using IBM-SPSS software (version 24). The results indicate that caregivers have low levels of Burnout and that there is a low risk of violence against the elderly. However, significant correlations were found between these two dimensions. There is a need for intervention in this professional group, focusing on the promotion of workers' health in the prevention of, and combat against, Burnout Syndrome, with the adoption of coping strategies. This could reduce the effects of prolonged stress levels experienced by formal caregivers of the elderly, in order to then reduce the possibility of acts of violence against the elderly.

Keywords: Formal caregivers · Burnout · Violence · Elderly

1 Introduction

1.1 Aging in Portugal and Institutionalisation

Increased longevity is now a reality that marks all developed and developing societies. In Portugal, the process of population aging, which has happened rapidly, has revealed the importance of developing and adapting structures (health services and social

F. Mendes—Researcher Responsible for the Project ESACA- Ref.ª: ALT20-03-0145-FEDER-000007.
J. A. Pereira—Project Fellow ESACA- Ref.ª: ALT20-03-0145-FEDER-000007.

© Springer Nature Switzerland AG 2019
J. García-Alonso and C. Fonseca (Eds.): IWoG 2018, CCIS 1016, pp. 327–333, 2019.
https://doi.org/10.1007/978-3-030-16028-9_29

support) that meet the health and social needs of the population [2]. Another of the great challenges that the aging of the population brings to society is the increasing need for professionals trained in the care of the elderly [3].

In addition to population aging, families increasingly need to put their elderly relatives in residential care homes, in order to ensure them the best care, quality of life and well-being. Thus, residential care homes are one of the temporary or permanent social responses to elderly people or others who have lost or are at risk of losing their independence and autonomy [4]. These residential care homes promote social support activities and provide health and nursing care. Their main objectives include: providing permanent and adequate services to the biopsychosocial problems of the elderly; cooperating to stimulate an active aging process; creating conditions to ensure and stimulate the intra-family relationship and enhance social integration [5]. When integrating into a residential care home where the elderly person stays 24 h a day, there is a change in people's lives that requires a complicated and difficult transition. The elderly people need to adapt to a different environment with new rules and routines and where they have to share the same area with people who they do not know, which may lead to some situations of anxiety and anger. However, institutionalisation also has some positive aspects, particularly in the case of elderly people who previously lived in isolation and without access to basic care. In these institutions, older people may feel more supported, more active and even happier than when they were alone in their homes [6]. Regarding the organisation and management of residential care homes, it is essential that professionals and employees work together in order to establish a hospitable, humanised and personalised environment that provides the elderly with a sense of satisfaction according to their desires and interests [6].

1.2 The Role of Formal Caregivers

Formal caregivers have a fundamental role in families that are not available to fulfil this role, but the lack of knowledge and inadequate working conditions makes this work difficult, and training and qualifications are essential for the provision of quality care and affection in order to meet the emotional needs of the elderly people in this process [7, 8]. An essential aspect in the success of the activity of formal caregivers is the quality of the services provided and the knowledge and the capacities required to respond to the needs of this group, in order to perform their role with competence and sensitivity [9]. Formal caregivers are cornerstones in any institution. They are the ones who help the elderly in their basic and instrumental activities of daily life. In general, the care provided to the elderly is an arduous and complex task, resulting from the needs of care tasks and some personal vulnerability factors, causing situations of stress at work. This process of work is characterised by variability and does not occur in all caregivers, since some feel satisfaction when they achieve good results, regardless of the physical and psychological efforts that are required [10]. Therefore, we can say that the professional, emotional and personal demands on the formal caregivers, in the care of the elderly during the aging process, are almost always a source of stress and friction. This work is considered stressful, both physically and mentally, which makes caregivers vulnerable to diseases related to occupational stress [11]. Providing formal care can thus become an arduous and complicated task, with impacts on the quality of life of these professionals. The caregiver's work overload can lead to health problems, both psychological and physical, in the caregiver as well as in the elderly person and their family.

1.3 Burnout in Formal Caregivers of the Elderly

The term Burnout was used for the first time in the United States in the nineteen-seventies by Freudenberger. This author has described Burnout as the breakdown, deterioration, or exhaustion due to excessive demands on energy, strength or resources, or when a member of the organisation becomes inefficient. The concept of burnout has been particularly emphasized in the human service professions, where work is based on the relationship between those who provide and those who receive the service. It is predominant in health professionals. Professionals involved in patient care, when trying to solve problems manifested by them, or when providing care to them, may develop a conflict between the profession they perform, occupational satisfaction and client responsibility [12, 13].

According to Maslach and Jackson [12], burnout can be characterised as a state of physical, emotional and mental exhaustion caused by long-term involvement in situations of high emotional demands in the workplace. These requirements are usually caused by a combination of very high expectations and chronic situational stress, which develop from experiences of stress at work where the individual is confronted with an incongruence between expectations and personal and professional motivations, and the resources available to satisfy them [14].

According to Montero-Marín and collaborators [15], burnout results from the subject's perception of a disagreement between the efforts made and what they achieve in their work. It is defined as a syndrome formed of three dimensions: emotional exhaustion, depersonalisation and reduced professional achievement [16]. The professional starts by feeling exhausted, then expressing a negative and dehumanised attitude towards the work and/or the people with whom they work, as well as negatively assessing their professional performance and feeling frustrated and that they lack professional achievement [17].

Emotional exhaustion (the central quality of burnout) consists of an exhaustion of the individual's emotional, moral, and psychological resources. Depersonalisation characterises an affective distance or emotional indifference towards others, namely those who are the very reason for the professional activity (patients, clients, among others). It is an involuntary emotional defence manifested in cold, cynical attitudes that are devoid of affection and are inhumane. Finally, personal fulfilment expresses a reduction of feelings of competence and pleasure related to the fulfilment of a professional activity [18].

According to the data provided by the European Agency for Safety and Health at Work [19], about 51% of EU industry emphasizes the existence of stress in their work, a figure that before 2010 was around 20% [20]. One of the consequences of chronic stress at work is burnout [21], a phenomenon that has already been considered a public health problem, especially in caregivers, and has been the subject of extensive research since the 1970s until today [1, 16].

2 Objective of the Study

The main objective of this article is to analyse how Burnout in formal caregivers may be related to the risk of violence against institutionalised elderly people.

3 Method

The sample consisted of professional caregivers of both sexes, from residential care homes for elderly people and which collaborated with the project Aging in Safety in the Alentejo - Understanding to Act, at the University of Évora, with a total of 82 caregivers. The study had as its only exclusion criterion that employees must be doing an internship at the institution. Three instruments were used: the sociodemographic characterisation questionnaire, the Copenhagen Burnout Inventory (CBI) and the Caregiver Abuse Screen (CASE).

The CBI consists of nineteen (19) items, distributed on three scales: personal Burnout, consisting of six items that assess the degree of physical and psychological fatigue and exhaustion experienced by the person; work-related Burnout, consisting of seven items that examine the degree of physical and psychological fatigue and exhaustion that is perceived by the person in relation to their work; and customer-related Burnout, which encompasses six items that analyse the degree of physical and psychological fatigue and exhaustion perceived by the individual in relation to client work [22].

The CASE consists of eight items and the response categories take the dichotomised form. It is composed of questions about situations that fall under the dimensions of physical, psychosocial and financial violence and neglect, without, however, directly affecting violent behaviours or acts. The different items of the CASE focus more on interpersonal and psychological relationships than on the social context [23].

In the statistical analysis, the SPSS 24 software was used for data processing and analysis. The statistical test was Pearson's correlation, which was used to correlate the score data of each dimension of the Copenhagen Burnout Inventory with the total score of the Caregiver Abuse Screen (CASE). The significance level was set at $p \leq 0.05$.

All the ethical procedures of human research were followed. All the authorisations required for the study, such as the informed consent of the elderly people, were requested and all conditions of anonymity and confidentiality of the answers obtained were also guaranteed. The project was approved by the Ethics Committee of the Health and Welfare Area of the University of Évora under number 16012 of 05/19/2016.

4 Results

It was found that of the 82 caregivers participating in the study, 80 were female and 2 were male. The participants' ages ranged from 25 to 68, with a mean of 46.05 and a standard deviation of 10.85. Regarding the academic qualifications of the 82 participants, 13 (15.9%) had completed the 1st Cycle, 16 (19.5%) had completed the 2nd Cycle, 20 (24.4%) had completed the 3rd Cycle, 19 (23.2%) attended secondary school and 14 (17.1%) had higher education. The average duration to have been practising their profession was 12.15 years (SD = 9.164), ranging from 0 to 35 years.

The data obtained on the CBI scale dimensions revealed that in the personal Burnout dimension, the sample mean was 42.01 (SD = 18.11), ranging from 0 to 95.83. In work-related Burnout, participants' scores ranged from 0 to 85.75, with a mean of 32.71 and a standard deviation of 19.84. In customer-related Burnout, the sample mean was 22.61 (18.13), ranging from 0 to 83.33.

Regarding the CASE, the participants' results ranged from 0 to 8, with an average of 3.02 and a standard deviation of 1.92.

In the relationship between CBI data and CASE data, significant correlations were found in three dimensions. The CASE is positively correlated with personal Burnout, r = .24, ρ = .03. It has been found that a higher CASE score is associated with a higher score in the personal Burnout dimension. There is a significant positive correlation between the CASE score and the work-related Burnout dimension, r = .28, ρ = .01. Higher CASE scores are associated with a higher job-related Burnout dimension. The CASE score is also positively correlated with customer-related Burnout, r = .33, ρ = .003. Thus, a higher CASE score is associated with a higher client-related Burnout.

5 Discussion

The formal caregivers of the elderly are, above all, female, which can be explained by historical, cultural and affective factors. However, this propensity is changing, and it seems an increase in male caregivers is beginning to be seen [6].

In terms of academic training, most of the subjects in the sample have 3rd cycle education, followed by secondary education, second cycle education, and finally higher education, which leads to the conclusion that a large part of the sample did not have access to higher education, or to some professional qualification for the job they are performing. The results on the training of formal caregivers of older people validate what was stated by Smith, Kerse and Parsons [24], who emphasize that the elderly population is often cared for by professionals with no minimum professional qualifications showing that they perform their functions based on the practical experience and observation of other colleagues. According to Carvalho [9], in Portugal there are several studies that indicate that most formal caregivers begin their career as professionals without any training in the area that enables them to deal with the elderly.

Most caregivers have low levels of Burnout in all three dimensions and also have a low risk of violence against the elderly. However, significant correlations were found between the different dimensions of Burnout and the risk of violence, as already mentioned. The understanding of the reasons for violence against the elderly is inseparable from the understanding of the different theoretical approaches that attempt to explain this phenomenon. There are several theoretical explanatory models, most of which were constructed from theories proposed to understand the origins of child abuse and domestic violence [19]. From the explanatory theories most referenced, for the explanation and interpretation of behaviours leading to situations of violence against the elderly, it is worth noting that the Situational Stress Model seems to be the most adequate to explain the relation between Burnout and the risk of violence against institutionalised elderly people.

According to this model, the act of violence plays a situational phenomenon, boosted by the stress experienced by the caregiver. This state of stress can be boosted by the physical or mental incapacity of the elderly person, as well as unfavourable socioeconomic conditions and low coping strategies of the caregiver [25].

6 Conclusion

Despite the sample size, this study allowed us to understand the dynamics of the association between the Burnout of formal caregivers of residential care homes for elderly people, and violence against institutionalised elderly people. The stress and work overload experienced daily by formal caregivers can contribute to environments that are conducive to the occurrence of acts of violence against the elderly. It was verified that the data validated Ferreira's [6] suggestions for the implementation of training programmes that focus on emotional support, on stress and the emotional overload of formal caregivers. The acquisition of skills and knowledge (specific training) by this professional group is another advantage in order to promote the quality of care provided to the elderly. Also, the intervention aimed at the health of the formal caregivers is very important, focusing on the promotion of the health of the workers, on the prevention of and the combat against, Burnout Syndrome, with the adoption of coping strategies that reduce the effects that are always evident when the employees experience prolonged stress levels. This is essential in reducing the risk of violence against the elderly in these residential care homes.

Acknowledgements. The authors thank all the participants and institutions for their contribution to this work, namely the University of Évora, the National Confederation of Solidarity Institutions (CNIS); the Regional Health Administration of the Alentejo, IP, (ARS Alentejo) and the programmes that financed the project Envelhecer em Segurança no Alentejo/Ref: ALT20-03-0145-FEDER-000007: Alentejo 2020, Portugal 2020 and the European Union.

References

1. Lin, L.P., Lin, J.D.: Job burnout amongst the institutional caregivers working with individuals with intellectual and developmental disabilities: utilization of the Chinese version of the Copenhagen Burnout Inventory survey. Res. Autism Spectr. Disord. 7(6), 777–784 (2013)
2. Azeredo, Z.: Cuidados continuados no domicílio: Cuidar o utente no seu habitat. Hospitalidade ano 73, 25–28 (2009)
3. Conceição, L.F.S.D.: Saúde do idoso: orientações ao cuidador do idoso acamado (2010)
4. Lima, M.: Políticas e respostas sociais de apoio à terceira idade em Portugal: O caso do concelho de Vila Verde. Braga. Tese de Mestrado, Universidade do Minho, Portugal (2013)
5. Instituto da Segurança Social. *Guia prático: Apoios sociais - idosos.* Acedido em fevereiro 2, 2014, em (2013). http://www.seg-social.pt

6. Ferreira, M.E.M.M.: Ser cuidador: um estudo sobre a satisfação do cuidador formal de idosos (Doctoral dissertation, Instituto Politécnico de Bragança, Escola Superior de Educação) (2012)
7. dos Santos Colomé, I.C., et al.: Cuidar de idosos institucionalizados: características e dificuldades dos cuidadores. Revista Eletrônica de enfermagem 13(2), 306–312 (2011)
8. Batista, M.P.P., Barros, J.D.O., Almeida, M.H.M.D., Mangia, E.F., Lancman, S.: Acompanhantes de idosos: reflexão sobre sua prática. Rev. Saude Publica 48(5), 732–738 (2014)
9. Carvalho, A.F.J.: Ajudantes de acção directa: percepções sobre formação profissional e impacto da formação na prestação de cuidados a idosos dependentes internados. Doctoral dissertation, Faculdade de Ciências Médicas. Universidade Nova de Lisboa (2012)
10. Freitas Ribeiro, M.T.D., Conceição Ferreira, R., Silami de Magalhães, C., Nogueira Moreira, A., Ferreira e Ferreira, E.: Processo de cuidar nas instituições de longa permanência: visão dos cuidadores formais de idosos. Revista Brasileira de Enfermagem 62(6) (2009)
11. Testad, I., Mikkelsen, A., Ballard, C., Aarsland, D.: Health and well-being in care staff and their relations to organizational and psychosocial factors, care staff and resident factors in nursing homes. Int. J. Geriatr. Psychiatry 25(8), 789–797 (2010)
12. Maslach, C., Jackson, S.E.: The measurement of experienced burnout. J. Organ. Behav. 2(2), 99–113 (1981)
13. Richardsen, A.M., Burke, R.J.: Models of burnout: implications for interventions. Int. J. Stress Manag. 2(1), 31–43 (1995)
14. Maslach, C.: Job burnout: new directions in research and intervention. Curr. Dir. Psychol. Sci. 12(5), 189–192 (2003)
15. Montero-Marín, J., García-Campayo, J., Mera, D.M., del Hoyo, Y.L.: A new definition of burnout syndrome based on Farber's proposal. J. Occup. Med. Toxicol. 4(1), 31 (2009)
16. Maslach, C., Schaufeli, W., Leiter, M.: Job burnout. Ann. Rev. Psychol. 52, 397–422 (2001)
17. Monteiro, B., Queirós, C., Marques, A.: Empatia e engagement como preditores do burnout em cuidadores formais de idosos. Psicologia, Saúde & Doenças 15(1), 2–11 (2014)
18. Maroco, J., Tecedeiro, M.: Inventário de Burnout de Maslach para estudantes portugueses. Psicologia, Saúde & Doenças 10(2), 227–235 (2009)
19. Perel-Levin, S.: World Health Organization. Discussing screening for elder abuse at primary health care level by Silvia Perel-Levin (2008)
20. Pereira, A.M., Queirós, C., Gonçalves, S.P., Carlotto, M.S., Borges, E.: Burnout e interação trabalho-família em enfermeiros: Estudo exploratório com o Survey Work-Home Interaction Nijmegen (SWING). Revista Portuguesa de Enfermagem de Saúde Mental 11, 24–30 (2014)
21. Gil-Monte, P.R.: Algunas razones para considerar los riesgos psicosociales en el trabajo y sus consecuencias en la salud pública (2009)
22. Kristensen, T.S., Borritz, M., Villadsen, E., Christensen, K.B.: The Copenhagen Burnout Inventory: a new tool for the assessment of burnout. Work Stress 19(3), 192–207 (2005)
23. Reis, M., Nahmiash, D.: Validation of the caregiver abuse screen (CASE). Can. J. Aging/La Revue Canadienne Du Vieillissement 14(S2), 45–60 (1995)
24. Smith, B., Kerse, N., Parsons, M.: Quality of residential care for older people: does education for healthcare assistants make a difference? J. New Zealand Med. Assoc. 118(1214), 1–13 (2005)
25. Moya, A., Barbero, J.: Malos tratos a personas mayores: guía de actuación. Ministerio de Trabajo y Asuntos Sociales, Madrid (2005)

Intervention Proposal of the Rehabilitation Nursing Care to the People in the ICU: Systematic Review of the Literature

Marco Jacinto[1]([✉]), Tânia Leite[2], and César Fonseca[3] [iD]

[1] Rehabilitation Nursing, Polytechnic Institute of Setúbal, Setúbal, Portugal
marco.jacinto1992@gmail.com
[2] Rehabilitation Nursing, Beatriz Angelo's Hospital, Loures, Portugal
[3] Évora University, Investigator POCTEP 0445_4IE_4_P, Évora, Portugal

Abstract. The increase of the average life expectancy led to an increase in acute diseases requiring hospitalization in the ICU.

Goal: Identify the cares in rehabilitation nursing in the ICU to people under IMV and/or in prolonged rest in bed.

Methodology: Articles were selected between January 2010 and September 2018, and the research was carried out in the databases present at EBSCO. Six articles were selected that met the inclusion criteria, and the inclusion grid of JBI, FAME was also applied. Two further studies were included that did not fit the temporal limit, but which were included by their pertinence, obtaining a total of eight articles.

Interventions: The interventions that the rehabilitation nurse plans and executes can be divided into two categories that complement each other, the interventions of the physical domain and the cognitive domain.

Results/Discussion: Early rehabilitation in the ICU is a fundamental tool in maintaining autonomy, as many people acquire complications during hospitalization. To reverse these complications requires the intervention of a multidisciplinary team, where the Rehabilitation Nurse develops a prominent role in the articulation of the team and in the realization of a structured plan involving the person, their relatives and the rest of the care team.

Conclusion: The studies presented in this review are unanimous about the achievement of early rehabilitation for people hospitalized in the ICU, and these programs have the potential to bring significant gains to people, both physically and cognitively.

Keywords: Rehabilitation Nurse · Intensive Care Unit · Early rehabilitation

1 Introduction

The increase in average life expectancy, increases the incidence of acute diseases [1]. In the last decades, advances in the treatment of this have significantly increased the survival of the critically ill person [1], these persons should preferably be hospitalized in an intensive care unit (ICU).

© Springer Nature Switzerland AG 2019
J. García-Alonso and C. Fonseca (Eds.): IWoG 2018, CCIS 1016, pp. 334–345, 2019.
https://doi.org/10.1007/978-3-030-16028-9_30

The ICU is a unit where the human and technical resources, necessary for an optimal monitoring and treatment of people with imminent or established failure of a vital function, affected by potentially reversible pathologies, are found [12].

The mean length of hospital stay in an ICU can vary from 6 to 13 days, during which approximately 68% of people undergo sedation for an average period of 2 to 6 days, and invasive mechanical ventilation (IMV), for an average period of 6 to 12 days [13].

In the ICU, people often develop acute dysfunctions at the cognitive level, with delirium being the most common [1]. This affects about 60% to 80% of people undergoing IMV, causing an increase in ventilation time, an increase in hospitalization and consequent delay in hospital discharge, resulting in an increased risk of death [1].

IVM is a procedure that implies that the person is intubated (with an endotracheal tube, laryngeal mask or tracheostomy cannula) and connected to a ventilatory prosthesis, improving gas exchange when spontaneous ventilation is ineffective [14].

These present ineffective airway clearance conditioned by the presence of the endotracheal tube, responsible for airway permeability [9]. In these people, the inefficacy of mucociliary transport, the displacement of pathogens from the oropharynx and the absence of cough, may lead to the accumulation of secretions that lead to several complications such as pulmonary atelectasis and pneumonia associated with IMV, leading to an increase time of weaning and consequent extubation [6, 9].

In the course of this therapy, many people remain immobile in bed, resulting in a whole range of other complications (OE, 2018). Immobility can lead to a significant decrease in the person's quality of life, making rehabilitation increasingly important in order to promote a better quality of life after hospital discharge [1, 5, 7].

The elderly submitted to VMI develop a greater incapacity at the level of their daily life activities (ADLs), compared to those who were hospitalized without this therapy [1, 7].

In this context, survivors of acute diseases, particularly the elderly, may develop new deficits acquired during hospitalization [1]. For them, the new deficits have a dramatic effect on their lives, causing changes in their daily routines and their autonomy [1]. Frustration and depression are quite common, because of the state of dependence in which the person is [11].

The main causes of the deficits mentioned above are the problems associated with immobility and prolonged sedation, which may be physical and/or cognitive deficits [1, 8].

Physical deficits often manifest as severe muscle weakness, referred to as ICU acquired weakness, it affects about 25% to 60% of survivors [1].

The ICU acquired weakness is a syndrome that describes the muscular weakness in people with acute and severe pathology in which there is no other explanation for its appearance [1].

This presents as a symmetrical limb weakness, which can progress to severe paralysis with shortening of the reflex tendons and loss of associated muscle mass. This loss is about 1% to 1.5% per day, with a total loss of about 50% in just two weeks of hospitalization [1, 6]. Studies indicate that the first muscles to weaken, are the muscles of the lower limbs [10].

Risk factors for the onset of this syndrome include multi-organ failure, sepsis, prolonged immobility, hyperglycemia, systemic inflammation, prolonged use of corticosteroids and antibiotics, and administration of anesthetics and curarizers [1, 3, 6–8].

Despite early rehabilitation, 25% to 33% of people hospitalized in the ICU develop this syndrome, mainly due to the fact that rehabilitation exercises performed in the bed are of low intensity [2, 3].

With regard to cognitive deficits, these are not so visible to the person, however they are as limiting in the level of their ADLs as the physical deficits [1]. The most frequent examples are difficulty in solving problems, memory impairment, and changes in thinking construction [1].

Previously, people with acute illness hospitalized in the ICU were seen as "very sick" to tolerate rehabilitation exercises in the initial phase of their hospitalization, being submitted to high doses of sedatives and prolonged rest in bed, as already described [2, 4, 7]. However, in the last 10 to 15 years, there have been increasing studies that demonstrate the efficacy, safety and feasibility of initiating early rehabilitation of the person in the ICU [4, 6].

Several studies have described that early rehabilitation is associated with a reduction in IMV time, a decrease in hospital admission, a decrease in the appearance of wounds and pressure ulcers, a reduction in pneumonia associated with IMV, and a decrease in delirium, and of other cognitive changes [3–7, 10].

These refer that the rehabilitation programs initiated in the ICU can be associated with a functional improvement of the person, translating into a greater autonomy in their self-care [5, 6].

Concerning the incidence of adverse events associated with early rehabilitation, these are very low, and the benefits should always be evaluated versus the risks to the person, using the multidisciplinary team whenever necessary [4].

However, despite the low incidence of adverse events during early rehabilitation, the lack of knowledge of the team, the level of sedation of the person and the reduced number of professionals and/or equipment, have been major obstacles to the early rehabilitation of people hospitalized in the ICU [6]. In this sense, technology has been increasingly used to overcome some of the shortcomings, namely through methods of cognitive stimulation, and it is also a driver of increased muscle strength, improved cardiopulmonary function and improved functionality, through devices such as the tilt table for example [6].

The severity of the pathology and the innumerable invasive techniques can contribute to the dehumanization and isolation of the person and his/her family, being central the role of the Rehabilitation Nursing (RN) in the inclusion of the family in the rehabilitation program [10]. These programs allow the family to learn and intervene with the person with acute pathology, showing that they also play a key role in the stimulation of the same [10].

In this sense, it was necessary to carry out a systematic review of the literature, with the objective of identifying the nursing care of rehabilitation in the ICU and its benefits in the person submitted to IMV and/or in prolonged bed rest. It was then elaborated the question delineating this review "What are the benefits of rehabilitation nursing care provided to people hospitalized in the ICU under IMV and/or in prolonged rest in bed?", Following the PICO methodology.

2 Methodology

To reach the mentioned objective, the systematic review was developed.

The research was carried out on the EBSCO platform, having selected all available databases: CINAHL Complete; MEDLINE Complete; Nursing & Allied Health Collection: Comprehensive; Cochrane Central Register of Controlled Trials; Cochrane Database of Systematic Reviews; Cochrane Methodology Register; Library, Information Science & Technology Abstracts; MedicLatina.

In order to start the selection of articles of interest, the descriptors were used using their combination in the English language "Rehabilitation", "Rehabilitation Nursing", "Self-Management", "Intensive Care Unit", "Quality of Life", "Artificial Respiration" and "Respiratory", using the intersection between them through the Boolean operators "AND" and "OR" and the truncation system with "*". The descriptors were all confirmed and validated in the DeCS platform, referring to the Descriptors in Health Sciences.

The following inclusion criteria were defined: articles whose publication date is between January 1, 2010 and September 10, 2018; all studies of a quantitative and qualitative nature, whether primary or secondary, to maximize the spectrum of the literature already produced.

From the research carried out in the databases, using the interconnection between the various discriminators, a total of 1204 articles were obtained. When entering search delimiters, we obtained 803 results. From these were selected only those in which it was possible to have access to the complete article having been deleted duplicate articles.

After reading all the titles, 50 articles were selected and, through the analysis of the summary of these, 37 were excluded. Of the 13 articles selected, after read in full, 7 more were excluded, obtaining a total of 6 articles which meet the defined inclusion criteria.

However, when reading the articles in full, two studies were found that were used as reference in the same ones, although they did not meet the inclusion criteria initially defined, because they were published before of 2010, we opted for include those.

In preparing the review, we considered that for the studies to be included, they would have to be identified with more than 50% of the items contained in the respective Joanna Briggs Institute (JBI) inclusion grids.

In all our studies, the methodological quality was evaluated through the "FAME" grid of JBI, and we used the same assumption above, that is, that they present a strong methodological quality, they would have to present more than 50% positive responses in the grids applied.

Finally, the level of scientific evidence was evaluated, considering the type of study included, using as a guide the grids of scientific evidence of efficacy, prognosis and significance of 2014 of JBI. The selected articles are outlined in the following table (Table 1).

Table 1. Identification of the selective articles

	Title of article	Type of study level of evidence
1	A Combined Early Cognitive and Physical Rehabilitation Program for People Who Are Critically Ill: The Activity and Cognitive Therapy in the Intensive Care Unit (ACT-ICU) Trial	Randomized Controlled Study Level 1.C
2	Comparison of Exercise Intensity During Four Early Rehabilitation Techniques in Sedated and Ventilated Patients in ICU: A Randomized Cross-Over Trial	Randomized Study Level 1.D
3	Effect of Physical Therapy on Muscle Strength, Respiratory Muscles and Functional Parameters in Patient with Intensive Care Unit- Acquired Weakness	Randomized Controlled Study Level 1.C
4	Expert Consensus and Recommendations on Safety Criteria for Active Mobilization of Mechanically Ventilated Critically Ill Adults	Experts Opinion Level 5.B
5	Standardized Rehabilitation and Hospital Length of Stay Among Patients With Acute Respiratory Failure	Randomized Controlled Study Level 1.C
6	Progressive Mobility Program and Technology to Increase the Level of Physical Activity and its Benefits in Respiratory, Muscular System, and Functionality of ICU Patients	Quasi-Experimental Study Level 2.D
7	Early Activity is Feasible and Safe in Respiratory Failure Patents	Cohort Study Level 3.B
8	Early Intensive Care Unit Mobility Therapy in the Treatment of Acute Respiratory Failure	Cohort Study Level 3.B

3 Interventions

As maintenance of the functionality seems to depend mainly on the muscular and cardiorespiratory systems, their importance should be recognized in early rehabilitation, however cognitive rehabilitation should not be neglected in order to care the person as a whole, that is, taking care holistically [6].

We must therefore plan a set of interventions with the objective of achieving the maximum possible functionality, and it is important that the plan be structured, to include not only the person in need of care, but also his family [10].

This brings us to what Orem (2001) says, that the capacity of each human being to engage in self-care involves a physical, cognitive, emotional/psychosocial and behavioral domain.

3.1 Interventions of the Physical Domain

Each rehabilitation session should be guided by the level of consciousness of the person, with the goal of always reaching their maximum potential during each session [1].

Daily rehabilitation should include a respiratory component, to control the fatigue easier, associated with the person's current health situation and the immobility to which he was subjected, associating this with muscular rehabilitation, focusing on muscle strengthening techniques to maintain the amplitude and to prevent muscle and tendon shortening [3].

The most commonly used exercise in people who are indicated for rest in bed, who are sedated or in coma, are the passive mobilizations, the passive cycle ergometer and the muscular electrostimulation of the quadriceps, this can be used for a maximum of 20 min [2, 6].

Once the person regains consciousness or ceases to be sedated, exercises with progressive resistance should be started [5].

Initially, passive mobilizations should be performed in all segments, not neglecting the mobilization also at the level of the cervical segment [1]. Sets with about six repetitions per movement should be performed until the person has an improvement in strength, as assessed by the scale that the NR finds most appropriate [3, 6].

Teachings regarding respiratory rehabilitation should be reinforced so that the person can control symptoms such as pain or tiredness [3]. To achieve this, awareness and dissociation of breathing times should be carried out and reinforced, as well as the frenolabial breathing in those who are not under IMV, if possible carrying out all the active cycle of respiratory techniques [3]. In those under IMV, a manual hyperinflation of the lungs should be performed, and aspiration of secretions should be performed to clean the airway, which by the presence of the endotracheal tube becomes physiologically ineffective [3].

In case the person already has muscle stimulus, with associated contractions, or if he/she can perform small movements, they should be encouraged to perform them, followed by series of passive mobilizations and also initiating series of active-assisted mobilizations [1, 3]. To achieve a progressive increase of the resistance in the mobilizations, elastic bands with different levels of resistance can be used [5].

If there are no contraindications, it is possible to initiate ball-bearing exercises in the bed, assisted rotation exercises and elevation of the basin, the so-called "bridge" [3, 6].

At this stage, changes in the balance in sitting position should be evaluated, if there are changes, we should train the static and later dynamic equilibrium.

At the end of each session, the person should sit in bed for about 2 h [1, 3]. As the rehabilitation program evolves, the number of sets and repetitions per exercise should increase, seeking to progressively exceed those initially performed, according to the tolerance of the person [1, 3].

3.2   Interventions of the Cognitive Domain

Cognitive rehabilitation focuses on specific interventions for a specific cognitive deficit, such as attention and memory, proving to be quite effective, since normally people hospitalized in the ICU are cognitively inactive for long periods [1].

According to the author, this rehabilitation goes through a progressive program with increasingly challenging exercises in sessions of about 20 min, 2 times a day, directed towards the person's orientation, attention and memory [1].

The program begins as soon as the person is more awake, with spontaneous ocular opening to the verbal stimulus, being that at that time, the person should be oriented alopsychically whenever approached. Later, when she is fully conscious, she will be invited to advance through the remaining exercises, including intellectual games such as puzzles and Sudoku, reading the newspaper, simple mathematical calculations, among others [1].

The person should be asked about their life history (having a family member nearby, so you can confirm and assist in some detail), numbering, alphabet, and recognition of identical patterns [1].

At the end of each session, the family should always be encouraged to talk about the person's main interests, be it animals, sports, games, among others [1].

Video games can also be used as one of the methods of cognitive stimulation, since they increase the level of cognitive reach through speed alerts, such as divert objects, moving movement and/ or need multitasking simultaneously. In addition, there are various visual and auditory stimuli that can trigger multiple memories [6].

The following table (Table 2) shows a summary of the main interventions carried out by E EER.

The RN may decide to use any other treatment, namely therapeutic massage or other devices such as the tilt table, in order to progressively put the person in orthostatic position [1].

In the last phase of the rehabilitation program, all exercises of the previous phases should be incorporated, with a greater number of sets and repetitions, and the use of weights of 0.5 kg to 1 kg may be used to increase resistance and increase muscular strength [3, 6].

At this stage, the daily life activities should star being trained, such as the transfer training (with transfer from the sitting position to the orthostatic position), the static and dynamic balance training in orthostatic position and the training of walking, with running gear if necessary, always respecting the tolerance and fatigue that the person presents [1, 3, 5].

Rehabilitation sessions should be performed daily until the person is able to perform his daily life activities with supervision only and is able to walk about 60 m with supervision for two consecutive days or until the date of hospital discharge [1].

Table 2. Summary table of the main RN interventions

Domain		Interventions
Interventions of the Physical Domain	Muscular	Passive Mobility of all the corporal segments [1–8]
		Active-assisted Mobility of all the corporal segments [1–8]
		Resisted Mobility with the use of elastics or weights [3, 5, 6]
		Use of a passive Cycle Meter [2]
		Muscular Electro-stimulation [2]
		Practice of static and dynamic sitting [1, 3]
		Static and dynamic balance training in orthostatic position [1, 3, 5]
		Bearings in bed [3, 6]
		Rotation and elevation of the pelvis [3, 6]
		Therapeutic massage [1]
		Transfer training [1, 3–5]
		Training of ADL's [3, 6]
		Training of March [1, 3–5]
	Respiratory	Consciousness and dissociation of respiratory time [3, 5, 6, 8]
		Pursed-Lip Breathing [3, 5, 6, 8]
		Active Cycle of the respiratory techniques [3, 5, 6, 8]
		Manual hyperinflation of the lungs in people submitted to IMV [3, 5, 6, 8]
		Suction of Secretions [3, 5, 6, 8]
Interventions in the Cognitive Domain		Alopsychic Orientation [1, 6]
		Stimulation through the familiar [1, 6]
		Recognition of symmetric patterns [1]
		Intellectual Games (puzzles, Sudoku) [1]
		Exercises of simple calculus [1]
		Videogames [6]

4 Results/Discussion

According to the study by Brummel et al. (2012), after 3 months of physical and cognitive rehabilitation interventions, the intervention group demonstrated significant improvements at functional level and fewer deficits in activities of daily living, compared to the control group [1].

The earlier the rehabilitation, the greater the functional and cognitive gains related to the deficits acquired during the health situation [1]. These also have less delusional time as compared to those who are not subject to early rehabilitation [1].

The author also states that people undergoing early rehabilitation are more likely to return to their functional status after hospital discharge [1]. Nonetheless, the author suggests that these results, while encouraging, require large-scale validation to generalize care, with the certainty that these programs will bring about functional and cognitive improvements, thus increasing the quality of life of the person [1].

Medrinal et al. (2018) in their study, affirmed that most of the exercises performed in the bed are of low intensity, inducing only a low level of muscular work, being that only the cycle ergometer produced an increase of the heart rate and improvements in the level of the cardiorespiratory system [2]. This suggests that early rehabilitation to be effective should be more intense to induce muscle contractions in bed rest sedated persons [2].

Passive mobilizations can be used to prevent ankyloses, but for this author further studies are needed to evaluate the effectiveness of early rehabilitation [2].

To Yosef-Brauner et al. (2015), early rehabilitation demonstrated a decrease in the number of days of hospitalization in the ICU in the intervention group when compared to the control group [3]. According to the study, the duration of hospitalization in the intervention group was considerably shorter, with about 13 days, compared to the control group in which the duration was 18 days [3].

Regarding the days of invasive mechanical ventilation, the group undergoing early rehabilitation presented an average of 9 days while the other group presented an average of 16 days of IMV [3].

Regarding the ability to walk during hospitalization, the author states that there were no differences between the two groups, but in terms of force scales and inspiratory time measurement, the intervention group showed significant improvements showing that people submitted early rehabilitation, show significant and faster improvements when compared to those who do not receive it [3], going against the study of Brummel et al. (2012).

Most of the time, people submitted to IMV tend to stay in bed longer due to sedation and IMV, however according to Hodgson's et al. (2014) study, the endotracheal tube is not a contraindication for performing early rehabilitation and should only be monitored if there is no displacement of the tube and if the person remains well oxygenated and well perfused at the peripheral level [4].

However, despite early rehabilitation, the number of complications associated with IMV and immobility, namely the number of people diagnosed with IMV-associated pneumonia, pulmonary embolism and deep venous thrombosis were not statistically different between the two groups [8].

Morris et al. (2016) states that during the study there were no significant differences between the two intervention groups, contrary to the results obtained in the studies presented previously. However, after 6 months, the group undergoing early rehabilitation presented a significant improvement compared to the control group, a situation that was not evident at the time of hospital discharge [5].

Bailey et al. (2007), in his study initiated the early rehabilitation program shortly after hemodynamic stabilization of the person, and continued rehabilitation interventions throughout the ICU stay [7]. This program was carried out without an increase of the UCI team, and should ideally be carried out by a multidisciplinary team [7].

In their study, the author showed that early rehabilitation has a low risk of complications, about 1%, even if people are under IMV, stating that delaying the rehabilitation process until discharge from the ICU can limit functional capacity that the person will reach, being able to be with permanent deficits [7], being therefore feasible and safe the beginning of the early rehabilitation in the people already hemodynamically stable.

The author also shows in his study that all people, including the elderly, were able to participate in the program, performing activities and interventions equivalent to the younger ones, demonstrating that age cannot be an exclusion factor in early rehabilitation programs [7].

However, the same author points out as a weak point of his study, the fact that no scales were used for the measurement of strength, only the functional objectives were evaluated, in terms of walking distance that each person walked [7]. This indicates that future studies should focus on interventions that can reduce complications of the ICU, improving the quality of life of people after a critical event [7].

For Morris et al. (2008), the most frequent reason to interrupt rehabilitation is the person's fatigue, evidenced by changes in vital signs [8]. Also for this author, length of stay in the ICU and hospitalization was significantly lower in the group undergoing early rehabilitation compared to the control group [8]. This is because early rehabilitation programs result in more exercise sessions and activities for the individual, leading to more functional and cognitive gains [8].

This study demonstrates that performing early rehabilitation is a prelude to the decrease of adverse events during subsequent rehabilitation sessions [8].

This is in line with other studies, demonstrating that early rehabilitation is safe and viable and is associated with a significant decrease in immobility and days of hospitalization, also reducing the costs associated with prolonged hospitalization [1, 5, 7, 8].

According to the same author, the early rehabilitation initiated in the ICU under the direction of a multidisciplinary team (nursing team, RN and physiotherapists), brings more gains for the person compared to the sessions performed only by physiotherapists, since these always depend on a medical prescription, thus being more efficient the approach of the person by a multidisciplinary team [8].

5 Conclusion

Physical and cognitive deficits are common in people who survive acute illness, and so far, most interventions focus on physical rehabilitation to recover the functionality lost during hospitalization [1]. However, although cognitive rehabilitation is common in other pathologies, it is rarely associated and performed after a critical incident requiring prolonged hospitalization in the ICU [1].

Passive mobilizations, whose main objective is to maintain mobility and joint range in the early rehabilitation phase, where there is still no hemodynamic stability for the performance of active interventions, the latter being mainly responsible for the increase in strength and muscle mass in the early rehabilitation programs [2].

As previously mentioned, ICU acquired weakness is a frequent complication during hospitalization, however if this syndrome is diagnosed early, early rehabilitation programs may intervene bringing more benefits and fewer problems to the person [3]. It is essential that the person is kept under surveillance, thus it is easier to identify motor, respiratory, cognitive and emotional changes during hospitalization, since after the initial recovery phase, functional improvements are slower and gradual [3].

Early rehabilitation is feasible and safe, even in people with respiratory failure under IMV, and most people undergoing early rehabilitation can walk short distances before transferring the ICU. This can be considered with a therapy or treatment for the muscular complications associated to the critical pathologies, presenting a reduction of the days of hospitalization, with consecutive reduction of the costs associated to the same [7, 8].

However, although most authors point to early rehabilitation as a set of interventions effective in the treatment and functional rehabilitation of the person hospitalized in the ICU, all refer that more studies should be developed in this area to generalize this procedure in a viable and safe way, with gains for people in need.

As a response to the question initially defined at the beginning of this review, the interventions that can be used are many, the RN should assess and intervene in all aspects, having a central role in the achievement and motivation of the person, in order to participate in the program outlined for her.

References

1. Brummel, N., Jackson, J., Girard, T., et al.: A combined early cognitive and physical rehabilitation program for people who are critically ill: the activity and cognitive therapy in the intensive care unit (ACT-ICU) trial. Phys. Ther. **92**(12), 1580–1592 (2012)
2. Medrinal, C., Combret, Y., Prieur, G., et al.: Comparison of exercise intensity during four early rehabilitation techniques in sedated and ventilated patients in ICU: a randomized cross-over trial. Crit. Care **22**(110), 1–8 (2018)
3. Yosef-Brauner, O., Adi, N., Shahar, T., Yehezkel, E., Carmeli, E.: Effect of physical therapy on muscle strength, respiratory muscles and functional parameters in patients with intensive care unit-acquired weakness. Clin. Respir. J. **9**(1), 1–6 (2015)
4. Hodgson, C., Stiller, K., Needham, D., et al.: Expert consensus and recommendations on safety criteria for active mobilization of mechanically ventilated critically ill adults. Crit. Care **18**(658), 1–18 (2014)
5. Morris, P., Berry, M., Files, C., et al.: Standardized rehabilitation and hospital length of stay among patients with acute respiratory failure: a randomized clinical trial. JAMA **315**(24), 2694–2702 (2016)
6. Schujmann, D., Lunardi, A., Fu, C.: Progressive mobility program and technology to increase the level of physical activity and its benefits in respiratory, muscular system, and functionality of ICU patients: study protocol for a randomized controlled trial. Trials **19**(274), 1–10 (2018)
7. Bailey, P., Thomsen, G., Spuhler, V., et al.: Early activity is feasible and safe in respiratory failure patients. Crit. Care Med. **35**(1), 139–145 (2007)
8. Morris, P., Goad, A., Thompson, C., et al.: Early intensive care unit mobility therapy in the treatment of acute respiratory failure. Crit. Care Med. **36**(8), 1–6 (2008)
9. Rose, L., Adhikari, N., Poon, J., Lease, D., McKim, D.: Cough augmentation techniques in the critically Ill: A Canadian national survey. Respir. Care **61**(10), 1360–1368 (2016)

10. Hopkins, R., Mitchell, L., Schafer, M., Thomsen, G., Link, M., Brown, S.: Implementing a mobility program to minimize post-intensive care syndrome. AACN Adv. Crit. Care **27**(2), 187–203 (2016)
11. Trees, D., Smith, J., Hockert, S.: Innovative mobility strategies for the patient with intensive care unit-acquired weakness: a case report. Phys. Ther. **9**(2), 237–247 (2013)
12. Ministry of Health: Evaluation of the National Situation of Intensive Care Units (2013). https://www.sns.gov.pt/wpcontent/uploads/2016/05/A3o-national-of-the-situation-of-units-of-care-intensive.pdf. Accessed 5 Oct 2018
13. Júnior, B., Martinez, B., Neto, M.: Braz. J. Intensive Ther. **26**(1), 65–70 (2014)
14. Cordeiro, M., Menoita, E.: Manual of Good Practices in Respiratory Rehabilitation: Concepts, Principles and Techniques, 1st edn. Luso-science, Loures (2014)

Public Health Initiatives

An Approach to Help Identifying Optimized Service Areas of Integrated Continuous Care Teams (ECCI): A Case Study in Alentejo - Portugal

Henrique Oliveira[1]([⊠]) [iD], Manuel José Lopes[2] [iD], César Fonseca[2] [iD],
Margarida Goes[3] [iD], David Mendes[2] [iD], and José Caeiro[4] [iD]

[1] Instituto de Telecomunicações,
IST Torre Norte - Piso 10, Av. Rovisco Pais, Lisbon, Portugal
hjmo@lx.it.pt
[2] Universidade de Évora, Escola Superior de Enfermagem de São João de Deus,
Évora, Portugal
[3] Instituto Politécnico de Beja, Escola Superior de Saúde, Beja, Portugal
[4] Instituto de Engenharia de Sistemas e Computadores,
INESC-ID, Lisbon, Portugal

Abstract. Objectives: To find how many elderly persons with 65 years and older are within a service area of each Integrated Continuous Care Team (Equipa de Cuidados Continuados Integrados - ECCI), with each area computed around the geographic location of each ECCI headquarters and encompassing all accessible streets that can be reached within a certain travel time spent on driving a vehicle.

Methods: A Geographic Information Systems (GIS) was developed, based on the geographical location of the elderly persons residing in the Alentejo region of Portugal (the study area), whose data was derived from the last National population census. Then, a network dataset model was also added to the GIS system, corresponding to a model of the real street network of the study area. After that, the GIS Service Area Solver was applied to determine all the ECCI service areas (one service area per each ECCI). Finally, the aim was to identify the several residing areas that overlap each ECCI service are, in order to compute the total number of elderlies residing within each ECCI service area.

Results: The number of elderly residents covered by ECCI teams for two ARS sub-regions increased, notably from 36725 to 40841 in relation to the ARS Alentejo Central, as well as from 19264 to 31429 in relation to the ARS Baixo Alentejo, when considering the ECCI service areas instead of the geographic division based on the Municipalities.

Discussion: The increase in elderly resident population that can be covered by ECCI teams in ARS Alentejo, based on the calculation of GIS services areas, was set in 14.6%.

Keywords: Integrated Continuous Care Teams · Elderly ·
Geographic Information Systems

© Springer Nature Switzerland AG 2019
J. García-Alonso and C. Fonseca (Eds.): IWoG 2018, CCIS 1016, pp. 349–358, 2019.
https://doi.org/10.1007/978-3-030-16028-9_31

1 Introduction

Regarding the provision of healthcare services to the Portuguese population by the National Healthcare System (Serviço Nacional de Saúde – SNS), the Portuguese main territory (not including the Madeira and Azores islands), is subdivided into five Regional Health Administrations (Administrações Regionais de Saúde – ARS), namely [1]: (i) ARS Norte; (ii) ARS Centro; (iii) ARS Lisboa e Vale do Tejo; (iv) ARS Alentejo; (v) ARS Algarve.

The study area adopted in this research paper was the ARS Alentejo, chosen because it is the one that present the major geographic area, as well as the one that shows the highest aging indexes in comparison to the others, notably: 72.9, 162.7 and 178.1 elderly person per 100 young, whose data were respectively derived from the three last National Population Census: 1991; 2001; 2011 [2]. Moreover, it is also the one that presents the lowest density population (only 24 residents per Km^2) [3].

Geographically, the ARS Alentejo is subdivided into four sub-regions, namely (see Fig. 1(a)): ACES of Alto Alentejo; ACES of Alentejo Central; ACES of Alentejo Litoral; ACES of Baixo Alentejo, where ACES means Groups of Health Centers. The entire administrative division of the ARS Alentejo, was extracted from the Official Administrative Cartography of the Portuguese Territory (Carta Administrativa Oficial de Portugal – CAOP), which was made publicly available by the Direcção Geral do Território (DGT), and it is represented in Fig. 1 [4].

Each ARS incorporates a certain number of Integrated Continuous Care Team (Equipa de Cuidados Continuados – ECCI), and according to the Portuguese Decree-law n° 1001/2006 from six of June, an ECCI is defined as "... *a multidisciplinary team, whose responsibility belongs to Primary Health Care (Cuidados de Saúde Primários – CSP) and social assistance entities, aiming to provide home services resulting from the full evaluation of, medical, nursing, rehabilitation and social support, or others types of cares, to persons in situations of functional dependence, terminal illness, or in convalescence process, whose situation does not require hospitalization but cannot move autonomously.*" [5]

According to the data listed in Table 1, obtained from the National Health Service, the ARS Alentejo comprises 47 Municipalities but only 37 ECCIs, with each of these ECCI teams been addressed to an Health Center located into a the respective Municipality [6]. Thus, the analysis of the data listed in the respective table below allows concluding that not all Municipalities present one ECCI, notably for the following ARS: Alentejo Central (missing 3 ECCIs); Baixo Alentejo (missing 7 ECCIs).

Table 1. Number of ECCIs and Municipalities per ARS Alentejo sub-region.

ARS Alentejo (sub-regions)	Number of ECCIs	Number of municipalities
Alto Alentejo	15	15
Alentejo Central	11	14
Alentejo Litoral	5	5
Baixo Alentejo	6	13

Based on the actual scenario of geographical distribution of ECCI teams in the ARS Alentejo (see Fig. 1 and also Table 1), the authors of the present study propose the following research question: Adopting the actual number of ECCI teams and their respective geographical distribution, especially in areas where the number of ECCIs is lower than the number of Municipalities, can their scope of geographic coverture be expanded, thus providing the effective delivery of cares to a more elderly residing population by those teams?

The next sections of this paper will describe the necessary procedure to allow for a proficient reply to the proposed research question.

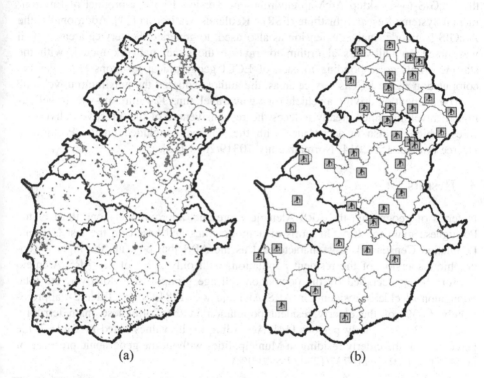

(a)   (b)

Fig. 1. The darker lines (see (a)) show the administrative division between ARS regions (Alto Alentejo (top); Alentejo Central (middle); Alentejo Litoral (bottom-left); Baixo Alentejo (bottom-right)), while the gray ones show the municipalities division included within each ARS sub-region, with the small gray areas (also in (a)) representing the geographical locations of the residing population. The green rectangular symbols in (b) show the geographic locations of all the ECCI headquarters identified within the ARS Alentejo sub-regions.

2 Methods

All the entire work described in this paper was developed under a geographic information system environment, which was composed by the following data layers: (i) demographic data (referred only number of the elderly residing in the ARS Alentejo), extracted from the National Population Census data of 2011, with reference to the polygon geo-information database designated "Base de Geográfica de Referenciação da Informação" (BGRI, see the top right link named «Importação (BGRI)» of the webpage listed on reference 7) [7, 8]; (ii) a street network model of the entire study area provided by ESRI-PORTUGAL [9]; (iii) the geographic location of all the ECCI teams provided from the National Health Service (SNS) [10]; (iv) part of the official administrative cartography of Portuguese territory (Carta Administrativa Oficial de Portugal – CAOP), the one corresponding to the administrative division of ARS Alentejo region, including the respective municipalities [4].

The Geographic Information System considered in this paper was developed under the ArcGIS-for-Desktop ArcMap environment, version 10.5.1, a product of Environmental Systems Research Institute (ESRI), Redlands, California [11]. Additionally, the ArcGIS Network Analyst extension as also used, to generate the service areas, which was based on Dijkstra's algorithm to traverse the street network model, with the starting points corresponding to each of ECCI geographical locations [12]. For the computation of the ECCIs service areas, the authors adopted the maximum travel time of 60 min spent on driving a vehicle (one way travel, thus 120 min tow-way travel), as higher travelling times greatly reduces the responsiveness of the effective delivery of cares, which is also in accordance with the statement included on the Portuguese Decree law no. 153/2014, Normative no. 10319/2014 [13].

3 Results

In terms of geography, the ARS Alentejo represents approximately one third of the Portuguese main territory. In terms of demographics and based on the last National Population Census [7], it is characterized as the ARS that presents the highest geographic dispersion of the resident population, with only 3.2% of the ARS Alentejo territory being occupied by the population (all age groups) [3]. Moreover, the total population of elderly residents in ARS Alentejo was 128427 (see Table 2), approximately 6.63% of the elderly resident population in the Portuguese main territory, notably 1937788 elderly persons [14]. According to the values listed in Table 2, the percentage of the elderly residing in Municipalities without the geographic presence of an ECCI is 13.03% (16737/128427 × 100%).

Table 2. Elderly persons residing in the ARS Alentejo sub-regions in Municipalities with/without ECCIs, whose data was extracted from the last National Population Census [7].

ARS Alentejo (sub-regions)	Total of elderly residents [7]	Elderly residents in Municipalities with ECCI	Elderly residents in Municipalities without ECCI
Alto Alentejo	32258	32258	0
Alentejo Central	40841	36725	4116
Alentejo Litoral	23443	23443	0
Baixo Alentejo	31885	19264	12621
Total	128427	111690	16737

Using the geographical locations of all the 37 ECCIs as input to the GIS Service Area Solver, developed under the ArcGIS ArcMap environment, as well as the complete street network or the entire ARS Alentejo region, and taking into account the maximum travel time of 60 min (one way) on driving a vehicle, as explained earlier in this paper, (see these geographic data represented in Fig. 2(a)), 37 service areas were computed, whose results are shown in Fig. 2(b).

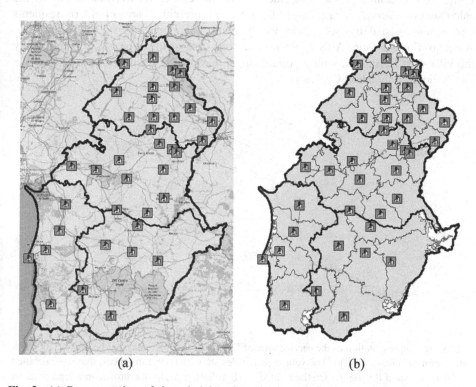

(a)   (b)

Fig. 2. (a) Representation of the administrative division of the four health sub-regions that compose the ARS Alentejo, superimposed to street network used as input data into the GIS Service Area Solver, to compute all the 37 ECCI service areas (one area per each ECCI). (b) Results of the 37 ECCIs service areas calculated by the GIS Service Area Solver, which was based on Dijkstra's algorithm to traverse the street network model. All the green rectangular symbols represent the geographical locations of ECCIs headquarters.

During the computation of these ECCIs service areas, some circumstances occurred, and some decisions had to be made by the authors. Moreover, the geographic boundaries of all the GIS service areas in an ARS sub-region were delimited by the boundary of the respective ARS sub-region.

In Fig. 3(a) two special cases were signaled. The first one, signaled by a rectangle in yellow color with label "1", represent a case of an area of elderly residents (shown in brown color) that is not completely overlaid by a service area, in this case corresponding to the service area calculated for the Serpa's ECCI. For cases similar to this one, the following rule was adopted by the authors: if the area of elderly residents (taken from the BGRI) presented an overlapping area more than its original half area with a given GIS service area, then the entire area of elderly residents will be addressed to that service area, which was the decision taken for the case labelled "1". Otherwise, if the overlapping area is lower than its original half area, the area of elderly residents is then addressed to the neighboring GIS service area. Regarding the case shown on Fig. 3(b-2), it exhibits an area of elderly residents that is not overlaid to any of the calculated GIS service areas. Cases like this one represent an area of elderly residents that is not assisted by any of the ECCI teams integrated into the ARS of Baixo Alentejo. For the entire ARS Alentejo, only one case of this type was found, namely the village of Barrancos, with a population of 456 elderly residents, according to the last National Population Census [15].

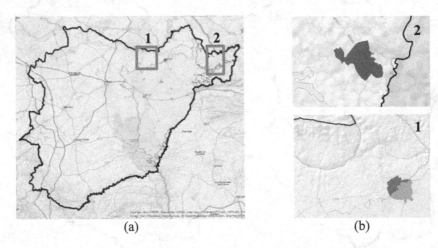

(a)   (b)

Fig. 3. (a) Representation of the service area of ECCI Serpa (blue area) that belongs to the ARS sub-region of Baixo Alentejo. The yellow rectangles show two circumstances, that were detailed on the right side if this figure. On the right side, (b-1, bottom-right) the brown area represents an elderly residing area that is not completed overlaid to the service area of ECCI Serpa, while (b-2, top-right) shows another elderly residing area (now depicted in red color), but in this case it is completely out of the range of any ECCI service area, since the 60 min of travel time (one-way) previously set on the GIS Service Area Solver was exceeded. (Color figure online)

Table 3 lists the results of the elderly population respectively to each ECCI team, based on the Municipalities geographic distribution, as well as based on the ECCI service areas computed by the GIS Service Area Solver. For the two ARS Alentejo sub-regions, notably: Alto Alentejo e Alentejo Litoral, the geographic distribution of the ECCI service areas is similar to the geographical distribution of the respective Municipalities, as can be seen by a visual comparison between the two results shown, respectively in Figs. 2(b) and 1(b). For these two ARS areas, there is no difference between the health care coverage provided to the elderly resident population, either based within the range of each Municipality or even in terms of the geographic distribution of each ECCI service areas.

Table 3. Elderly persons residing in the ARS Alentejo sub-regions based on Municipalities versus ECCI service areas, with demographic data extracted from the last National Population Census [7].

ARS (sub-regions)	Municipalities	ECCI Name	Elderly residents based on ECCI's Municipalities	Elderly residents in GIS Service Areas
Alto Alentejo	Alter do Chão	Alter do Chão	1189	1189
	Arronches	Arronches	1069	1069
	Avis	Avis	1406	1406
	Campo Maior	Campo Maior	1832	1832
	Castelo de Vide	Castelo de Vide	1129	1129
	Crato	Crato	1303	1303
	Elvas	Elvas	5103	5103
	Fronteira	Fronteira	960	960
	Gavião	Gavião	1685	1685
	Marvão	Marvão	1160	1160
	Monforte	Monforte	955	955
	Nisa	Nisa	2826	2826
	Ponte de Sor	Ponte de Sor	4246	4246
	Portalegre	Portalegre	5813	5813
	Sousel	Sousel	1582	1582
Total	–	–	*32258*	*32258*
Alentejo Central	Alandroal	–	–	*
	Arraiolos	Arraiolos	1932	3514
	Borba	Borba	1951	2359
	Estremoz	Estremoz	4082	3280
	Évora	Évora	11167	9893
	Montemor-o-Novo	Montemor-o-Novo	5003	4442
	Mora	–	–	*
	Mourão	–	–	*
	Portel	Portel	1773	2134
	Redondo	Redondo	1811	1900
	Reguengos de Monsaraz	Reguengos de Monsaraz	2614	4756
	Vendas Novas	Vendas Novas	2974	4008
	Viana do Alentejo	Viana do Alentejo	1467	1652
	Vila Viçosa	Vila Viçosa	1951	2903
Total	–	–	*36725*	*40841*
Alentejo Litoral	Alcácer do Sal	Alcácer do Sal	3280	3280
	Grândola	Grândola	3788	3788
	Odemira	Odemira	6835	6835
	Santiago do Cacém	Santiago do Cacém	7036	7036
	Sines	Sines	2504	2504
Total	–	–	*23443*	*23443*

(*continued*)

Table 3. (*continued*)

ARS (sub-regions)	Municipalities	ECCI Name	Elderly residents based on ECCI's Municipalities	Elderly residents in GIS Service Areas
Baixo Alentejo	Aljustrel	–	–	**
	Almodôvar	Almodôvar	2241	5128
	Alvito	–	–	**
	Barrancos	–	–	**
	Beja	Beja	7562	6943
	Castro Verde	–	–	**
	Cuba	–	–	**
	Ferreira do Alentejo	Ferreira do Alentejo	2210	5702
	Mértola	–	–	**
	Moura	–	–	**
	Ourique	Ourique	1759	1742
	Serpa	Serpa	4037	8474
	Vidigueira	Vidigueira	1455	3440
Total	–	–	*19264*	*31429*
Totals	–	–	111690	127971

For the case of Alentejo Central and Baixo Alentejo, two of ARS Alentejo sub-regions, it is clear that the number of elderly residents that are within the range of ECCI service areas is higher than the number of those that are within the scope of those teams based the Municipality division, respectively from 40841 to 36725 in relation to the ARS Alentejo Central, as well as from 31429 to 19264 in relation to the ARS Baixo Alentejo.

4   Discussion

The GIS Service Area Solver allowed calculating service areas of each ECCI team lager than the respective Municipalities, notably for the ARS sub-regions where the number of ECCI teams area lower in relation to the number of Municipalities that divide each ARS sub-region.

These larger ECCI service areas also allow an increased coverture of health care home services to a larger number of elderly resident population. Based on the results achieved and listed in Sect. 3 of this research paper, the number of elderly residents covered based on the calculated service areas, for the entire ARS Alentejo region, is 127971 (see Table 3, last line of fifth column). This results is lower that the number of elderly residents into the ARS Alentejo area, because one region, notably the village of Barrancos, with a population of 456 elderlies, was not reach by any ECCI service area, due to the limitation of 60 min of time on driven a vehicle.

The increasing in elderly resident population that can be covered by ECCI teams, based on the calculation of services areas, can be set in 14.6% {(127971-111690)/ 111690×100%}.

The symbol "*" in the fifth column of Table 3 means that the elderly population of the respective Municipality is included in another ECCI teams of the same ARS sub-region, in this case the ARS Alentejo Central. The same occurs regarding the symbol "**" in the same column of Table 3, with the respective elderly population being covered by one of the ECCI belonging to the ARS Baixo Alentejo. Due to de limitations of paper size, it is impossible to detail all these situations, which are represented and clearly identified in the GIS developed under the scope of this paper, because the BGRI database has approximately 19360 polygons (residential areas).

Taking into account all the results achieved in this research paper, the authors suggest the relocation of some ECCI teams, especially in ARS Baixo Alentejo, in order to ensure that none have routes longer than 60 min, an analysis that should be undertaken in a further research paper based on this topic. Moreover, the allocation in terms of the adequate number of health professionals to each ECCI team is an issue that should also be discussed in a future paper on the subject, since some ECCI teams may cover a larger number of elderly resident populations.

Acknowledgements. This work was supported by 4IE project (0045-4IE-4-P) funded by the Interreg V-A España-Portugal (POCTEP) 2014-2020 program.

Conflict of Interest. The authors declare that they have no conflicts of interest.

References

1. SNS. https://www.sns.gov.pt/institucional/entidades-de-saude/. Accessed 10 Sept 2018
2. PORDATA Homepage. https://www.pordata.pt/DB/Municipios/Ambiente+de+Consulta/ Tabela/5777883. Accessed 18 Oct 2018
3. INE, Population´s density (No./ km^2) by Place of residence (at the date of Census 2011) and Sex; Decennial. https://www.ine.pt/clientFiles/x-1WBENtzmzX6YSS7A7mznjM_20018.xls . Accessed 18 Oct 2018
4. DGT, Carta Administrativa Oficial de Portugal. http://www.dgterritorio.pt/cartografia_e_ geodesia/cartografia/carta_administrativa_oficial_de_portugal_caop/. Accessed 14 Oct 2018
5. ACSS. http://www2.acss.min-saude.pt/Portals/0/Orienta%C3%A7%C3%B5es%20para% 20a%20consti.pdf. Accessed 14 Oct 2018
6. ARS do Alentejo; Perfil Regional de Saúde. http://www.arsalentejo.min-saude.pt/arsalentejo/PlaneamentoEstrategico/Documents/Perfil_Regional_Saude.pdf. Accessed 12 Aug 2018
7. INE, BGRI Censos 2011. http://mapas.ine.pt/map.phtml. Accessed 25 Sept 2012
8. Santos, A.: A Infraestrutura de Dados Espaciais do Instituto Nacional de Estatística. Revista de Estudos Demográficos **51–52**, 55–71 (2013)
9. ESRI, New OpenStreetMap Vector Basemap Available. https://www.esri.com/arcgis-blog/ products/arcgis-living-atlas/mapping/new-osm-vector-basemap/. Accessed 07 Oct 2018
10. Serviço Nacional de Saúde. https://www.sns.gov.pt/sns/reforma-do-sns/cuidados-continuados-integrados-2/. Accessed 17 Sept 2018

11. ESRI-PORTUGAL, Homegape. https://dre.pt/pesquisa/-/search/55606457/details/normal?p_p_auth=fhLc2GFn. Accessed 12 May 2018

12. ESRI, ArcGIS Network Analyst. https://www.esri.com/en-us/arcgis/products/arcgis-network-analyst/overview. Accessed 17 Sept 2018

13. Diário da República Electrónico, DRE. https://dre.pt/pesquisa/-/search/55606457/details/normal?p_p_auth=fhLc2GFn. Accessed 17 Oct 2018

14. INE, Instituto Nacional de Estatística (Census 2011). https://www.ine.pt/clientFiles/x-1WBENtzmzX6YSS7A7mznjM_16349.xls. Accessed 17 Sept 2018

15. INE, Instituto Nacional de Estatística, Village of Barrancos, (Census 2011). https://www.ine.pt/clientFiles/x-1WBENtzmzX6YSS7A7mznjM_28394.xls. Accessed 17 Sept 2018

The Effect of Religious Identity on Optimism Across the Lifespan

Lisete dos Santos Mendes Mónico[✉][iD]
and Valentim António Rodrigues Alferes[iD]

Faculty of Psychology and Educational Sciences,
University of Coimbra, Coimbra, Portugal
lisete.monico@fpce.uc.pt

Abstract. *Background*: It is acknowledged that religious traditions prescribe not only a framework of values but also a set of guidelines for personal life. Furthermore, people often report that their system of values endorses or are influenced by their religious trends.

Objective: Given the changes in religious identity resulting from secularization and the growth of religious minorities in Portugal, this paper investigates the effect of Portuguese religious identity (minority versus majority) in the relationship between religiosity and optimism across the lifespan, given the mediation by individual's life satisfaction.

Method: We conducted an empirical study, based on a self-report questionnaire to 329 members of religious minorities in Portugal and 408 Portuguese Catholics (major religion in Portugal).

Results: We found a positive correlation between religiousness and optimism in both majority and minority religious groups. However, the mediation effect of life satisfaction was only significant among Portuguese religious majority; in Portuguese religious minorities religiosity had a direct effect on optimism. A correspondence factor analysis showed mainly that participants with high levels of religiosity and optimism have a minority religious identity and high life satisfaction.

Conclusions: The establishment of a self-regulating system is discussed as are beliefs and religious practices as perpetuators. Confrontation with personal frailty, powerlessness and fear were discussed as predetermining factors to disembedding, as described by Giddens (1991, 1997), and factors that facilitates the engagement in a religious system, while reembedding occurs with the individual regaining self-control, as a outcome of divine factors prone to optimism.

Keywords: Religiosity · Optimism · Religious identity · Lifespan · Life satisfaction

1 Introduction

"Religion is a powerful social force" (McCullough and Willoughby 2009, p. 1). It performs vital functions in such a way that it becomes in separable from human existence. Considering the analysis of the roles of religiosity and its impact on health,

© Springer Nature Switzerland AG 2019
J. García-Alonso and C. Fonseca (Eds.): IWoG 2018, CCIS 1016, pp. 359–377, 2019.
https://doi.org/10.1007/978-3-030-16028-9_32

risk behavior sand well-being as classic (v.g., Buck et al. 2009; Carver et al. 2010; Dezutter et al. 2006; Kirchner and Patiño 2010; Koenig et al. 2001; Luquis et al. 2012; Mónico et al. 2016), research about the impact of religiosity on optimism are less well understood. Given the influence of the secularization boundaries in current religious beliefs and practices, we consider that it is important to distinguish the effect of religious identity in the association between religiosity and optimism. Thus, this study aims to evaluate the existence of a relationship between religiosity and optimism, differentiating it according to religious identity, minority or majority in Portugal, and analyze the role of life satisfaction in this association.

1.1 Religiosity

It is understood that religiosity is the individual level of commitment to beliefs, doctrines and practices of a religion (Barker and Warburg 1998; Mookherjee 1994). Counterpart expression of religious experience (Geerts 1990), concerns the extent to which an individual believes, follows, and practices a religious doctrine, considering its two regulating poles: Beliefs and rites. In the classic work of William James (1902/1985), religiosity is defined as "the feelings, acts, and experiences of individual men in their solitude, so far as they apprehend themselves to stand in relation to whatever they may consider the divine" (p. 31). This can be introduced either in a traditional way, in a formal and non-reflective way that follows the customs, or in an individual way, looking for answers to questions, needs, ideas, and ideals (Grom 1994).

Both religion and religiosity have an expression resulting in spirituality, namely, the recognition of an on-material force materialized in the search for meaning, unity, and human transcendence (Hill and Pargament 2003; Pargament 1997). The concepts of spirituality and religion share a considerable overlap (Taylor 1998). Although many authors refer to religiosity using the term spirituality, the first differs from the latter by reference to a specific doctrinal system of worship of a god and/or other deities, shared with a group (Koenig 1997, 1998; Yuen 2007).

1.2 Optimism

Also regarded as a belief, optimism refers to expectations of good outcomes (Carver et al. 2010): "optimists are people who expect good experiences in the future. Pessimists are people who expect bad experiences" (Carver and Scheier 2000, p. 31). The tendency for the positive, the expectation of future success, and the explanation given to negative events generally characterize optimism, detected in such diverse areas of life as health, academic or professional achievement, interpersonal relationships, and security (Alarcon et al. 2013; Hoorens 1994; McKenna 1993; Peterson 2000; Segerstrom 2007; Simonds 2005). The positive expectations are usually generalized and stable, demonstrating that people consider themselves, generally, slightly happier than others; they show appositive asymmetry in respect to distribution of positive experiences, whereas an opposite asymmetry for the experiencing of negative events (Alarcon et al. 2013; Carver et al. 2010; Scheier and Carver 1985, 1987, 1992; Weinstein 1980, 1983, 1984, 1989).

Regarding to the subject, when we speak about "stable tendency to believe that good instead of bad situations will happen" (Scheier and Carver 1985, p. 219), we refer to the absolute or dispositional optimism, that is, to the wide spread expectations of achieving good outcomes in the individual confrontation with problems in important life areas, differentiating from social or situational optimism (Carver et al. 2010; Hjelle et al. 1996; Fischer and Chalmers 2008). Having influence on the set of expectations, in a stable and consistent way across situations, this kind of optimism is seen as a personality trait, a disposition or attitude that positive outcomes will arise for the individual (Carver and Scheier 2000; Scheier and Carver 1985).

The conception of dispositional optimism, dealing with general event sand not focusing on specific perceived differences between the self and the others (Chang 1998, 2000; Scheier and Carver 1985), emerges as the most present in, in concomitance with the observation that people predict, in comparison with others, that they will experience a greater number of positive situations (Alarcon et al. 2013; Peeters et al. 2001; Shepperd et al. 2002). This trend is known as comparative optimism (Weinstein 1980, 1984, 1989).

1.3 Religious Identity and Secularization

In no period of human history was there only one religion. Religious groups are sought for several reasons, summarized in search for meaning, solutions and identities, as also in control, comfort, and life transformation (Craig 2007; Martin 2007).

If social identity corresponds to that "part of the individual's self-concept which derives from the recognition of membership to one (or several) social(s) group(s), along with the emotional significance and value attached to that membership" (Tajfel 1981, p. 63), religious identity is the part of the self-concept that coming from the membership of a religious group (Closs et al. 2013).

To understand religious behavior, it is essential to consider the role of religious groups. Particularly in the western world, religion as an institution was moved from its central role and lost hegemony (Berger 1999; Haught 1995; Martin 1996; Vanderwoerd 2011). The secularization thesis states that the beliefs and religious practices become more individualized, fragmented, privatized, and personal (Ecklund et al. 2008; Martelli 1995; Reynolds 1995; Rodrigues 2004; Wallis and Bruce 1991). The concept of religion, mimetic associated to the institutions that represent a doctrinal tradition of the world, a sacred cosmovision legitimated a priori, stops to predominate (Heelas and Woodhead 2000; Hervieu-Léger 1997; Taylor 1998). However, secularization does not state a process of religion deficit, but rather the institutionalization and influence of tradition and State reduction, giving freedom for religious option and expression. Therefore, the religious tendency of human beings persists. The concept of "invisible religion" arises (Luckmann 1967), because now religion is not being more recognized and manifested in institutions, but transferred to the invisible and autonomous individual privacy. The "privatization of religion, away of 'anthropomorphic religion' occurs, where the religious becomes purely private, an individual choice among the many offerings available" (Rodrigues 2004, p. 44).

1.4   Religious Minorities in the Post-modern Period

As a social, cultural, and historical phenomenon, religious movements find themselves in continuous transformation (Deneulin and Rakodi 2011; Stausberg 2009). Portugal is not exception to this reality (Cabral et al. 2000; Mónico et al. 2010, 2011). The search for the spiritual and the emotional religiosity characterizes social identity of religious minorities. Religion becomes progressively more performative, symbolic and subjective (Mónico et al. 2010, 2011).

In the pluralistic and secularized Western world, it is possible to see a transmutation of the monopoly of a unique religion to a religious pluralism (Cabral et al. 2000; Deneulin and Rakodi 2011; Rodrigues 2004). Here we find that the approach to life is in no way related to the traditional religious manifestations (Stausberg 2009). The increase in these new movements potentiates the decline in religious compromise of people, leading to associations and identities that are progressively ephemeral, and that sometimes, convert religion into a type of pragmatic utilitarianism (Taylor 1998). There are cases, however, in which the religious experience of minority groups develops a routine, an institutional, doctrinal and liturgical adaptation over time, leading to a process of expansion (Grigoropoulou and Chryssochoou 2011; Mariz 2004). Sometimes the religion is used to define the boundaries of group identities and relationships, to include or exclude people and to enhance or block cooperation (Lichterman 2008).

Given the multiplicity of religions, the individual is led to follow a combination of religions (Noddings 2008), consistent with the contemporary notion of choice, given that in post-secular societies, the religion and the domains of social life are dissociated (Caputo 2007; Hervieu-Léger 1997; Martellii 1995). When a ritual, a symbolism, and an institutional structure are radically modified, a new religious movement emerges (Barker and Warburg 1998), whose members easily enter or leave according to their needs or personal wishes (Mariz 2004). Consequently, religious minorities become unequal in theological and even sociological terms (Mónico and Edições Vercial 2011).

1.5   Aims and Hypotheses

In the search for a model that analyzes the relationship between religiosity and optimism, we sought to know the reality in which religious phenomena manifest and life satisfaction of Portuguese citizens with a minority religious identity, in comparison with Portuguese Catholics (majority religious identity), across the lifespan.

There is a long tradition of research that points for the connection between religiosity and optimism (v.g. W. James, Freud, Weber, Durkheim, Allport; Mattis et al. 2003; Mónico et al. 2010, 2011). Despite the posited link between religiosity and optimism, we unknown literature that analyzes the link between religiosity and optimism attending the differential effect of religious identity.

In light of the current state of lack of definition of the role of minority religions in Portugal, we sought to analyse how optimism is supported by religiosity (Mónico 2012), given the differential effect of religious identity and the mediation through life satisfaction. We also don´t know how life satisfaction is related with these three variables. Given the above review of research, we formulated two hypotheses. The first one (H1) is based on the supposition that the search to religiosity may be a powerful coping strategy in the promotion of optimism, mainly in adverse life situations in which the individuals, realistically, could be led to pessimism (Chang 2000; Closs et al. 2013; Norem 2000). The H1 states that there is a positive relationship between religiosity and the individuals' optimism.

The knowledge obtained from the interviews with religious minority group leaders in Portugal (see Mónico et al. 2010) led us to the perception that integration into religious minorities essentially occurs in difficult and sometimes extremely painful life situations. Despite the diversity in each of these situations, individual's self-confidence to deal with the problems seems reduced. In these circumstances, religiosity may function as a support for personal optimism, although this link is mediated by life satisfaction. Our second hypothesis (H2) states that the link between religiosity and optimism is mediated by the self-perception of life satisfaction. By life satisfaction we consider the cognitive dimension of subjective well-being, namely, the psychological balance that each individual makes about his own life based on his unique experience of the world (Clemente et al. 2012; Mónico et al. 2016; Parreira et al. 2016). Effect of nurses' mobilization in satisfaction at work and turnover: An empirical study in the hospital setting. BMC Health Services Research, 16(3), 40–41. https://doi.org/10.1186/s12913-016-1423-5). Subjective well-being refers to "an individual's own assessment of his or her own life — not the judgments of experts — and includes satisfaction (both global and satisfaction with specific domains), pleasant affect, and low negative affect" (Diener et al. 2004, p. 189).

2 Method

2.1 Sample

Our sample in composed by 737 participants, aged 18 to 77 years old. 329 (32.4%) are members of religious minority groups in Portugal (Christians but not Catholics) and 408 (67.6%) are national citizens belonging to Catholicism (major religion in Portugal). Among males (n = 237; 32.2% of the overall sample), 127 (17.2%) are members of minority religious groups and 110 (15.0%) are Catholic. For females (n = 500; 67.8% of the overall sample), 187 (25.4%) are members of minority religious groups and 313 (42.5%) are Catholic.

Considering the educational level, with the 1st cycle of Basic Education we found 125 participants (17.7%), followed by 79 (11.2%) with the 2nd cycle, 224 (31.8%) with the 3rd cycle, and 84 (11.9%) with higher education. Most of the participants are single or married (n = 636; 90.6%), with only 38 respondents (5.4%) divorced, separated or widowed.

2.2 Measures

We developed the CROP Questionnaire (Portuguese acronym for Religious Beliefs, Optimism and Pessimism), which measures were analysed with reliability and factorial analyses in Mónico et al. (2010, 2011). The measures are classified into three indexes: Religiosity, Life Satisfaction and Optimism.

For the first index – Religiosity – we considered the Likert questions retrieved from Cabral et al. (2000) Belief in God (BIG; 1 = never believed to 4 = always believed) and Religiosity level (REL; 1 = absolutely not religious to 7 = extremely religious). We built the dummy measures (0 = does not apply to me; 1 = applies to me) Attitudes and religious practices (ARP; 16 items; Kuder Richardson reliability coefficient KR-20 = .93), Types of religious beliefs (TBE –19 items, KR-20 reliability = .82), Approach to God in moments of happiness and easiness (AGH – 3 items, KR-20 reliability coefficient = .87) and Approach to God in moments of difficulty and uncertainty (AGD –7 items, KR-20reliability coefficient = .83), all analyses in Mónico (2010, 2011).

Life Satisfaction index was measured using the Life Satisfaction Rating (Neugarten et al. 1961); each item was rated by yes or no (scored 1 or 0). Additionally, we considered the Likert questions Self-evaluation of the current life (1 = very bad to 5 = very good) and Experiencing hard life situations (EHS; 1 = never to 5 = constantly; reversal score), as well as the dummy measures Favorability of the current personal experiences (FCE –15 items, KR-20 reliability coefficient = .84, adapted from Mónico 2003), all psychometric analysed in Mónico (2010, 2011).

For the Optimism index, we considered the following measures: a) Estimate of positive future occurrences (EPO; adapted from Wiseman 2006; 24 items, measured from 0 to 100%, Cronbach α = .76); b) two factors of the scale Luck profile (Wiseman 2006, evaluated from 1 – strongly disagree to 5 – strongly agree):Intuition-propulsive action (IPA; 3 items, alpha reliability coefficient = .73) and Expectancy-optimism (EOP; 2 items, r = .30); and c) two dummy measures adapted from Scheier et al. (1994): Optimism in times of happiness and ease (OHE; 3 items, KR-20 reliability coefficient = .68) and Optimism in times of difficulties and uncertainty (EPO; 5 items, KR-20 reliability coefficient = .71).

2.3   Procedures

The data was collected in the Centre of Portugal. We conducted a preliminary contact with religious leaders (priests, pastors, and holy fathers), in order to collect information on the topic under study and explain the purpose of our research. After obtaining consent of the majority and minority religious leaders, the administration of the CROP Questionnaire occurred at the end of the religious cults. The procedure adopted was the same. The presentation of the research aims (to study the religiosity in everyday-life) was made orally by the researcher, in the presence of the religious leader of each group. After guaranteeing the anonymity and confidentiality of the answers, we asked for informed and voluntary consent of the members of each group to fill in the questionnaire.

3   Results

3.1   Test of Hypothesis 1

Hypothesis 1 points out the existence of a positive correlation between religiosity and optimism. We resorted to the measures of Religiosity and Optimism indexes and we proceeded to the canonical correlation (Härdle and Simar 2012). We found statistically significant linear correlations between the set of measures of each index: rcanonical = .75, Wilks' Λ = .25, $F(208, 3855) = 2.71$, $p < .001$. The study of the predictive skills of the measures that comprise the index of religiosity reinforces this outcome. By standardizing and grouping the measures of optimism in one unique index, making it the criteria variable, the analysis of multiple regression points to a predictive effect of the measures of the index Religiosity: the association obtained is rmultiple = .486, $F(14, 183) = 4.04$, $p < .001$. We concluded that the correlation between the measures of the indexes of religiosity and optimism is positive, indicating that more intense religiosity levels are associated with stronger levels of optimism. Thus, we found empirical support for the Hypothesis 1.

3.2   Test of Hypothesis 2

We build a path model, considering the prediction of optimism by religiosity and the mediation of this link by life satisfaction. After specifying the measure model, we proceeded to the estimation and evaluation of the degree of adjustment, using AMOS 20.0 program.

The dependency relationships, developed between the latent constructs and observed variables, were based on the Hypothesis 1, that points to a positive relationship between religiosity and optimism. We build a path diagram and we specified the model (Byrne 2010; Kline 2005; Schumacker and Lomax 1996), fixing the residual variance at zero (Hatcher 1996). Figure 1 shows a non-recursive model of the proposed measure, where the latent constructs and the observable variables are seen, as well as the respective structural and directional links.

Table 1 shows the outcomes of normality and exploratory factor analysis (see factorial loadings from the Principal Component Analysis, Varimax rotation). The solution found pointed to the existence of three factors, corresponding to the latent variables of the proposed model: religiosity, optimism and life satisfaction. The factorial loadings are high, comprising between .46 and .92 (Bentler 1990; Osborne and Costello 2009; Schumacker and Lomax 1996). The reliability indexes – standardized alphas and composite reliability (CR) – are acceptable (CR > .40), allowing us to consider (together with the factorial loadings of the subjacent variables of each construct) that there is convergent validity (see Table 2). With regards to the extracted variance (EV), the more explanatory latent variable concerns to religiosity of Catholics (majority religious identity), followed by life satisfaction, and, lastly, optimism (see Table 2).

The exploratory PCA was followed by a confirmatory one, taking into account the convergent and discriminant validities (Byrne 2010; Luque 2000). Regarding the latter, we consider to have a good index, in the sense that the average score calculated from

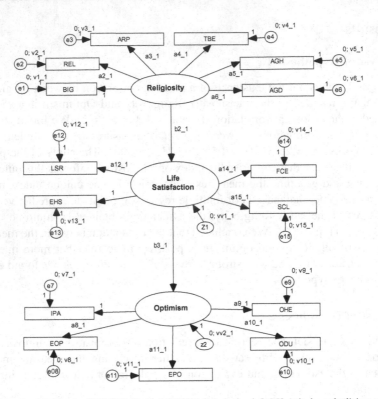

Legend: *Measures of Religiosity:* [BIG] Belief in God; [REL] Religiosity level; [ARP] Attitudes and religious practices; [TBE] Type of religious beliefs; [AGH] Approach to God in times of happiness and ease; [AGD] Approach to God in times of difficulty and uncertainty;
Measures of Life Satisfaction: [LSR] Life Satisfaction Rating; [FCE] Favorability of the current personal experience. [SCL] Self-evaluation of current life; [EHS] Experiencing hard life situations (reversed score);
Measures of Optimism: [OHE] Optimism in times of happiness and ease; [ODU] Optimism in times of difficulties and uncertainty; [EPO] Estimate of positive future occurrences; [IPA] Luck profile, Intuition-propulsive action; [EOP] Luck profile, Expectancy-optimism.

Fig. 1. Path model for exploratory structural model testing religiosity and optimism mediated through life satisfaction

the extracted variances from the variables in analysis (.21 and .30, respectively, for religious identity majority and minority) is higher than the values of the correlation coefficients between each pair of constructs (Bollen 1989). Given the reference values of the goodness of fit (Bentler 1990; Byrne 2010; Schumacker and Lomax 1996), we concluded that the proposed model is adjusted: CMIN/DF(188) = 2.17 (*p* < .001), NFI = .788, CFI = .868, and RMSEA = .050.

The outcomes obtained in the structural model are graphically represented in Fig. 2. Excluding the multiple regression coefficient between religiosity and life satisfaction for the minority religious identity, the remaining coefficients βy e λx are all significant (*p* < .01) and positive.

The direct, indirect and total effects between the three latent variables of the model are presented in Table 3. The religious identity of the Portuguese citizens affects the

Table 1. Exploratory factor analysis and normality: Factorial loadings, asymmetry and kurtosis for the religious identity (RI) majority and minority.

Latent constructs	Observable variables*	Factorial loadings			Normality			
		F1	F2	F3	RI Majority		RI Minority	
					Asymmetry	Kurtosis	Asymmetry	Kurtosis
Religiosity (C1)	[ARP] Attitudes and religious practices	.915	−.058	.004	−0.70	−1.05	−0.73	1.47
	[AGD] Approach to God in times of difficulty and uncertainty	.883	−.062	.025	−0.50	−1.30	−1.70	3.84
	[BIG] Belief in God	.828	.064	−.090	−1.24	−0.06	−1.40	2.71
	[REL] Religiosity level	.760	.023	−.028	−0.82	−0.23	−0.91	0.31
	[AGH] Approach to God in times of happiness and ease	.722	.004	−.161	−0.74	1.19	−0.11	0.39
	[TBE] Type of religious beliefs	.528	−.027	.305	0.69	0.55	0.44	0.05
Life Satisfaction (C2)	[LSR] Life Satisfaction Rating	.182	.721	,238	0.47	−0.66	0.17	−0.68
	[FCE] Favorability of the current personal experience	.026	.689	.025	−0.31	0.78	−0.23	0.06
	[SCL] Self-evaluation of current life	−.078	.614	.063	0.30	1.24	0.99	0.29
	[EHS] Experiencing hard life situations*	−.094	.594	−.271	0.88	3.33	−0.18	−0.40
Optimism (C3)	[EPO] Estimate of positive future occurrences	.230	.067	.683	0.50	0.26	0.20	−0.08
	[OHE] Optimism in times of happiness and ease	.031	.052	.593	−0.94	0.95	−0.78	−0.17
	[EOP] Luck profile, Expectancy-optimism	−.251	.050	.554	−0.63	1.35	−0.59	0.50
	[ODU] Optimism in times of difficulties and uncertainty	.019	.151	.467	−0.72	0.26	−0.89	1.50
	[IPA] Luck profile, Intuition-propulsive action	−.218	.400	.460	−0.13	−0.11	−0.29	0.24

* Reversed score

links between the three latent variables. If for majority religious identity (Portuguese Catholics) the latent variable Life Satisfaction has a mediator effect of the link between Religiosity and Optimism ($\beta C1C2 = .13$ e $\beta C2C3 = .87, p < .001$), for the Portuguese with a minority religious identity the effect is null ($\beta C1C2 = .06$, p = .41); However,

Table 2. Confirmatory factor analysis: Ratios F, standardized alphas (αs), extracted variance (EV) and composed reliability (CR).

Latent constructs	F		α_s		EV (%)		CR	
Religious identity (RI):	RI Majority	RI Minority	RI Majority	RI Minority	RI Majority	RI Minority	RI Majority	RI Minority
Religiosity (C1)	426.98***	2780.18***	.869	.722	.525	.280	.837	.630
Life Satisfaction (C2)	3482.89***	2714.35***	.417	.444	.228	.214	.458	.432
Optimism (C3)	208.61***	339.45***	.427	.506	.140	.139	.418	.432

*** $p < .001$

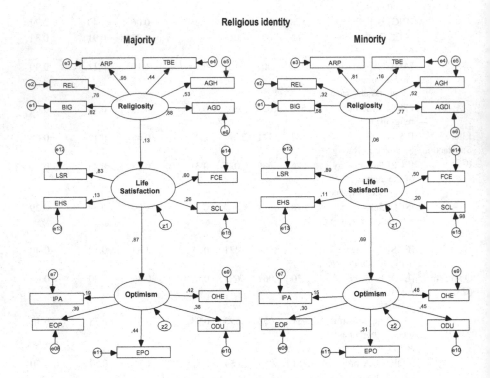

Religious identity

Legend: *Measures of Religiosity:* [BIG] Belief in God; [REL] Religiosity level; [ARP] Attitudes and religious practices; [TBE] Type of religious beliefs; [AGH] Approach to God in times of happiness and ease; [AGD] Approach to God in times of difficulty and uncertainty;
Measures of Life Satisfaction: [LSR] Life Satisfaction Rating; [FCE] Favorability of the current personal experience. [SCL] Self-evaluation of current life; [EHS] Experiencing hard life situations (reversed score);
Measures of Optimism: [OHE] Optimism in times of happiness and ease; [ODU] Optimism in times of difficulties and uncertainty; [EPO] Estimate of positive future occurrences; [IPA] Luck profile, Intuition-propulsive action; [EOP] Luck profile, Expectancy-optimism.

Fig. 2. Path models for the association between religiosity and optimism mediated through life satisfaction: Standardized regression coefficients for the multigroup structural model

the positive link between life satisfaction and optimism are maintained ($\beta C2C3 = .69$, $p < .001$), although slightly lower. We concluded that the self-perception of life satisfaction mediates the positive association between religiosity and optimism only for Portuguese citizens with a majority religious identity. For the Portuguese citizens with

Table 3. Estimates of direct, indirect and total effects: Standardized multiple regression coefficients

Religious Identity (RI):	Religiosity (C1)						Life Satisfaction (C2)					
	RI Majority			RI Minority			RI Majority			RI Minority		
Effects:	Direct	Indirect	Totals	Direct	Indirect	Totals	Direct	Indirect	Totals	Direct	Indirect	Totals
Optimism (C3)	.00	.03	.03	.00	.41***	.41***	.87***	.00	.87***	.69***	.00	.69***
Life Satisfaction (C2)	.13**	.00	.13**	.06	.00	.06	–	–	–	–	–	–

** $p < .01$ *** $p < .001$

a religious minority identity, an increase in religiosity directly promotes optimism, and this link is not influenced by the self-perception of their life satisfaction. Hypothesis 2, which refers to the mediation of the link between religiosity and optimism by life satisfaction, only found empirical support for the Portuguese citizens with a majority religious identity, in other words, for the Portuguese Catholics.

The analysis of the standardized multiple regression coefficients in Table 3 allows us to corroborate the Hypotheses 2 for the participants with a majority religious identity. For the minorities, the religiosity has a significant effect on optimism (see indirect effects), not being necessary individuals are satisfied with their lives.

3.3   Religiosity and Optimism in Relation to Life Satisfaction: Correspondence Factor Analysis

Considering the mediation effect of life satisfaction, we intended to analyze a structure of associations between this index and the levels of religiosity and optimism in participants with religious identities minority or majority. We established two aggregate variables:

(1) Religious Identity (RI) x Life Satisfaction (LS): RI majority (RI maj) vs. RI minority (RI min) x LS low (Life Satisfaction Rating <30 percentile), medium (from 30 to 70 percentile), and high (>70 percentile); 6 categories: RI min_LS low, RI min_LS medium, RI min_LS high, RI maj_LS low, RI maj_LS medium, and RI maj_LS high;
(2) Optimism (OPT) xReligiosity (REL): OPT low (scores below average in the Optimism measures) vs. OPT high (scores above average in the Optimism measures) x REL low (scores below average in the Religiosity measures) vs. REL high (scores above average in the Religiosity measures);4 categories: OPT low_REL low, OPT low_REL high, OPT high _REL low, and OPT high _REL high.

We proceeded to a correspondence factor analysis (symmetric normalization). Of the factorizations, through the table of contingencies of life satisfaction in the two religious identities, using the low and high levels of religiosity and optimism, three dimensions were extracted, accounted for the total amount of inertia: 70.4% for the first, 23.3% for the second and only 6.3% for the third, $\chi^2(15) = 47.66$, p < .001. Retaining the first two, we obtain a two axes solution, whose outcomes are presented in Table 4 and Fig. 3.

Table 4. Correspondence factor analysis: Projection in two dimensions of Religious Identity (Majority-Maj vs. Minority-Min) and Life Satisfaction (low, medium, and high), and Optimism (OPT low vs. high) and Religiosity (REL low vs. high)

Religious Identity (RI)	Life Satisfaction (LS)					
	Dimension 1			Dimension 2		
	LS Low	LS Medium	LS High	LS Low	LS Medium	LS High
Majority (RI maj)	1.03	0.73	−0.15	−0.10	0.02	0.67
Minority (RI min)	−0.05	−0.37	−0.99	−0.56	−0.81	0.11
Optimism (OPT)	Religiosity (REL)			
	Dimension 1		Dimension 2	
	REL low	REL high	REL Low	REL High
Low (OPT low)	0.76	−0.06	0.05	−0.75
High (OPT high)	0.58	−0.79	0.68	0.28

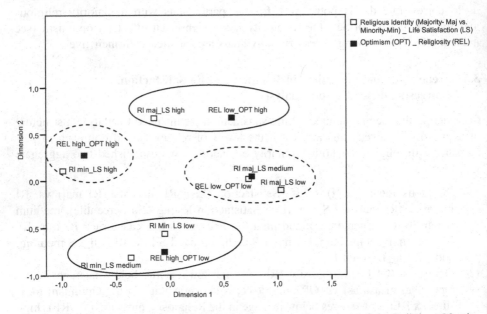

Fig. 3. Correspondence factor analysis: Projection in two dimensions of the Religious Identity (Majority-Maj vs. Minority-Min) and Life Satisfaction (low, medium, and high), and the Optimism (OPT low vs. high) and Religiosity (REL low vs. high) levels

As we can see, participants with high levels of religiosity and optimism are grouped in the negative pole of Dimension 1, integrated in the religious identity minority (RI min), who are satisfied with their lives. These participants oppose themselves to those who belong to the religious majority (RI maj), have a low or medium life satisfaction, and low levels of religiosity and optimism. Given Dimension 2, the negative pole reflects the minority members who show high religiosity and low optimism and have a low or medium life satisfaction. In the positive pole, we find the participants who belong to the majority religious group and that present low levels of religiosity and high levels of optimism and life satisfaction.

4 Discussion and Conclusions

There is some evidence that some particular aspects of social context may promote or mitigate optimism (Mattis et al. 2003; Mónico et al. 2010, 2013). The primary purpose of this study was to examine the potential prediction of religiosity and life satisfaction attending to one of them: The religious identity of Portuguese citizens. Portugal constitutes a mono-religious society that has gradually become religiously diverse in the last years.

In this article it was seen that a more intense religiosity is associated to higher optimism, providing empirical support to Hypothesis 1. The differentiation in terms of antecedent and consequent was evaluated in the multiple regression analysis and in the structural model, in which we expressed the possibility of anticipating optimism levels from individuals' religiosity.

Given the declining hegemony of the Catholic religion, concomitantly with dominant religions in other societies, we have seen in Portugal a growing pluralism in religious beliefs, expressed in new doctrines associated with new proselytisms, new religious markets, new adherents, and new conversions. The current religious revival is reinforced by the individuals unsatisfaction with life (Vásquez-Borau 2008), which led us to assign to life satisfaction in this research the role of mediator in religiosity–optimism link (Mónico et al. 2016).

In recent decades, researchers in positive psychology have come to recognize the self-regulation as an important aspect of several attributes of self, such as resilience, adaptation adversity (Bosacki et al. 2011; Higgins et al. 1999), or even the spiritual and religious development (McCullough and Boker 2007; McCullough and Willoughby 2009). We consider that individuals can use beliefs and religious behaviours as a self-regulatory mechanism, which confers them stability and promotes optimism. As McCullough and Boker (2007) refer, "to a certain point, spiritual and religious changes can also be caused by self-regulatory processes that are intrinsic to the functioning of the individual" (p. 385). The importance that each one gives to religion is, in some way, ruled by the functioning of an internal orientation system that seeks to find a balance level.

Hypothesis 2, which announces the mediation of self-perception of life satisfaction in the relation between religiosity and optimism, was only supported in Portuguese citizens with a majority religious identity: Religiosity only anticipates a higher level of optimism when they are satisfied with their lives. For Portuguese citizens with a minority religious identity, the mediator effect of life satisfaction was insignificant, since religiosity had a direct implication on optimism. It seems that in the Portuguese citizens with a majority religious identity, the link religiosity-optimism works manly through the self-perception of life satisfaction, opposing itself to the performing mechanism in Portuguese citizens with a minority religious identity, in which religiosity is expressed as a vehicle of optimism, regardless of how much they are satisfied with their lives at a given time.

The correspondence analysis of the religious identity and low and high levels of religiosity and optimism contrasts Portuguese members of religious minorities with high life satisfaction and religiosity and optimism levels with Catholics citizens, with low religiosity and optimism and medium life satisfaction. At last, minority religious members very religious and slightly optimistic, with low or medium life satisfaction, contrast with majority religious members with low religiosity, high optimism and life satisfaction.

Giddens (1991, 1997) draws attention to the disorientation of individuals that currently form social organizations, as if they found themselves involved in a number of situations that do not fully understand. For the author, in modern societies, time and space do not blend, as social space is no longer confined by the set of boundaries of space in which people move. Given this distinction, the events are ever changing and occur at a fast rhythm; there are feelings of discomfort, fear and anxiety, consequences that Giddens called disembedding, in other words, "dislocation of social relationships of local interaction contexts and their restructuring by means of undefined extensions of time-space" (Giddens 1991, p. 29). Thus, the need to re-establish balance occurs, through which individuals develop mechanisms that seek to acquire security and reduce anxiety, by getting closer to other people or (religious) groups. These mechanisms, which Giddens calls reembedding, consist in "a way to establish trust in reliability and integrity of familiar people" (p. 90).

In order to restore individuals' cognitive balance, between the reembedding actions, we signaled the search for new religious movements and/or a new religious understanding. The individual fragility against the mundane adversities is anchored in divine factors that promote optimism, necessary to re-establish self-confidence and self-esteem. A cycle is established, that begins with a feeling of impotence, fear and cognitive imbalance (disembedding), followed by an optimism based on divine intercessions which come from these new religious cults or from these new religious understanding. Consequently, the self-confidence in overcoming the adversities of life is re-established, now basing itself on a new doctrinal system (reembedding), which contributes directly to the individual optimism in minority religions, contrasting with the indirect effect felt by the majority, mediated by life satisfaction.

Limitations and Future Directions

This study has some limitations. First, religiosity, life satisfaction, and optimism were paper-pencil self-reported measures, prone to social desirability (Roberts 2007). Second, this study involved cross-sectional and correlational data, thus limiting our ability to draw causal inferences. Upcoming studies should include longitudinal data, to further establish temporal ordering and causality concerning the relation between religiosity and optimism. Third, it is necessary to enlarge the sample to other religious minorities, in order to guarantee the representativeness of the sample in terms of minority religious identity. Thus, future research is necessary to explore the links between religiousness and optimism in several religious minority affiliations. Fourth, it is necessary to analyze the extent to which the link between religiosity and optimism are moderated by some demographic variables such as gender, age, and ethnicity. Fifth, this it is important to identify a range of socio-contextual and socio-cultural factors that influence the religious identity among Portuguese citizens, and to analyze the extent to which these factors interact to promote or limit the optimism of Portuguese citizens.

References

Alarcon, G.M., Bowling, N.A., Khazon, S.: Great expectations: a meta-analytic examination of optimism and hope. Personality Individ. Differ. **5**(7), 821–827 (2013)

Barker, E., Warburg, M. (eds.): New Religions and New Religiosity. Aarhus University Press, Springfield (1998)

Bentler, P.: Multivariate analysis with latent variables: Causal modeling. Annu. Rev. Psychol. **31**, 419–456 (1990)

Berger, P.L.: The Desecularization of the World: Resurgent Religion and World Politics. William B. Eerdmans Publishing, Washington, DC (1999)

Bollen, K.A.: Structural Equations with Latent Variables. Wiley, New York (1989)

Bosacki, S.L., Moore, K., Talwar, V., Park-Satzman, J.: Preadolescents' gendered spiritual identities and self-regulation. J. Beliefs Values Stud. Relig. Educ. **32**(3), 303–316 (2011). https://doi.org/10.1080/13617672.2011.627679

Buck, A.C., Williams, D.R., Musick, M.A., Sternthal, M.J.: An examination of the relationship between multiple dimensions of religiosity, blood pressure, and hypertension. Soc. Sci. Med. **68**(2), 314–322 (2009). https://doi.org/10.1016/j.socscimed.2008.10.010

Byrne, B.M.: Structural Equation Modeling with AMOS: Basic Concepts, Applications and Programming, 2nd edn. Lawrence Erlbaum, London (2010)

Cabral, M.V., Vala, J., Pais, J.M., Ramos, A.: Atitudes e práticas religiosas dos portugueses. ISCTE, Lisboa (2000)

Caputo, J.D.: Atheism, A/theology, and the postmodern condition. In: Martin, M. (ed.) The Cambridge Companion to Atheism, pp. 267–282. Cambridge University Press, New York (2007)

Carver, C.S., Scheier, M.F.: Optimism, pessimism, and self-regulation. In: Chang, E.C. (ed.) Optimism and Pessimism: Implications for Theory, Research, and Practice, 1st edn, pp. 31–51. American Psychological Association, Washington, DC (2000)

Carver, C.S., Scheier, M.F., Segerstrom, S.C.: Optimism. Clin. Psychol. Rev. **30**, 879–889 (2010)

Chang, E.C.: Does dispositional optimism moderate the relation between perceived stress and psychological well-being: a preliminary investigation. Personality Individ. Differ. **25**, 233–240 (1998)

Chang, E.C.: Introduction: optimism and pessimism and moving beyond the most fundamental question. In: Chang, E.C. (ed.) Optimism & Pessimism: Implications for Theory, Research, and Practice, 1st edn, pp. 3–12. American Psychological Association, Washington, DC (2000)

Clemente, D.F., Frazão, A.A., Mónico, L.S.: Bem-estar subjetivo em idosos institucionalizados e não institucionalizados. In: Pocinho, R., et al. (eds.) Envelhecer em tempos de crise: Respostas sociais, pp. 39–50. LivPsic, Porto (2012)

Closs, S.J., Edwards, J., Swift, C., Briggs, M.: Religious identity and the experience and expression of chronic pain: a review. J. Relig. Disabil. Health **17**(2), 91–124 (2013). https://doi.org/10.1080/15228967.2013.778515

Osborne, J.W., Costello, A.B.: Best practices in exploratory factor analysis: four recommendations for getting the most from your analysis. Pan-Pac. Manag. Rev. **12**(2), 131–146 (2009)

Craig, W.L.: Theistic critiques of atheism. In: Martin, M. (ed.) The Cambridge Companion to Atheism, pp. 69–85. Cambridge University Press, New York (2007)

Deneulin, S., Rakodi, C.: Revisiting religion: development studies thirty years on. World Dev. **39** (1), 45–54 (2011). https://doi.org/10.1016/j.worlddev.2010.05.007

Dezutter, J., Soenens, B., Hutsebaut, D.: Religiosity and mental health: a further exploration of the relative importance of religious behaviors vs. religious attitudes. Personality Individ. Differ. **40**(4), 807–818 (2006). https://doi.org/10.1016/j.paid.2005.08.014

Diener, E., Scollon, C.M., Lucas, R.E.: The evolving concept of subjective well-being: the multifaceted nature of happiness. In: Costa, P.T., Siegler, I.C. (eds.) The Psychology of Aging, vol. 15, pp. 187–220. Elsevier, Amsterdam (2004). https://doi.org/10.1016/j.eurpsy. 2010.04.003

Ecklund, E.H., Park, J.Z., Veliz, P.T.: Secularization and religious change among elite scientists. Soc. Forces **86**(4), 1805–1939 (2008)

Fischer, R., Chalmers, A.: Is optimism universal? A meta-analytical investigation of optimism levels across 22 nations. Personality Individ. Differ. **45**(5), 378–382 (2008)

Geerts, H.: An inquiry into the meaning of ritual symbolism: Turner and Peirce. In: Heimbrock, H.-G., Boudewijnse, H.B. (eds.) Current Studies on Rituals: Perspectives for the Psychology of Religion, Amsterdam, Atlanta, pp. 19–32 (1990)

Giddens, A.: Modernity and Self-Identity: Self and Society in the Late Modern Age. Polity, Cambridge (1991)

Giddens, A.: Sociology, 3ª edn. Polity Press, Cambridge (1997)

Grigoropoulou, N., Chryssochoou, X.: Are religious minorities in Greece better accepted if they assimilate? The effects of acculturation strategy and group membership on religious minority perceptions. J. Commun. Appl. Soc. Psychol. **21**(6), 499–514 (2011). https://doi.org/10.1002/casp.1119

Grom, B.: Psicología de la religión. Editorial Herder, Barcelona (1994)

Härdle, W., Simar, L.: Applied Multivariate Statistical Analysis. Springer, Berlin (2012). https://doi.org/10.1007/978-3-642-17229-8

Hatcher, L.: A Step-by-Step Approach to Using the SAS System for Factor Analysis and Structural Equation Modelling. SAS Institute Inc., Cary (1996)

Haught, J.F.: Science and Religion: From Conflict to Conversation. Paulist Press, Mahwah (1995)

Heelas, P., Woodhead, L. (eds.): Religion in Modern Times. Blackwell Publishers, Oxford, Cambridge (2000)

Hervieu-Léger, D.: Representam os surtos emocionais contemporâneos o fim da secularização ou o fim da religião? Religião e Sociedade **18**(1), 31–48 (1997)

Higgins, E.T., Grant, H., Shah, J.: Self-regulation and quality of life: Emotional and non-emotional life experiences. In: Kahneman, D., Diener, E., Schwartz, N. (eds.) Well-Being: The Foundations of Hedonic Psychology, pp. 244–266. Russell Sage, New York (1999)

Hill, P.C., Pargament, K.: Advances in the conceptualization and measurement of religion and spirituality: implications for physical and mental health research. Am. Psychol. **58**(1), 64–74 (2003)

Hjelle, L.A., Busch, E.A., Warren, J.E.: Explanatory style, dispositional optimism, and reported parental behavior. J. Genet. Psychol. **157**(4), 489–499 (1996)

Hoorens, V.: Unrealistic optimism in social comparison of health and safety risks. In: Rutter, D. (ed.) The Social Psychology of Health and Safety: European Perspectives, pp. 153–174. Aldershot, Avesbury (1994)

James, W.: The Varieties of Religious Experience: A Study in Human Nature. Harvard University Press, Cambridge (1985). [Original Work Published 1902]

Kirchner, T., Patiño, C.: Stress and depression in Latin American immigrants: the mediating role of religiosity. European Psychiatry **25**(8), 479–484 (2010)

Kline, R.B.: Principles and practice of structural equation modeling, 2nd edn. The Guilford Press, New York (2005)

Koenig, H.G.: Is Religion Good for Your Health? Effects of Religion on Natural and Physical Health. Haworth Press, New York (1997)

Koenig, H.G. (ed.): Handbook of Religion and Mental Health. Academic Press, San Diego (1998)

Koenig, H.G., McCullough, M.E., Larson, D.B.: Handbook of Religion and Health. Oxford University Press, New York (2001)

Lichterman, P.: Religion and the construction of civic identity. Am. Sociol. Rev. **73**, 83–104 (2008)

Luckmann, T.: The Invisible Religion. McMillan, New York (1967)

Luque, T.: Técnicas de análisis de datos en investigación de mercados. Ediciones Pirámide, Madrid (2000)

Luquis, R.R., Brelsford, G.M., Rojas-guyler, L.: Religiosity, spirituality, sexual attitudes, and sexual behaviors among college students. J. Relig. Health **51**(3), 601–614 (2012)

Mariz, C.L.: A renovação carismática católica no Brasil: Uma revisão da bibliografia. In: Rodrigues, D. (ed.) Em nome de Deus: A religião na sociedade contemporânea, pp. 109–183. Edições Afrontamento, Porto (2004)

Martelli, S.: A religião na sociedade pós-moderna: Entre secularização e dessecularização. Edições Paulinas, São Paulo (1995)

Martin, D.: Remise en question de la théorie de la sécularisation. In: Gracie, D., Léger, D.H. (eds.) Identités religieuses en Europe. La Découverte, Paris (1996)

Martin, M.: Atheism and religion. In: Martin, M. (ed.) The Cambridge Companion to Atheism, pp. 217–232. Cambridge University Press, New York (2007)

Mattis, J.S., Fontenot, D.L., Hatcher-Kay, C.A.: Religiosity, racism, and dispositional optimism among African Americans. Personality Individ. Differ. **34**(5), 1025–1038 (2003). https://doi.org/10.1016/S0191-8869(02)00087-9

McCullough, M.E., Boker, S.M.: Dynamical modeling for studying self-regulatory processes: an example from the study of religious development over the life span. In: Ong, A.D., van Dulmen, M. (eds.) Handbook of Methods in Positive Psychology, pp. 380–394. Oxford University Press, New York (2007)

McCullough, M.E., Willoughby, B.L.: Religion, self-regulation, and self-control: associations, explanations, and implications. Psychol. Bull. **135**, 69–93 (2009)

McKenna, F.P.: It won't happen to me: unrealistic optimism or illusion of control? Br. J. Psychol. **84**, 39–50 (1993)

Mónico, L.S.: Autopercepção da beleza física e estratégias de auto-apresentação em contextos de sedução. Faculdade de Psicologia e de Ciências da Educação, Porto. Dissertação de Mestrado em Psicologia (especialidade em Psicologia Social) (2003). Accessed 9 May 2003

Mónico, L.S.: Religiosidade e optimismo: Crenças e modos de implicação comportamental. Coimbra: Faculdade de Psicologia e de Ciências da Educação. Dissertação de Doutoramento em Psicologia, especialidade em Psicologia Social (2010). Accessed 12 Oct 2010

Mónico, L.S.: Individualização religiosa e otimismo. Edições Vercial (2011)

Mónico, L.S.: Religiosity and optimism in ill and healthy elderly. Int. J. Dev. Educ. Psychol. **1**(2), 59–70 (2012)

Mónico, L.S.: Aging, health and disease: the effect of religiosity on the optimism of elderly people. In: Oliveira, A.L. (eds.) Promoting Conscious and Active Learning and Aging: How to Face Current and Future Challenges?, pp. 371–382. Imprensa da Universidade de Coimbra, Coimbra (2013). https://doi.org/10.14195/978-989-26-0732-0

Mónico, L., Alferes, V.R., Brêda, M.S., Carvalho, C., Parreira, P.M.: Can religiosity improve optimism in participants in states of illness, when controlling for life satisfaction? BMC Health Serv. Res. 16(3), 123 (2016). https://doi.org/10.1186/s12913-016-1423-5

Mookherjee, H.N.: Effects of religiosity and selected variables on the perception of well-being. J. Soc. Psychol. 134(3), 403–405 (1994)

Neugarten, B.I., Havighurst, R.J., Tobin, S.S.: The measurement of life satisfaction. J. Gerontol. 16, 134–143 (1961)

Noddings, N.: The new outspoken atheism and education. Harvard Educ. Rev. 78(2), 369–392 (2008)

Norem, J.K.: Defensive pessimism, optimism and pessimism. In: Chang, E.C. (ed.) Optimism & Pessimism: Implications for Theory, Research, and Practice, 1st edn, pp. 77–100. American Psychological Association, Washington, DC (2000)

Pargament, K.I.: The Psychology of Religion and Coping: Theory, Research and Practice. Guilford Press, New York (1997)

Parreira, P.M., Carvalho, C., Mónico, L., Pinto, C., Vicente, S., Brêda, M.S.: Effect of nurses' mobilization in satisfaction at work and turnover: an empirical study in the hospital setting. BMC Health Serv. Res. 16(3), 40–41 (2016). https://doi.org/10.1186/s12913-016-1423-5

Peeters, G., Czapinski, J., Hoorens, V.: Comparative optimism, pessimism, and realism with respect to adverse events and their relationship with will to live. Int. Rev. Soc. Psychol. 14(4), 143–162 (2001)

Peterson, C.: The future of optimism. Am. Psychol. 55(2000), 44–55 (2000)

Reynolds, V.: Secular change and religious inertia. In: Jones, E., Reynolds, V. (eds.) Survival and Religion: Biological Evolution and Cultural Change, pp. 187–205. Wiley, New York (1995)

Roberts, L.D.: Equivalence of electronic and offline measures. In: Reynolds, R.A., Woods, R., Baker, J.D. (eds.) Handbook of Research on Electronic Surveys and Measurements, pp. 97–103. Idea Group Reference, Hershey (2007)

Rodrigues, D.: O reencantamento do mundo: Modernidade, secularização e novos movimentos religiosos. In Rodrigues, D., (eds.) Em nome de Deus: A religião na sociedade contemporânea, pp. 43–52. Edições Afrontamento, Porto (2004)

Scheier, M.F., Carver, C.S.: Optimism, coping, and health: assessment and implications of generalized outcome expectancies. Health Psychol. 4, 219–247 (1985)

Scheier, M.F., Carver, C.S.: Dispositional optimism and physical well-being: the influence of generalized outcome expectancies on health. J. Pers. 55, 169–210 (1987)

Scheier, M.F., Carver, C.S.: Effects of optimism on psychological and physical well-being: theoretical overview and empirical update. Cogn. Ther. Res. 16, 201–228 (1992)

Scheier, M.F., Carver, C.S., Bridges, M.W.: Distinguishing optimism from neuroticism (and trait anxiety, self-mastery, and self-esteem): a reevaluation of the Life Orientation Test. J. Pers. Soc. Psychol. 67, 1063–1078 (1994)

Schumacker, R.E., Lomax, R.G.: A Beginner's Guide to Structural Equation Modeling. Lawrence Erlbaum Associates, Mahwah (1996)

Segerstrom, S.C.: Optimism and resources: effects on each other and on health over 10 years. J. Res. Pers. 41(4), 772–786 (2007). https://doi.org/10.1016/j.jrp.2006.09.004

Shepperd, J.A., Carroll, P., Grace, J., Terry, M.: Exploring the causes of comparative optimism. Psychologica Belgica 42, 65–98 (2002)

Simonds, M.G.: Optimism: a comprehensive psycho-educational program design: Social circumstances, inequalities and health. Dissertation Abstract, Dissertation Abstracts International: Section B: The Sciences and Engineering 65(10-B) (2005)

Stausberg, M.: The study of religion(s) in Western Europe III: Further developments after World War II. Religion 39(3), 261–282 (2009). https://doi.org/10.1016/j.religion.2009.06.001

Tajfel, H.: Human Groups and Social Categories. Cambridge University Press, Cambridge (1981)

Taylor, M.C.: Critical Terms for Religious Studies. The University of Chicago Press, Chicago and London (1998)

Vanderwoerd, J.R.: Reconsidering secularization and recovering Christianity in social work history. Soc. Work Christianity 38(3), 244–246 (2011)

Vásquez-Borau, J.L.: Os novos movimentos religiosos: Nova era, ocultismo e satanismo. Paulus, Lisboa (2008)

Wallis, R., Bruce, S.: Secularization: trends, data, and theory. In: Lynn, M.L., Moberg, D.O. (eds.) Research in the Social Scientific Study of Religion, vol. 3, pp. 1–31. Jai Press, London (1991)

Weinstein, N.D.: Unrealistic optimism about future life events. J. Pers. Soc. Psychol. 39, 806–820 (1980)

Weinstein, N.D.: Reducing unrealistic optimism about illness susceptibility. Health Psychol. 2, 11–20 (1983)

Weinstein, N.D.: Why it won't happen to me: Perceptions of risk factors and susceptibility. Health Psychol. 3, 431–457 (1984)

Weinstein, N.D.: Optimistic biases about personal risks. Science 246(8), 1232–1233 (1989)

Wiseman, R.: O factor sorte. Publicações Dom Quixote, Lisboa (2006)

Yuen, E.J.: Spirituality, religion, and health. Am. J. Med. Qual. 22(2), 77–79 (2007)

Author Index

Printed in the United States
By Bookmasters

Printed in the United States
By Bookmasters